INTRODUCTION TO
HEALTH POLICY

INTRODUCTION TO
HEALTH POLICY

Leiyu Shi

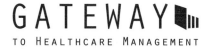

GATEWAY
TO HEALTHCARE MANAGEMENT

AUPHA

Health Administration Press, Chicago, Illinois
Association of University Programs in
Health Administration, Arlington, Virginia

Library of Congress Cataloging-in-Publication Data

Shi, Leiyu.
  Introduction to health policy / Leiyu Shi.
    pages cm
  Includes index.
  ISBN 978-1-56793-580-6 (alk. paper)
  1. Medical policy--History. 2. Health care reform. 3. Public health--International cooperation. I. Title.
  RA393.S473 2014
  362.1--dc23

                        2013005276

The paper used in this publication meets the minimum requirements of American National Standard for Information Sciences—Permanence of Paper for Printed Library Materials, ANSI Z39.48-1984.♾ ™

Acquisitions editor: Janet Davis; Project manager: Joyce Dunne; Cover designer: Marisa Jackson; Layout: Cepheus Edmondson

Found an error or typo? We want to know! Please email it to hapbooks@ache.org, and put "Book Error" in the subject line.

For photocopying and copyright information, please contact Copyright Clearance Center at www.copyright.com or (978) 750-8400.

Health Administration Press
A division of the Foundation
  of the American College of
  Healthcare Executives
One North Franklin Street
Suite 1700
Chicago, IL 60606-3529
(312) 424-2800

Association of University Programs
  in Health Administration
2000 North 14th Street
Suite 780
Arlington, VA 22201
(703) 894-0940

I dedicate this book to my wife, Ruoxian,
and my children, Sylvia, Jennifer, and Victor Shi.

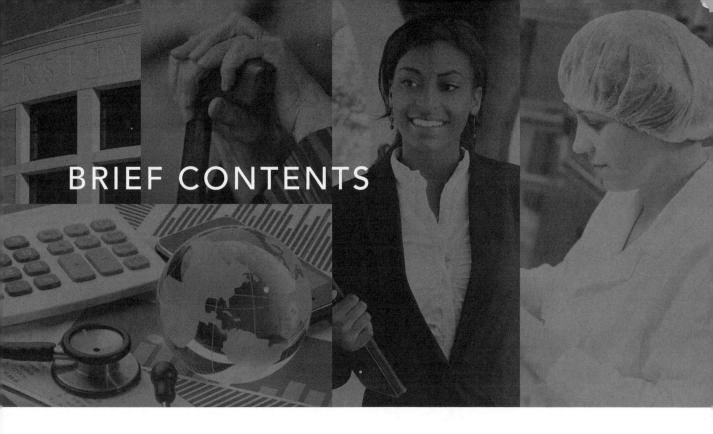

BRIEF CONTENTS

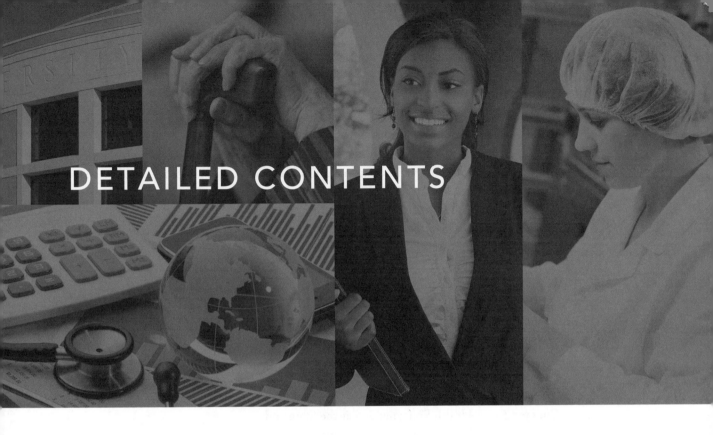

DETAILED CONTENTS

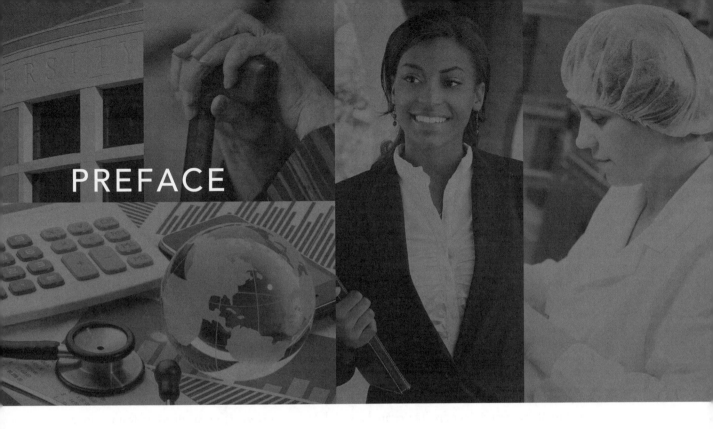

PREFACE

For decades, US policymakers have been struggling to find solutions to our healthcare challenges. Thus, healthcare reform is among the top priorities of almost every administration.

This introductory textbook on US health policy covers the related areas of health policymaking, critical health policy issues, health policy research, and an international perspective on health policy and policymaking.

The book offers the following features:

- ◆ Real-world cases to exemplify the theories and concepts presented from a variety of perspectives, including the hospital setting, public health, managed care, ambulatory care, and extended care
- ◆ Learning objectives and key points
- ◆ Discussion questions
- ◆ A glossary
- ◆ Boxes, including Learning Points, For Your Consideration, Key Legislation, and others, as well as exhibits to present background information on concepts, examples, and up-to-date information
- ◆ Instructor's materials, including PowerPoint slides and answers to the discussion questions that appear in each chapter

ORGANIZATION OF THE BOOK

This book is organized in four parts: an introduction, an overview of health policymaking, a health policy issues section, and a discussion of health policy research and analysis. Chapter 1, the sole chapter in Part I, introduces key terms related to, and the determinants of, health and health policy. It lists the key stakeholders in health policymaking and presents important reasons for studying health policy. The chapter lays the foundation for the rest of the book.

Part II examines the policymaking process at the federal, state, and local levels; in the private sector; and in international settings. Chapter 2 focuses on the policymaking process at the federal level of the US government. Important activities within the three policymaking stages—policy formulation, policy implementation, and policy modification—are described. The key characteristics of health policymaking in the United States are analyzed, and the role of interest groups in making that policy is discussed.

The focus of Chapter 3 is the US policymaking process at the state and local levels and in the private sector, which includes the research community, foundations, and private industry. Examples of policy-related research by private research institutes and foundations are described. The impact of the private sector's services and products on health and policy is illustrated using the fast-food industry and cigarette companies as examples.

Chapter 4 discusses international health policymaking. The World Health Organization is presented as an example of an international agency involved in policymaking related to health and major health initiatives. Five countries—Canada, the United Kingdom, Sweden, Australia, and China—are highlighted to illustrate diverse policymaking processes in various geographic regions. The experiences of these countries show that different political systems and policymaking processes lead to different approaches to population health and healthcare delivery.

In Part III, we discuss the policy issues related to social, behavioral, and medical care health determinants; to people from diverse populations; and to international health. Chapter 5 describes how US healthcare is financed and delivered. Private and public health insurance programs are summarized, and the subsystems of healthcare delivery—managed care, the military system, care for vulnerable populations, the public health program, the long-term care system, and oral health delivery—are introduced. After summarizing the major characteristics of US healthcare delivery, the chapter provides examples of health policy issues related to financing (regulatory and market approaches) and delivery (healthcare workforce, certification and accreditation of healthcare organizations, antitrust regulations, access-to-care issues, and patient rights concerns).

Chapter 6 defines vulnerable populations and discusses the dominant healthcare policy issues related to those populations. People from diverse populations include racial or ethnic minorities, those with low income, the elderly, women and children, people with HIV/AIDS, the mentally ill, and the homeless. In each segment, the magnitude of the problem is summarized and a detailed discussion of the policies and strategies meant to address the problem is presented.

In Chapter 7, dominant health policy issues in the international community are discussed, with examples given for select countries. The chapter begins by discussing issues shared by developed countries, such as modifying health systems to better serve aging and diverse populations while maintaining high-quality care at a low cost. It then discusses challenges faced by developing nations, such as creating and maintaining high-functioning health systems with limited resources and dealing with the burdens of morbidity and mortality associated with poverty. Several emerging issues are also illustrated that could affect global health in the future.

Part IV presents an overview of policy analysis, focusing on examples of commonly used quantitative and qualitative methods. Chapter 8 introduces health policy research (HPR) and highlights the discipline's defining characteristics, including applied, policy-relevant, ethical, multidisciplinary, scientific, and population-based studies. The HPR process is summarized, and the chapter concludes with a discussion of ways to communicate findings and the challenges in implementing those findings in practice.

In Chapter 9, we illustrate commonly used methods in health policy research. Quantitative methods include experimental research, survey research, evaluation research, and cost–benefit and cost-effectiveness analysis. Because evaluation research is closely tied to policy research, the process involved in this type of research is described in greater detail. Qualitative methods include participant observations, in-depth interviews, and case studies.

Chapter 10 provides an example that illustrates the key steps in health policy analysis: assessing the determinants of a health problem, identifying policy intervention to the problem, critically evaluating the policy intervention, and proposing next steps in addressing the problem.

ACKNOWLEDGMENTS

My PhD advisee Sarika Rane Parasuraman contributed Chapter 10 (an applied example) and is hereby acknowledged. The preparation of this book was also aided by Xiaoyu Nie and Hannah Sintek, who served as my administrative assistants. The editorial staff of Health Administration Press, in particular Joyce Dunne and Janet Davis, have provided hands-on assistance in editing the manuscript to make it more compatible with the audience. Of course, all errors and omissions remain the responsibility of the author.

Leiyu Shi
Professor of Health Policy

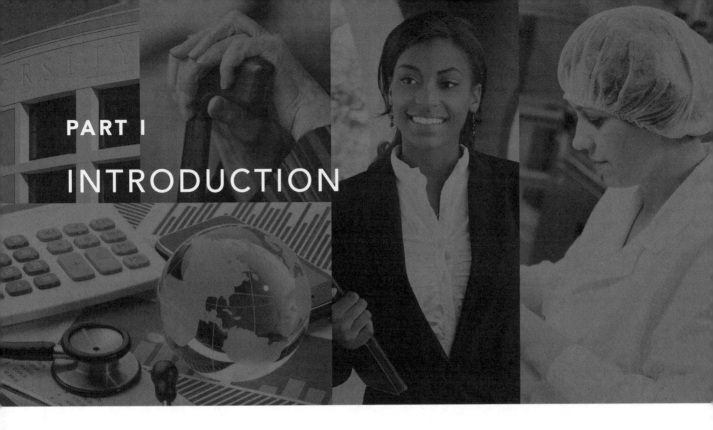

PART I

INTRODUCTION

The introduction, which consists of Chapter 1, provides an overview of health policy. It defines key terms related to health policy, reviews the frameworks of health determinants, and outlines the concept of health policy formulation. In addition, the chapter introduces topics related to health policy, including stakeholders, the major types of health policies, and the importance of studying health policy. The introduction should provide readers with a foundation for examining how health policy is set in the United States and elsewhere.

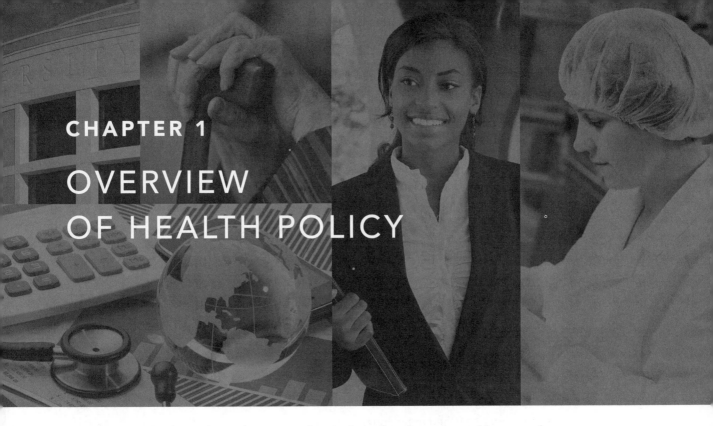

CHAPTER 1
OVERVIEW
OF HEALTH POLICY

I have never had a policy. I have simply tried to do what seemed best each day, as each day came.

— Abraham Lincoln

LEARNING OBJECTIVES

Studying this chapter will help you to

➤ define key terms related to health policy,

➤ appreciate the influence of health determinants,

➤ understand the framework of health policy formulation,

➤ identify the stakeholders in health policy,

➤ describe the major types of health policies, and

➤ discuss the importance of studying health policy.

CASE STUDY

HEALTHCARE REFORM: HILLARY CLINTON AND BARACK OBAMA

Two major healthcare reform initiatives have played out on the US political landscape in the last two decades: the Health Security Act, developed by the Clinton administration in the 1990s and spearheaded by then First Lady Hillary Clinton, which failed to pass into law, and the Patient Protection and Affordable Care Act (ACA), drafted by the Obama administration, which became federal law in March 2010.

The hallmark of the Clinton plan was its universal coverage mandate, which required all employers to contribute to a pool of funds intended to cover the costs of insurance premiums for their workers, with caps on total employer costs and subsidies for small businesses. Competition among private health plans and a cap on the growth of insurance premiums was to have held costs in check, and additional financing was to have been provided through savings from cuts in projected Medicare and Medicaid spending and increased taxes on tobacco (Oberlander 2007).

The Obama plan focused on reforming the private health insurance market, extending insurance coverage to the uninsured, providing better coverage for those with preexisting conditions, improving prescription drug coverage in Medicare, and extending the life of the Medicare trust fund accounts. The ACA is expected to be financed through taxes, such as a 40 percent tax on "Cadillac" insurance policies—policies that offer the richest benefits—taxes on pharmaceuticals, medical devices, and indoor tanning services (KFF 2011); and other offsets (provisions of the law that reduce the overall cost of enacting the legislation, such as penalties on uninsured individuals).

The political landscape in 2009, as President Barack Obama's healthcare reform initiative was being debated, was similar to that in the early 1990s: Both the Clinton and Obama administrations were affiliated with the Democratic Party, both chambers of the US Congress were controlled by Democrats, and national opinion strongly favored healthcare reform (Sack and Connelly 2009).

However, whereas the Obama reform initiative became law, the Clinton healthcare reform package was defeated in Congress. Although Americans supported healthcare reform in theory, the Clinton plan was derailed by the heavy opposition of the medical and insurance industries and by anti-tax rhetoric. The disenchantment of the electorate following that failed effort helped Republicans gain control of the House of Representatives and Senate in the 1994 election (Trafford 2010).

At 17.9 percent of the nation's total economic activity, also known as the **gross domestic product**, healthcare spending in the United States leads all countries in overall and per capita measures (KFF 2012). Yet its health system does not perform well compared to those of other industrialized countries. A 2010 World Health Organization (WHO) report ranks the US health system thirty-sixth among 191 countries, and a Commonwealth Fund study completed the same year ranks it last among six other countries—Australia, Canada, Germany, the Netherlands, New Zealand, and the United Kingdom—on the basis of quality, efficiency, access, equity, and healthy lives measures (Davis, Schoen, and Stremikis 2010).

> *Gross domestic product*
> Refers to the value of all goods and services produced within a country for a given period; a key indicator of the country's economic activity and financial well-being.

Why have health policies tended to fail in the United States while they appear to be succeeding in other countries? The answer might be found in the context—the United States—and the determinants of health and health policy in the United States.

The main purpose of this chapter is to present a framework of health policy determinants and discuss their impact in the United States. Understanding this framework helps the reader appreciate factors that contribute to health policy development in general and in the United States in particular. The chapter first defines key concepts related to health policy and later discusses the importance of studying health policy, including an awareness of the international perspective. The stakeholders of health policy are also presented and analyzed as key parts of the policy context.

HEALTH DEFINED

WHO (1946) defines health as "not merely the absence of disease or infirmity but a state of complete physical, mental and social well-being." This broad definition recognizes that health encompasses biological and social elements in addition to individual and community well-being. Health may be seen as an indicator of personal and collective advancement. It can signal the level of an individual's well-being as well as the degree of success achieved by a society and its government in promoting that well-being (Shi and Stevens 2010). This definition of health strikes a common chord among governments that allows policymakers at WHO, and others in the global health community, to build the case that issues such as poverty; lack of education; discrimination; and other social, cultural, and political conditions found around the world are essentially public health issues.

However, health is also the result of personal characteristics and choices. This concept is the source of the fundamental tension in public health and has been a major topic in the United States in the past few years. Major debates continue over whether people can be forced to take actions to ensure their own health, such as buying health insurance (the individual mandate in the Affordable Care Act), or be prohibited from performing actions that are unhealthy, such as limiting soft drinks in schools. Health policy in the United States must attempt to balance the good of the public health with personal liberty, often a difficult compromise to make. Indeed, the conflict between WHO's definition of health

KEY LEGISLATION
What Is the Status of Healthcare Reform in the United States?

In the United States, *healthcare reform* typically denotes a government-sponsored program that attempts to make health insurance available to the uninsured. Although universal health insurance is a difficult goal to realize, incremental reforms have been successful when the political and economic environments were favorable. The first such program came in the form of the Old Age Assistance program, which was enacted as part of the 1935 Social Security Act. It provided direct financial assistance to needy elderly persons.

Full health insurance for the elderly became available under the Medicare program, as did health insurance for the indigent under the Medicaid program. Both programs were created in 1965 under the Great Society reforms of President Lyndon Johnson in an era when civil rights and social justice had taken central stage in the United States. Later, authorized under the Balanced Budget Act of 1997, the State Children's Health Insurance Program (later renamed the Children's Health Insurance Program) was developed whereby states can use federal funds to cover children up to age 19 through the states' existing Medicaid programs.

One of the most significant healthcare reform efforts resulted in the Affordable Care Act of 2010, designed to bring about major changes to the delivery of US healthcare. The key objective of the ACA, to be implemented in full in 2014, is to provide most (if not all) Americans with health insurance coverage.

Life expectancy
Anticipated number of years of life remaining.

Mortality
Number of deaths in a given population within a specified period.

Morbidity
Incidence or prevalence of diseases in a given population within a specified period.

and much of the social, cultural, and political issues surrounding the US healthcare system is one of the most important areas of debate facing health policymakers.

PHYSICAL HEALTH

The most common measure of physical health is **life expectancy**—the anticipated number of remaining years of life at any stage. Exhibit 1.1 shows the ten countries ranking highest in their population's life expectancy as of 2006 and includes the US ranking for comparison.

Although good or positive health status is commonly associated with the definition of health, the most frequently used indicators measure the lack of health or the incidence of poor health—for example **mortality**, **morbidity**, **disability**, and various indexes that

Disability
A physical or mental condition that limits an individual's ability to perform functions generally characterized as normal.

EXHIBIT 1.1
Top Ten Countries with the Longest Life Expectancy, with the United States as Comparison

Rank	Country (state/territory)	Life expectancy at birth (years)		
		Overall	Male	Female
1	Japan	82.6	78.0	86.1
2	Hong Kong	82.2	79.4	85.1
3	Iceland	81.8	80.2	83.3
4	Switzerland	81.7	79.0	84.2
5	Australia	81.2	78.9	83.6
6	Spain	80.9	77.7	84.2
7	Sweden	80.9	78.7	83.0
8	Israel	80.7	78.5	82.8
9	Macau	80.7	78.5	82.8
10	France (metropolitan)	80.7	77.1	84.1
36	United States	78.3	75.6	80.8

SOURCE: Data from DESA (2007).

combine these factors. One such measure is **quality-adjusted life years**, which combines mortality and morbidity in a single index. The Learning Point box titled "Measures of Mortality, Morbidity, and Disability" lists categories by which each indicator is measured.

MENTAL HEALTH

In contrast to physical health, measures of mental health are limited. The major categories of mental health measures are mental conditions (e.g., depression, disorder, distress), behaviors (e.g., suicide, drug or alcohol abuse), perceptions (e.g., perceived mental health status), satisfaction (with life, work, relationships, etc.), and services received (e.g., counseling, drug treatment).

SOCIAL WELL-BEING

The most commonly used measure of relative social well-being is one's socioeconomic status (SES). An SES index typically considers such factors as education level, income, and occupation. Quality of life is another common measure and may include one's ability

Quality-adjusted life years
A combined mortality–morbidity index that reflects years of life free of disability and symptoms of illness.

LEARNING POINT
Measures of Morbidity, Mortality, and Disability

Morbidity measures
- Incidence (number of new cases in a defined population within a specified period) of specific diseases
- Prevalence (number of instances in a defined population within a specified period) of specific diseases

Mortality measures
- Crude (unadjusted for any other factors) death rate
- Age-specific death rate
- Condition-specific death rate
- Infant mortality
- Maternal mortality

Disability measures
- Restricted activity days (e.g., bed days, work-loss days)
- Limitations in performing activities of daily living (i.e., bathing, dressing, toileting, getting into or out of a bed or chair, continence, eating)
- Limitations in performing instrumental activities of daily living (i.e., doing housework and chores, grocery shopping, preparing food, using the phone, traveling locally, taking medicine)

Social contacts
The frequency of social activities a person undertakes within a specified period.

Social resources
Interpersonal relationships with social contacts and the extent to which the individual can rely on them for support.

to perform various roles (e.g., self-care, family care, social functioning), perceptions (e.g., emotional well-being, pain tolerance, energy level), and living environment (e.g., pollution levels, crime prevalence). A third set of social well-being measures, often used by sociologists, is composed of **social contacts** and **social resources**. Examples of social contacts include visits with family members, friends, and relatives and participation in social events, such as membership activities, professional conferences, and church gatherings. The social contacts factor can be used as an indicator of social resources by determining whether an individual can rely on his social contacts for needed support and company and whether these contacts meet the individual's needs for care and love.

PUBLIC HEALTH DEFINED

Winslow (1920) defined public health as "the science and the art of preventing disease, prolonging life, and promoting physical health and efficiency through organized community efforts for the sanitation of the environment, the control of community infections, the education of the individual in principles of personal hygiene, the organization of medical and nursing service for the early diagnosis and preventive treatment of disease, and the development of social machinery which will ensure to every individual in the community a standard of living adequate for the maintenance of health." It focuses on prevention and involves the efforts of society as a whole. Finally, public health is intended to protect lives and improve the health of populations around the globe.

Whereas healthcare is intended to treat, influence, and care for individuals, public health operates on a larger scale. The field is defined by the American Public Health Association (APHA n.d.) as (1) "the practice of preventing disease and promoting good health within groups of people" and (2) the research and surveillance conducted to better understand the health issues facing a group and, in turn, to craft good health policy.

Public health has broad implications for a population. Successful public health activities and initiatives can save money by promoting healthy living and prevention, thus reducing healthcare costs and disease burden. In addition, these activities can improve quality of life and reduce suffering caused by ill health in a population (APHA n.d.). The practice of public health leads to direct (e.g., healthier children, less chronic disease, less need for acute care) and indirect (e.g., fewer days missed from school and work; increased funding available for other initiatives, such as education) benefits for a society.

It is important to remember that public health, healthcare, and health policy are interconnected areas of study and of practice. All three have great influence on health.

WHAT ARE THE DETERMINANTS OF HEALTH?

Numerous theories related to assigning the **determinants of health** have been proposed over the past several decades. Blum (1974) offered a framework called Force Field and Well-Being Paradigms of Health, which suggests four major influences—the force fields—on health: environment, lifestyle, heredity, and medical care. According to Blum, the most important force field is the environment, followed by lifestyle and heredity; medical care has the least impact on health and well-being.

More recent models focus on socioeconomic context and health behaviors. For example, the Dahlgren and Whitehead (2006) model divides factors that influence health into two categories. *Fixed factors*, the first category, are unchangeable, such as age, sex, and genetic makeup. The second category is composed of *modifiable factors*, such as individual lifestyle choices; social networks and community conditions; the environment in which one lives and works; and access to important goods and services, such as education, sanitation, food, and healthcare. The factors in the second category form layers around the population, and modifying them positively can improve population health.

Ansari and colleagues (2003) propose a public health model of the determinants of health in which these factors are categorized into four major groups: social determinants, healthcare system attributes, disease-inducing behaviors, and health outcomes.

Determinants of health
Factors that influence one's health status. Typically, they include one's socioeconomic status, environment, behaviors, heredity, and access to medical care.

LEARNING POINT
Prominent Theories on the Causes of Disease

Many of the historically dominant theories related to health focus on disease rather than well-being. The three most prominent theories of disease causality are germ theory, lifestyle theory, and environmental theory.

Germ theory gained prominence in the nineteenth century with the rise of bacteriology (Metchnikoff, Pasteur, and Koch 1939). Essentially, the theory holds that every disease has a specific cause, which should be identifiable. Knowledge of that cause allows the discovery of a cure. Microorganisms, the general causal agent identified by germ theory, are thought to act independently of the environment. Furthermore, the individual who serves as host of the microorganism is the source of the disease, which then may be transmitted from one person to another (known as contagion). Strategies to address the disease focused on identifying people with symptoms and providing follow-up medical treatment. Much of biomedical research is still based on germ theory. The traditional concept of the agent, host, and environment as the epidemiological triangle (*epidemiology* is the study of factors controlling the presence or absence of a disease) also is based on the single-cause, single-effect framework of germ theory.

Lifestyle theory tries to isolate specific behaviors (e.g., exercise, diet, smoking, drinking) as causes of a disease and identifies solutions on the basis of changing these behaviors. As with germ theory, lifestyle theory defines problems as they relate to individuals and focuses solutions on individual interventions.

Environmental theory considers the general health and well-being of individuals more so than disease. It maintains that health is best understood by examining the larger context of community. Traditional environmental approaches focused on poor sanitation, which was connected to certain infectious diseases. With industrialization and its byproducts of overcrowding and filth, contemporary environmental approaches examine the impact of production and consumption on emerging health problems. Environmental theory considers disease to be influenced by environmental and social factors. It contends that solutions should be developed through policy and regulation and be systems focused rather than focused on individuals and medical treatment.

A conceptual framework developed by the WHO Commission on Social Determinants of Health (2008) focuses on the socioeconomic and political context; structural determinants and socioeconomic position; intermediary determinants, such as material circumstances, socioenvironmental circumstances, behavioral and biological factors, social cohesion, and the healthcare system; and the impact on health equity and well-being measured as health outcomes.

Similarly, the US Department of Health and Human Services (HHS) publication *Healthy People 2020* embraces a holistic approach by considering the range of personal, social, economic, and environmental factors that determine the health status of individuals or populations (HHS 2010).

Exhibit 1.2 provides an overview of the health determinants—environment, health status, medical care, and individual characteristics (discussed in more detail below)—as they interact to influence health. For example, while individual characteristics and medical care each affect health on their own, they also interact to become another type of factor influencing health.

ENVIRONMENT

The environment in this context is composed of physical and social dimensions of an individual's existence over which he or she has little or no control. These dimensions exert influence at the family, community, and policy levels of society. Environmental determinants have a greater impact on health than does the medical care system.

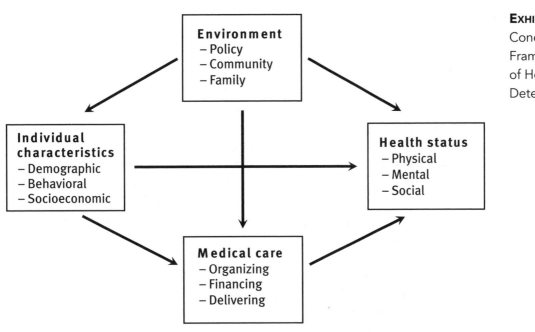

EXHIBIT 1.2
Conceptual Framework of Health Determinants

Physical Dimension

The use of energy sources (e.g., oil, coal) by a population creates certain health hazards in the physical environment. Those hazards can present themselves in the form of air, noise, or water pollution, resulting in hearing loss, infectious disease, gastroenteritis, cancer, emphysema, and bronchitis.

Social Dimension

The social environment is reflected in a nation's political, economic, and cultural preferences, which exert significant influence on the health of the population. Characteristics of an environment's social dimension include behavioral health factors and demographic trends. In the United States, for example, rates of psychological stress, homicide, suicide, and other behavioral health indicators can be attributed in part to crowding, isolation, and other social environmental factors. In terms of population trends, the increase in the number of elderly (those aged 65 years or older) as a proportion of the total population will place increasing pressure on healthcare systems around the world.

INDIVIDUAL CHARACTERISTICS RELATED TO HEALTH

Demographic, behavioral, and socioeconomic conditions shape individual characteristics, which explain much of the variation in health status within populations. As discussed in the following paragraphs, these factors interact with and are influenced by the environment, thereby affecting individuals' health.

Demographics

Age, gender, race, and ethnicity are strongly associated with health. Advancing age, for example, contributes to arthritis, diabetes, atherosclerosis, and cancer. Gender health is influenced in part by the social construct of gender characteristics, such as in the association between masculine identity and risk taking.

People also experience significant differences in health status depending on their race or ethnic origin. Explanations for these differences include socioeconomic status, behaviors, social circumstances, level of access to healthcare services (CDC 2005a; Shi 1999; Shi and Stevens 2010), and differences that are associated with particular ethnic or racial groups (CDC 2012).

Behaviors

The leading causes of death in the United States have shifted over the past 100 years. In 1900, infectious diseases, such as diphtheria, tuberculosis, measles and pneumonia, caused

797 per 100,000 deaths in the United States. Today, infectious diseases cause fewer than 100 per 100,000 deaths, and chronic diseases, such as heart disease and cancer, cause significantly higher mortality (Armstrong, Conn, and Pinner 1999). This "epidemiologic transition" supports the idea that the presence of behavioral risk factors, including poor dietary habits, cigarette smoking, alcohol abuse, lack of exercise, and unsafe driving, tends to predict higher risk for certain chronic diseases and mortality. See Exhibit 1.3 for examples of the association between risk factors and leading causes of death.

The level of behavioral risk factors exhibited by a population is related to socioeconomic status. For example, the prevalence of smoking is greater among those with less education than those with more education; in 2008, 41.3 percent of Americans who have obtained a GED (General Educational Development) certificate reported being a current cigarette smoker, compared to only 5.7 percent of those who held graduate degrees (CDC 2009). Behavioral risk factors are divided into three categories: leisure activity risks, consumption risks, and employment participation and occupational risks (Dever 2006). These categories are determined in part by the collection of decisions made by individuals in a particular group that affect their health. The degree of control they have in these decisions varies by category: Individuals have least control over employment and occupational

	Heart disease	Cancers	Stroke	Diabetes	Cirrhosis	Homicide
Health behaviors						
Smoking	X	X				
High blood pressure	X		X			
High cholesterol	X					
Poor diet	X	X		X		
Obesity	X			X		
Lack of exercise	X					
Stress	X					X
Alcohol abuse		X			X	X
Drug misuse	X					X

EXHIBIT 1.3
The Association Between Health Behaviors and Leading Causes of Death

factors, more control over consumption factors, and greatest control over leisure activity–related factors.

Destructive behaviors related to employment and occupational risks are usually difficult for individuals to control. To offset such risk, the federal government created regulatory agencies (e.g., the Occupational Safety and Health Administration) that force employers to maintain safe workplaces and practices.

Individuals have more control over consumption than over occupation-related behaviors; however, environmental factors, such as availability of affordable, healthy foods, play a significant role in the extent of their control. Consumption risks include overeating (resulting in obesity), high cholesterol intake (heart disease), alcohol consumption (motor vehicle accidents), alcohol addiction (cirrhosis of the liver), cigarette smoking (chronic bronchitis and emphysema, lung cancer, aggravating heart disease), drug dependency (suicide, homicide, malnutrition, accidents, social withdrawal, acute anxiety), and excessive glucose (sugar) intake (dental caries, obesity, hyperglycemia).

Unlike the risks related to employment and occupation, those that accompany leisure and consumption activities are relatively unregulated, with the exception of efforts to control the use of illegal drugs and the purchase of tobacco and alcohol products by underage youth. Leisure-related destructive behaviors include sexual promiscuity and unprotected sex, which can result in sexually transmitted diseases, including AIDS, syphilis, and gonorrhea, and limited or no exercise, which may lead to overweight and obesity.

Socioeconomic Status

The major components of SES are income, education, and occupational status. SES is a strong and consistent predictor of health status. Individuals with low SES suffer disproportionately from most diseases and experience higher rates of mortality than those with mid- or high-level SES. For example, after controlling for access to medical care, studies show that countries providing universal health insurance, such as England, report the same SES–health relationships as those found in the United States, which does not offer universal health insurance (Acheson 1998).

SES influences health in the extent to which individuals and populations are exposed to physical and social threats; have knowledge of health conditions; encounter adverse environmental conditions, such as pathogens and carcinogens; and are exposed to undesirable social conditions, such as crime.

MEDICAL CARE

Most items that we buy and sell are commodities, which are defined as goods and services whose worth can be captured as a monetary value, that serve a specific (rather than an intrinsic or esoteric) purpose, and that can be exchanged with other similar products (Doty 2008). Medical care differs from traditional commodities in four important ways. First, the demand for medical care is *derived*; that is, it stems from the demand for a more fundamental commodity—health itself.

The second difference is the presence of the **agency relationship**. Because patients generally lack the technical knowledge to make health-related decisions, they delegate this authority to their physicians with the expectation that physicians will act for patients as patients would for themselves if they had the appropriate expertise.

Agency relationship
The consumer, or the patient in healthcare, delegates some authority to make decisions and perform actions on his behalf to an expert agent (in the case of healthcare, the physician or other healthcare provider).

If physicians were to act solely in the interests of patients, the agency relationship would be virtually indistinguishable from normal consumer behavior. However, physicians' decisions typically reflect the physicians' self-interests as well as the interests of the patients. Those self-interests may arise from pressures imposed by professional colleagues and institutions, adherence to medical ethics, or a desire to make good use of available resources.

One implication of the agency relationship is that medical care may or may not be provided depending on the payer of services for the patient. For example, physicians who treat members of health maintenance organizations (HMOs) may have an incentive to restrict the number of hospital admissions they order because HMO patients' care is prepaid; that is, the physician will not be paid more to provide more services. Acting on this incentive means the physician is acting as an *imperfect agent*.

The third difference between medical care provision and the provision of other products and services is that healthcare pricing varies according to who pays the fees. Because most patients are covered by insurance, the amount paid by patients out-of-pocket at the point of care for most medical services is often significantly lower than the total payment made to the provider.

The fourth difference is that medical care service provision is influenced by the environment in which it takes place, whereas other commodities are not. In other words, the social, economic, demographic, technological, political, and cultural contexts dictate how, when, where, and to whom healthcare services are offered, which is not true of other products and services. For example, of the forces currently reshaping the healthcare industry, the growing number of uninsured (social context) is a major factor driving health insurance reform debates.

POLICY DEFINED

A *policy* is a decision made by an authority about an action—either one to be taken or one to be prohibited—to promote or limit the occurrence of a particular circumstance in a population. In the public sector, the authority charged with making policy is a legislative, executive, or judicial body operating under the purview of a federal, state, or local public administration. Public policy—decision making that affects the general population or significant segments of the general population—is meant to improve the conditions and general welfare of the population or subpopulations under its jurisdiction.

Although public policies are intended to serve the interests of the public at large, the term *public* has different interpretations according to the political context in which it is applied. For example, policymakers tend to be most responsive to the views and wishes of constituents who are politically active and communicate directly with their representatives.

In the private sector, authority is conferred to the executive or board of directors of an organization. Private policy—that which affects the private organization only—is meant to improve the conditions and general welfare of the employees of that organization. Because private organizations function in the larger social (public) environment, private policies must take into account the spirit of public policies.

HEALTH POLICY

Miller (1987, 15) defines health policy as "the aggregate of principles, stated or unstated, that . . . characterize the distribution of resources, services, and political influences that impact on the health of the population." This definition and others focus on US federal or public-level health policy and do not reflect non-US political systems or account for the fact that private-sector policy also influences health.

Health policy

Legislation over individuals, organizations, or the society whose goal is to improve health for the population or subpopulations.

Therefore, we define **health policy** as policy that pertains to or influences the attainment of health. In terms of the determinants-of-health framework, health policy refers to legislation that may influence, directly or indirectly, social and physical environments, behaviors, socioeconomic status, and availability of and accessibility to medical care services. Health policies affect groups or classes of individuals, such as physicians, the poor, the elderly, and children. They can also affect types of organizations, such as medical schools, HMOs, nursing homes, medical technology producers, and employers. On the basis of this broad definition, health consequences may result from virtually all major policies, such as Social Security mandates, national defense–related guidelines, labor policy, and immigration policy.

Furthermore, in the United States, each branch and level of government can influence health policy. For example, both the executive and legislative branches at the federal, state, and local levels can establish health policies, and the judicial branch at each level can uphold, strike down, or modify existing laws affecting health and healthcare. Examples of public, or government, health policy include legislative and regulatory efforts to ensure air and water quality and support for cancer research.

Health policies can also be made through the private sector. Examples of private-sector health policies are the decisions made by insurance companies regarding their product lines, pricing, and marketing and by employers regarding health benefits, such as leave policies, worksite health promotion, and insurance coverage.

Health policy must be distinguished from **healthcare policy**, which refers to that part of health policy pertaining to the financing, organization, and delivery of care. Healthcare policy may cover the training of health professionals; licensing of health professionals and facilities; administration of public health insurance programs, such as Medicare and Medicaid; deployment of electronic health records; efforts to control healthcare costs; and regulation of private health insurance. Whereas the predominant goal of health policy is to improve population health, the goals of healthcare policy are typically to provide equitable and efficient access to and quality of needed healthcare services.

> *Healthcare policy*
> Part of health policy but with a focus on healthcare. Specifically, it is related to the financing, delivery, and governance of health services for the populations or sub-populations within a jurisdiction.

TYPES OF HEALTH POLICY

The scope of health policy is determined by the political and economic system of a country. In the United States, where pro-individual and pro-market sentiments tend to dominate (see the For Your Consideration box titled "The United States as an Individualist Culture"), health policies are likely to be fragmented, incremental, and noncomprehensive. National policies and programs are typically crafted to reflect the notion that local communities are in the best position to identify strategies to address their unique needs. However, the type of changes that can be enacted at the community level are clearly limited. Next, we summarize the two major types of health policies: regulatory and allocative.

> **(?) FOR YOUR CONSIDERATION**
> The United States as an Individualist Culture
>
> The American political culture is characterized by some as being rooted in a distrust of power—particularly government power—and a preference for volunteerism and self-rule in small, homogeneous groups with limited purposes. How would you describe the political culture of average Americans? Do you agree or disagree with the characterization posed here? Provide examples to support your answer.

Regulatory Health Policies

Health policies may be used as regulatory tools that call on government to prescribe and control the behavior of a particular target group by monitoring the group and imposing sanctions if it fails to comply. Examples of **regulatory policies** include prohibition of smoking in public places, licensure requirements for medical professions, and processes related to the approval of new drugs. State insurance departments across the country regulate health insurance companies in an effort to protect customers from default on coverage in the case of a company's financial failure, excessive premiums, or deceptive practices.

Private health policies can also be regulatory. For example, physicians set standards of medical practice and hospitals undergo accreditation assessments from accreditation service organizations, such as The Joint Commission, to ensure compliance with all standards.

> *Regulatory policies*
> Regulations or rules that impose restrictions and are intended to control the behavior of a target group by monitoring the group and imposing sanctions if it fails to comply.

Distributive policy
Regulations that provide benefits or services to targeted populations or sub-populations, typically as entitlements.

Redistributive policy
Deliberate efforts to alter the distribution of benefits by taking money or property from one group and giving it to another.

Allocative Health Policies

Allocative health policies involve the direct provision of income, services, or goods to certain groups of individuals or institutions. They can be distributive or redistributive. **Distributive policies** spread benefits throughout society. Examples include the funding of medical research through the National Institutes of Health, provision of public health and health promotion services, training of medical personnel, and construction of health-care facilities. **Redistributive policies** take money or power from one group and give it to another. This approach typically creates visible beneficiaries and payers. Examples include means-tested social insurance programs such as Medicaid, which takes tax revenue from the more affluent residents and spends it to provide free or low-cost health insurance to the poor, to subsidize the welfare program, and to fund public housing.

DETERMINANTS OF HEALTH POLICY

As noted earlier, the framework for health determinants includes four major categories: environment, health status, medical care, and individual characteristics (see Exhibit 1.2). The framework for *health policy determinants* is presented in Exhibit 1.4. Broad determinants include the nature of the health problem, the sociocultural norms that influence the perception of the problem, and the political system within which policy is formulated. The inner circle of the framework shows the narrower determinants:

♦ Potential solutions to the identified health problem

♦ Views and efforts of the stakeholders

♦ Demonstrated leadership of the policymakers

♦ Available resources needed to implement the policy

This general framework may be applied to health policies at the national, state, or local level, to public and private policies, and to health policies within the United States and elsewhere. The remainder of this section describes these components in greater detail, and chapters 2 through 4 illustrate the application of this framework in various settings.

BROAD DETERMINANTS OF HEALTH POLICY

Health Problem

The nature of the health problem is typically the first consideration of policy, the significance of which is determined by its magnitude and severity. *Magnitude* indicates the reach

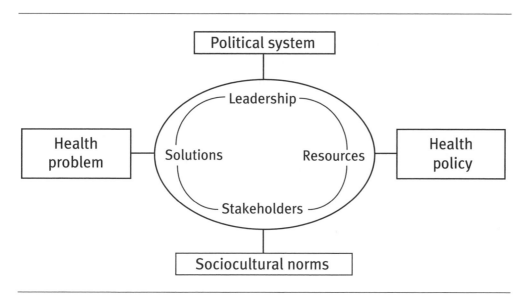

EXHIBIT 1.4
A Conceptual
Framework of
Health Policy
Determinants

of the problem. If the health problem affects a large segment of the population (e.g., heart disease, diabetes), it is considered widespread. *Severity* denotes the extent to which the problem is urgent. See the Learning Point box titled "Severe Acute Respiratory Syndrome (SARS)" for an example.

Sociocultural Norms

Sociocultural norms reflect the accepted values, beliefs, attitudes, and behaviors of a society or group. These norms play a significant role in the public's perception of the nature of a health problem, the role of government versus individuals in addressing that problem, and the type of solution or policy implemented to manage it. For example, mental illness carries a social stigma in many cultures. Although poor mental health has long been a pervasive problem in the United States and elsewhere, relatively little public action has been taken to promote improvements in mental health status, care, and treatment.

 LEARNING POINT
Severe Acute Respiratory Syndrome (SARS)

SARS is a serious form of viral pneumonia that can result in acute respiratory distress and, sometimes, death. SARS first came to the attention of Asian health officials in February 2003. In just a few months, SARS had spread throughout North America, South America, Europe, and Asia, sickening 8,098 individuals in more than 25 countries. Of those infected, 774 died. The 2003 epidemic demonstrates how quickly an infectious respiratory disease can spread across the world and registers among the most severe health problems in recent history.

SOURCE: CDC (2005b).

Political System

Although a democratically governed country is more likely to develop health policies that reflect public interest (officials are publicly elected and presumably represent the electorate's interests), the process of policy development is typically more difficult in democratic systems than in single-rule governments not only because the development of legislation in a democracy is arduous but also because the public's interests are rarely coherent. In authoritarian (single-party) countries, policies can be developed quickly but may not truly reflect the public's interests.

NARROW DETERMINANTS OF HEALTH POLICY

Solutions

Potential solutions to a health problem facilitate policy development. If solutions do not emerge, policymakers may direct their efforts away from full-fledged policy consideration and toward finding a solution, likely by initiating a research study. If a health problem has more than one potential solution, policy research and analysis is conducted to identify the optimal solution given the political climate, available resources, and expectations of prominent stakeholders.

Stakeholders

Entities or individuals who have a direct or indirect role in the development of policy are considered stakeholders. The influence of stakeholders is particularly strong in a democracy, as elected officials often cater to the interests of their constituency—either to fulfill a campaign promise or to gain reelection. Policy is more likely to be enacted when the positions of the various stakeholders converge. The next major section in this chapter describes the key stakeholders in US health policy.

Leadership

No matter how significant the problem or how determined the stakeholders, health policy addressing a particular problem will not appear on the policy agenda without the approval of the governing body's leader. The case study at the beginning of this chapter demonstrates the contrasting leadership styles of President Barack Obama and former First Lady Hillary Clinton.

Resources

Not even the most effective policy can be implemented without the availability of financial and administrative resources. Financial feasibility tests are conducted during the policy development process to ensure adequate funds are available and to verify that the benefits will outweigh the costs. Administrative feasibility studies examine how the policy can be translated into programs and carried out under an existing or a new infrastructure.

STAKEHOLDERS OF HEALTH POLICY

As shown in the framework of health policy determinants (Exhibit 1.4), stakeholders frequently exert powerful influence on health policy development. Indeed, as shown in later chapters, stakeholders influence not only the formulation of health policy but also its implementation and modification.

One type of stakeholder is the **interest group**. Interest groups are composed of individuals or entities that at least nominally present a unified position on their preferences regarding a particular health problem or its solution. **Lobbying** by organized interest groups is a common component of the political process in a democracy. Because stakeholders often differ in their positions and preferences and coalition building is usually specific to an issue, interest groups are not always static, and their formations typically depend on the particular health problem under policy consideration. The following paragraphs introduce the major stakeholders in US health policy.

Consumers and patients. Consumers and patients are typically the intended beneficiaries of health policy because they suffer the consequences of a health problem that could be the target of health policy. However, consumers have diverse health problems, and the prioritization of those problems is not always determined by consumers. Furthermore, consumers with the same health problem may have diverse interests and different cultural norms. The more their interests converge and the more organized they become as a collective, the more likely consumers are to influence policy development.

Healthcare providers. Healthcare providers—those individuals who provide direct patient care—include physicians, nurses, dentists, pharmacists, and other health professionals. Traditionally, healthcare providers value autonomy and have an interest in preserving the prestige and expertise that have been associated with their careers in recent decades.

Healthcare organizations. Healthcare organizations are the institutional settings in which healthcare providers work or provide care to patients. Traditional settings include hospitals (inpatient and outpatient) and community-based offices. Organizational settings now also include diagnostic imaging centers, occupational health centers, psychiatric outpatient centers, and many others. Administrators of those institutions may share an

Interest group
A collective of individuals or entities that hold a common set of preferences on a particular health issue and often seek to influence policymaking or public opinion.

Lobbying
Activities seeking to influence an individual or organization with decision-making authority.

Health maintenance organization (HMO)
A managed care organization that focuses on wellness care and requires use of a specified panel of providers.

Preferred provider organization (PPO)
A managed care organization that offers unrestricted provider options to enrollees and discounted fee arrangements to providers.

interest, for example, in serving their customers and maintaining the financial well-being of their institutions at the same time.

Payers and insurers. Payers and insurers can be private (commercial or other private enterprise) or public (government-operated entity). Private insurance is offered by commercial insurance companies (e.g., Aetna, Prudential); Blue Cross/Blue Shield; self-insured employers; and managed care organizations (MCOs), such as **health maintenance organizations** and **preferred provider organizations** (PPOs). Public insurance includes federally funded programs such as **Medicare**, which provides insurance for the elderly and certain disabled individuals; **Medicaid**, for the indigent; TRICARE, for Department of Defense active military service personnel and their families; and Veterans Affairs programs, for former armed forces personnel. One interest that private insurance companies and MCOs have in common is maintaining their share of the health insurance market; in contrast, a main interest of public payers is ensuring coverage for vulnerable populations at reasonable costs.

Regulators. In addition to providing public insurance for the elderly and indigent, the government functions as a regulator, seeking to make sure that basic services are provided and their quality maintained by the providers and that the overall cost of providing care in the community or sector is contained.

Medical device and pharmaceutical manufacturers. Manufacturers of medical equipment and drugs have a vested interest in health policy, especially with regard to payments for the use of their products. With the rapid advancement of science and technology, numerous devices and types of equipment have been developed for medical use, such as fetal monitors, computerized electrocardiography, and magnetic resonance imaging. The equipment is useful in the diagnosis of diseases but is expensive.

Educational and research institutions. Health policy affects the type and quantity of healthcare providers to be trained, making educational institutions another significant stakeholder. Similarly, research facilities are affected by health policy that directs the types of research to be conducted.

Businesses and corporations. American businesses and corporations have a keen interest in health policy that, among other issues, mandates healthcare coverage levels. These stakeholders seek to minimize the cost they incur for providing health insurance as a benefit to their employees.

WHY IS IT IMPORTANT TO STUDY HEALTH POLICY?

Understanding how health policy is developed is the first step toward influencing policy. And only by knowing the health policy determinants and how they manifest in particular contexts can one appreciate the key features of policy development.

In addition, the study of health policy allows an individual or a group the ability to engage in efforts to improve it. For example, *policy entrepreneurs*—those who work from outside the government to introduce and implement innovative ideas into public-sector practice—are instrumental in bringing new ideas and fundamentally changing the usual way of practice.

Furthermore, the importance of health policy itself is another reason to study it. As shown in the framework of health determinants (see Exhibit 1.2), policy is an integral component of environmental health determinants. Improvements to policy development, such as ensuring that a policy truly addresses a critical health problem and that it is developed in an expeditious manner, can significantly improve a population's overall health. In addition, policy influences other determinants of health and therefore must be thoroughly understood to enhance the country's health system.

Medicare

Federal government insurance plan for persons aged 65 years or older, disabled individuals who are entitled to Social Security benefits, and people who have end-stage renal (kidney) disease.

Medicaid

Joint federal and state insurance plan for the indigent.

(?) FOR YOUR CONSIDERATION
Why Is an International Perspective of Health Policy Useful?

Countries vary in their demographics, population health needs, and social norms, but they share commonalities, such as population aging and leading causes of death. Learning from the best practices of other countries—compared to a country developing its own evidence-based approaches—can significantly shorten the time in which the country improves healthcare delivery. Just as the US experience and lessons can benefit other countries as they consider healthcare delivery reform, so can the United States learn from the experiences of other countries in expanding health policy options. One result of this convergence of international health policies is the increase in similarity of global trends.

Industrialized countries need not limit their examination to other developed countries; the experiences of developing countries can also be instructive (Dixon and Alakeson 2010). Such countries tend to focus on basic and community-oriented public health and primary care, which may prove instructive for developed countries as they struggle to control costs and improve outcomes.

KEY POINTS

➤ Health determinants, such as environment and social structure, interact with biological factors and medical care to determine an individual's health status.
➤ Health policy formulation is influenced by broad determinants—health problems, sociocultural norms, and political system—and by narrow determinants—solutions, stakeholders, leadership, and resources.
➤ The major stakeholders in US health policy include consumers and patients, healthcare providers, healthcare organizations, payers and insurers, regulators, medical device and pharmaceutical manufacturers, educational and research institutions, and businesses and corporations.
➤ US health policy has evolved over time and will continue to change in response to new health concerns and interests.

CASE STUDY QUESTIONS

After researching the events surrounding the healthcare reform initiatives undertaken by the Clinton and Obama administrations, answer the following questions:

1. What factors might explain why the Obama plan succeeded? What events may have caused the Clinton plan to fail?
2. How do you think the failure of the Clinton healthcare reform effort influenced the outcome of the congressional election that followed?
3. Why does health reform continue to be controversial despite widespread opinion in favor of change?

FOR DISCUSSION

1. How is health defined?
2. What are the major determinants of health? How do they interact?
3. What is health policy, and what are its determinants?
4. Who are the stakeholders of health policy? What kinds of concerns does each stakeholder have about the current US healthcare system?
5. What are the major types of health policies? Cite an example of each type.
6. Why is it important to study health policy?

REFERENCES

Acheson, D. 1998. *Independent Inquiry into Inequalities in Health Report.* Accessed February 5, 2013. www.archive.official-documents.co.uk/document/doh/ih/ih.htm.

American Public Health Association (APHA). n.d. "What Is Public Health?" Accessed March 4, 2013. www.apha.org/NR/rdonlyres/C57478B8-8682-4347-8DDF-A1E24E82B919/0/what_is_PH_May1_Final.pdf.

Ansari, Z., N. J. Carson, M. J. Ackland, L. Vaughan, and A. Serraglio. 2003. "A Public Health Model of the Social Determinants of Health." *Sozial und Präventivmedizin [Social and Preventive Medicine]* 48 (4): 242–51.

Armstrong, G. L., L. A. Conn, and R. W. Pinner. 1999. "Trends in Infectious Disease Mortality in the United States During the 20th Century." *Journal of the American Medical Association* 281 (1): 61–66.

Blum, H. 1974. *Planning for Health.* New York: Human Sciences Press.

Centers for Disease Control and Prevention (CDC). 2012. "Racial and Ethnic Minority Populations." Accessed February 5, 2013. www.cdc.gov/minorityhealth/populations/remp.html.

———. 2009. "Cigarette Smoking Among Adults and Trends in Smoking Cessation—United States, 2008." *Morbidity and Mortality Weekly* 58 (47): 1227–32.

———. 2005a. "Health Disparities Experienced by Black or African Americans—United States." *Morbidity and Mortality Weekly* 54 (1): 1–3.

———. 2005b. "Severe Acute Respiratory Syndrome (SARS)." Accessed December 10. www.cdc.gov/sars/about/fs-SARS.html.

Commission on Social Determinants of Health, World Health Organization. 2008. *Closing the Gap in a Generation: Health Equity Through Action on the Social Determinants of*

Health. Accessed November 2010. www.who.int/social_determinants/thecommission/finalreport/en/index.html.

Dahlgren, G., and M. Whitehead. 2006. *European Strategies for Tackling Social Inequities in Health: Levelling Up Part 2*. World Health Organization Europe. Accessed December 13, 2012. www.euro.who.int/__data/assets/pdf_file/0018/103824/E89384.pdf.

Davis, K., C. Schoen, and K. Stremikis. 2010. *Mirror, Mirror on the Wall: How the Performance of the U.S. Health Care System Compares Internationally, 2010 Update*. Pub. No. 1400. New York: Commonwealth Fund.

Department of Economic and Social Affairs of the United Nations Secretariat (DESA). 2007. "World Population Prospects: The 2006 Revision." United Nations. Accessed December 6, 2012. www.un.org/esa/population/publications/wpp2006/WPP2006_Highlights_rev.pdf.

Dever, G. 2006. *Managerial Epidemiology: Practice, Methods, and Concepts*. Sudbury, MA: Jones & Bartlett.

Dixon, J., and V. Alakeson. 2010. "Reforming Health Care: Why We Need to Learn from International Experience." Nuffield Trust for Research and Policy Studies in Health Services. Published in September. www.nuffieldtrust.org.uk/sites/files/nuffield/publication/Reforming_health_care_international_experience.pdf.

Doty, T. 2008. "Healthcare as a Commodity: The Consequences of Letting Business Run Healthcare." Accessed February 5, 2013. www.ucalgary.ca/familymedicine/system/files/Resident+Research+Review+Report.pdf.

Health Careers Center. 2004. "Health Care Administrator." Copyright 2004. www.mshealthcareers.com/careers/healthcareadmin.htm.

Kaiser Family Foundation (KFF). 2012. "Health Care Costs: A Primer." Published in May. www.kff.org/insurance/upload/7670-03.pdf.

———. 2011. "Focus on Health Reform: Summary of New Health Reform Law." Modified April 15. www.kff.org/healthreform/upload/8061.pdf.

Metchnikoff, E., L. Pasteur, and R. Koch. 1939. *The Founders of Modern Medicine: Pasteur, Koch, Lister*. New York: Walden.

Miller, A. 1987. "Child Health." In *Epidemiology and Health Policy*, edited by S. Levine and A. Lillienfeld. New York: Tavistock.

Oberlander, J. 2007. "Learning from Failure in Health Care Reform." *New England Journal of Medicine* 357: 1677–79.

Sack, K., and M. Connelly. 2009. "In Poll, Wide Support for Government-Run Health." *New York Times*. Published June 20. www.nytimes.com/2009/06/21/health/policy/21poll .html.

Shi, L. 1999. "Experience of Primary Care by Racial and Ethnic Groups in the United States." *Medical Care* 37 (10): 1068–77.

Shi, L., and G. Stevens. 2010. *Vulnerable Populations in the United States*, 2nd ed. San Francisco: Jossey-Bass.

Trafford, A. 2010. "Obama's Struggle with Health-Care Reform Echoes Clintons' Failure in 1994." *Washington Post*. Published February 2. www.washingtonpost.com/wp-dyn/ content/article/2010/02/01/AR2010020103200.html.

US Department of Health and Human Services (HHS). 2010. *Healthy People 2020*. Washington, DC: HHS.

Winslow, C. E. A. 1920. "The Untilled Field of Public Health." *Science* 51 (1630): 23–33.

World Health Organization (WHO). 2010. *The World Health Report—Health Systems Financing: The Path to Universal Coverage*. Geneva, Switzerland: WHO Press.

———. 1946. "Preamble to the Constitution of the World Health Organization." Geneva, Switzerland: WHO.

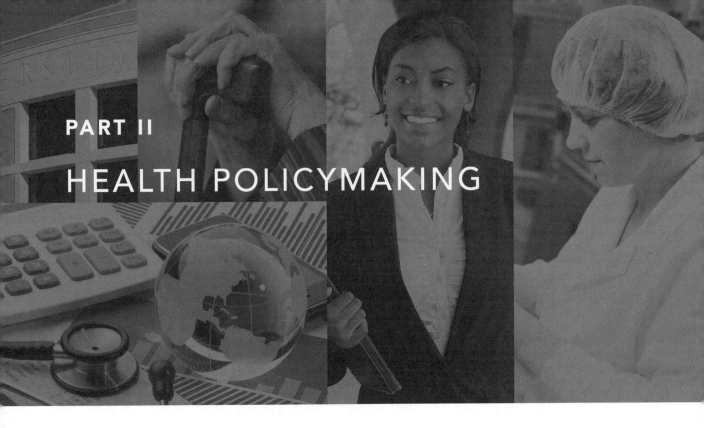

PART II

HEALTH POLICYMAKING

This section consists of three chapters that describe how health policy is made in the United States and elsewhere. Chapter 2 describes policymaking at the US federal level, and Chapter 3 illustrates the process at the US state and local levels and in the private sector. Chapter 4 covers health policymaking by international agencies such as the World Health Organization and provides examples of the process in selected countries. The spectrum of health policymaking presented in these chapters is intended to give students a comprehensive view of health policy development. This knowledge should prepare readers to examine the specific health issues commonly addressed by health policy in the United States and elsewhere.

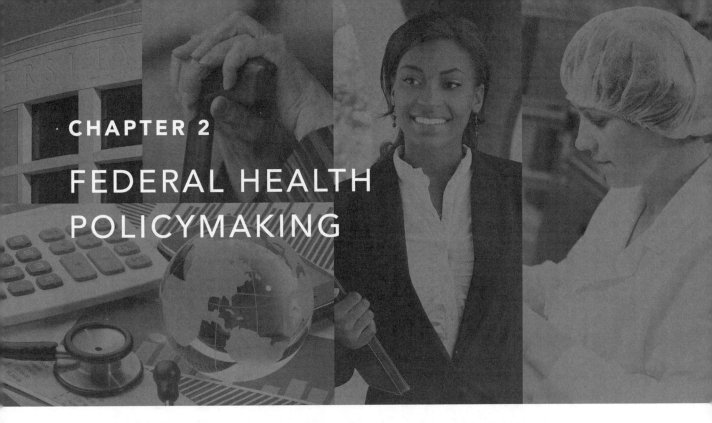

CHAPTER 2

FEDERAL HEALTH POLICYMAKING

In any moment of decision the best thing you can do is the right thing, the next best thing is the wrong thing, and the worst thing you can do is nothing.

— Theodore Roosevelt

LEARNING OBJECTIVES

Studying this chapter will help you to

➤ understand the US policymaking process at the federal level,

➤ discuss the policy formulation stage,

➤ provide examples of the types of health and healthcare policies developed,

➤ understand the policy implementation stage,

➤ describe the policy modification stage,

➤ analyze the characteristics of health policymaking in the United States, and

➤ appreciate the role of interest groups in US health policymaking.

CASE STUDY

THE DEVELOPMENT OF MEDICARE AND MEDICAID

In 1965, the US Congress passed amendments to the Social Security Act creating the Medicare and Medicaid programs. With this legislation, for the first time in US history, the government assumed direct responsibility for paying some healthcare costs on behalf of two vulnerable population groups: the elderly (Medicare) and the poor (Medicaid).

Prior to 1965, these populations were forced to rely on their own resources, limited public programs, or charity from hospitals and individual physicians to obtain healthcare services. The unemployed, too, received little assistance, as private health insurance—the only widely available source of payment for healthcare—was available primarily to middle-class working people and their families.

Government assistance for the poor and the elderly emerged as a solution when the market alone would not ensure access to care for these vulnerable populations. Most poor and elderly individuals could not afford the increasing costs of healthcare without assistance. Moreover, because the health status of these groups was significantly worse than that of the general population, the poor and the elderly required a higher level of healthcare services. The elderly, in particular, experienced higher incidence and prevalence of disease compared to younger groups.

Through the legislative process, a three-layered program was developed. The first two layers constituted Part A and Part B of Medicare, as outlined in Title XVIII of the Social Security Amendments. Medicare Part A finances hospital insurance and partial nursing home coverage for the elderly, and Part B covers their physicians' bills.

The third layer of publicly financed insurance, Medicaid, as set forth in Title XIX of the Social Security Amendments, extends federal matching funds to the states to cover healthcare costs for the poor. Recipients of Medicaid are deemed eligible on the basis of means testing—establishing financial need—administered by each state. Medicaid is available to the indigent of all age groups.

Although adopted simultaneously, Medicare and Medicaid reflect sharply different traditions. Medicare traditionally has seen broad grassroots support and has carried no inherent class distinction; Medicaid, on the other hand, is burdened by the stigma of public welfare. Medicare has uniform national standards for eligibility and benefits; Medicaid varies from state to state in terms of eligibility and benefits. Medicaid, in essence, has ushered in a two-tier system of government-funded medical care delivery whereby its recipients may experience limited access because the reimbursement fees set by the government are low and, as a consequence, some physicians refuse to accept Medicaid patients.

n the United States, health policymaking takes place at the federal, state, and local levels of government as well as in the private sector, but it is federal health policy that has the most profound impact on care delivery. This chapter presents health policymaking at the federal level. Looking ahead, Chapter 3 considers the process at other levels of government and in the private sector, and Chapter 4 discusses the processes adopted in the international arena.

THE US POLITICAL SYSTEM

The political system in the United States operates through three branches of government: the legislative, the executive, and the judicial branches (Exhibit 2.1).

LEGISLATIVE BRANCH

The legislative branch of the federal government is referred to as the US Congress and is composed of two chambers: the House of Representatives and the Senate. Congress is the most active of the three branches in policymaking by way of the statutes or laws it enacts. This body of **legislators** operates by virtue of three powers that drive its influence in health policymaking:

Legislator
Individual responsible for making or enacting laws.

◆ The US Constitution grants Congress the *power to use any reasonable means not directly prohibited by the Constitution to carry out the will of the people.* With this mandate Congress can enact laws influencing a broad array of health policy issues.

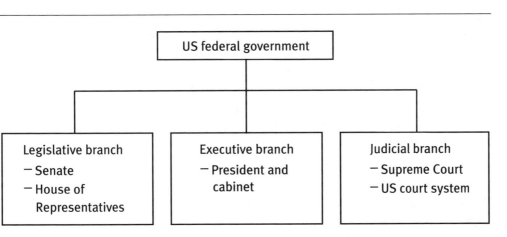

EXHIBIT 2.1
The US Political System—Federal Level

♦ Congress possesses the *power to tax*, which allows it to regulate—albeit indirectly—the health behavior of individuals, organizations, and states. Taxes on cigarettes, for example, are intended to reduce individuals' cigarette consumption; tax exemptions for employer health benefits are designed to promote increased insurance coverage for working people.

♦ Congress is granted the *power to spend*. It allocates funding as it deems appropriate to support the public's health through federal programs, such as Medicare. It also may restrict the manner in which states use those funds, such as establishing minimum requirements for basic services offered by the joint federal- and state-funded Medicaid program.

EXECUTIVE BRANCH

Legislation
Law made by government to achieve a particular objective.

The president of the United States and the department heads—referred to as cabinet members—within his or her administration comprise the executive branch of the federal government. This branch crafts **legislation** that reflects the administration's preferred policies and attempts to convince legislators to enact those policies. Executive branch members also make policy by establishing rules and regulations used to implement statutes and laws.

JUDICIAL BRANCH

Statutory authority
The capacity to enforce legislation on behalf of the government as granted by the US Constitution.

The judicial branch, made up of the US court system, influences health policy through its **statutory authority** to interpret the law. Whenever a court interprets a statute, establishes a judicial precedent, or interprets the US Constitution, it makes policy. The courts also have the power to declare that federal or state laws are unconstitutional. Because federal judges are appointed for life, they are generally not subjected to the types of conflicts of interest that may accompany the reelection efforts of legislators and the president.

POLICYMAKING PROCESS AT THE FEDERAL LEVEL

The three major stages of policymaking are policy formulation, policy implementation, and policy modification. Exhibit 2.2 displays a framework of health policymaking at the federal level (Longest 2010).

The relationships among the stages are not as straightforward as they may seem. On the one hand, the three stages are consecutive. Policy formulation, which includes setting the policy agenda and developing the related legislation, begins the policymaking process. That stage is followed by policy implementation, which includes making the rules and putting them into operation. Policy modification concludes the process. In this stage, policies are adjusted as necessary to accommodate real-world application.

On the other hand, the three stages are interactive and reinforcing. For example, the rules and regulations proposed in the implementation stage typically solidify the policy and often become the laws and policies themselves. Policymaking rarely forgos modification; as time passes, new priorities and needs arise, which in turn affect the formulation of new policies. The sections that follow describe the three stages of the policymaking process in more detail.

POLICY FORMULATION

The two main components of the policy formulation stage are agenda setting and legislation development.

> **? FOR YOUR CONSIDERATION**
> Public Policy as Health Policy
>
> Health policies often develop as a by-product of existing public policies. For example, important changes in the US healthcare system came about after the conclusion of World War II. At this time, policies were implemented to exclude fringe benefits from income or Social Security taxes, and the Supreme Court ruled that employee benefits, including health insurance, could be legitimately included in the collective bargaining process. Used as a strategy to compete for skilled workers, employer-provided health insurance benefits grew rapidly in the mid-twentieth century.
>
> What other health policy initiatives were developed as the result of public policy changes?

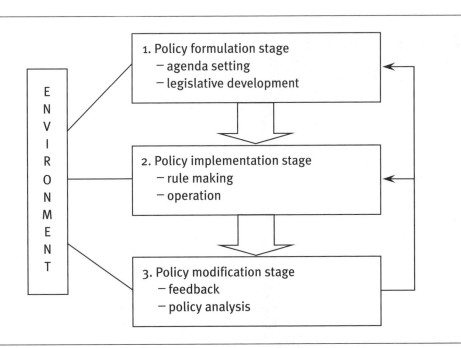

EXHIBIT 2.2
The Process of Health Policymaking

SOURCE: Information from Longest (2010).

Agenda Setting

Agenda setting refers to the selection of a health problem as a policy target. A health problem can come to the attention of policymakers through multiple pathways, and when several pathways converge on a health problem, its chances of appearing on the policy **agenda** are increased. Here we describe the most common pathways to agenda setting.

Impact of the health problem. The health problems that lead to legislative action typically either affect the general population or have a concentrated impact on a small but powerful subpopulation. For example, bioterrorism—the deliberate release of viruses, bacteria, or other germs (agents) used to cause illness or death in people, animals, or plants (Shi and Singh 2011; CDC 2007)—emerged as a health problem targeted for policymaking following 9/11 (September 11, 2001, when New York's World Trade Center and the Pentagon in Washington, DC, were attacked by terrorists). To help prevent, protect against, and respond to any future acts of terrorism in the United States, former President George W. Bush signed into law the Homeland Security Act of 2002, opening a new chapter in health protection in the United States.

Public opinion. The likelihood of policy action is greatest when public interest is high and the degree of conflict or dispute is low. Individuals tend to be concerned with the likely impact of any new healthcare bill on their personal lives and well-being. Policymakers must structure the issues they want to address in terms of the concerns of the public to achieve a high degree of relevance and support.

Presidential involvement. The president may form his or her **policy positions** on the basis of input from a variety of sources, including personal interests; recommendations of advisers, cabinet members, and agency chiefs; campaign information; expert opinions; and public opinion polls. He or she must firmly believe in the merits of an issue to be a strong advocate for a targeted policy. For example, President Barack Obama declared a major goal of his administration to be a drastic reduction in the number of Americans who have no health insurance coverage. His healthcare agenda was accepted as public policy through the passage of the Affordable Care Act in 2010, which was achieved by uniting the Democratic Party behind this cause.

Legislator interest. Legislators influence agenda setting by championing a health issue

FOR YOUR CONSIDERATION
Homeland Security Act

The Homeland Security Act (HSA) of 2002 was formulated following the 9/11 terrorist attacks. It created the US Department of Homeland Security and the new, cabinet-level position of secretary of Homeland Security. The primary mission of the department is to prevent terrorist attacks within the United States, reduce the vulnerability of the United States to terrorism, and minimize the damage and assist in the recovery from terrorist attacks that do occur within the United States.

The HSA has a significant impact on US foreign and domestic policies. How do you think it has affected health policy in the United States and abroad? Can you think of examples?

that either they personally embrace or their constituents demand. The late Senator Edward "Ted" Kennedy (D-MA), for example, became a national leader and advocate for improving mental healthcare following the diagnosis of his son Patrick with bipolar disorder.

Media coverage. In a democracy whose fundamental freedoms include freedom of the press, the media—newspapers, magazines, radio, television, websites—serve as a layer of checks and balances outside of the government's purview to guard against the abuse of power by public officials.

In addition, the media heighten awareness of issues through investigative reporting and frequent exposure of their findings, which may produce strong public reaction that leads to new regulations and laws. The reporting of Walt Bogdanich (1987) for the *Wall Street Journal* is just one example. Bogdanich documented evidence that poorly trained laboratory technicians were misreading Pap smear tests, leading to false diagnoses of cervical cancer or no diagnosis when the cancer was present (Otten 1992). His reporting prompted Congress to pass the Clinical Laboratory Improvement Amendments in 1988, prescribing minimum standards of training, testing, and workloads for laboratory technicians.

> **(?) FOR YOUR CONSIDERATION**
> Public Opinion and Policymaking: Universal Healthcare
>
> The repeated failure of the United States in creating a universal healthcare system is an example of the influence that the public holds over healthcare policy. Although US residents in general believe that offering healthcare to all is "the right thing to do," they also express concern that its implementation could adversely affect their own status.
>
> What do you think? Should the United States expand coverage mandated by the Affordable Care Act to all US residents as a universal approach to healthcare? How would you frame universal coverage legislation to reflect the concerns of the public at large?

Speaker of the House
The presiding officer of the US House of Representatives, typically chosen from the majority party of the House.

Legislation Development

Federal Legislative Process

Exhibit 2.3 summarizes the progression of US federal legislation, and the steps are described in more detail here.

A bill introduced in Congress—either the House of Representatives or the Senate—is assigned to a congressional committee by the **speaker of the House** or the **majority leader in the Senate**. The committee chair forwards the bill to the appropriate subcommittee, which in turn forwards it to agencies potentially affected by it; holds hearings and hears testimony; and may amend the bill. The subcommittee and full committee may recommend the bill for consideration by the entire body of Congress, not recommend it, or recommend **tabling the legislation**.

Senate majority leader
Senate leader elected by the party that holds majority in the Senate. He or she serves as the chief Senate spokesperson for the party and is responsible for scheduling the legislative and executive business of the Senate.

EXHIBIT 2.3

The Progression of
Federal Legislation

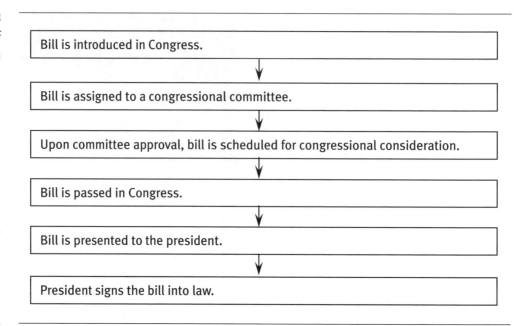

Bill is introduced in Congress.

Bill is assigned to a congressional committee.

Upon committee approval, bill is scheduled for congressional consideration.

Bill is passed in Congress.

Bill is presented to the president.

President signs the bill into law.

Tabling legislation
An action undertaken
by Congress to post-
pone consideration of
the legislation.

Amendment
Change or addition to a
current law or piece of
legislation.

Veto
Unilaterally stopping
an official action; as a
noun, the authority to
do so.

Assuming it is approved in committee, the full House or Senate hears the bill and may add **amendments**; the bill can be approved with or without these amendments and is then sent to the other chamber for consideration.

Once the House and Senate have approved an identical bill, it is presented to the president for his or her signature. The president has three options in acting on legislation:

♦ Sign the legislation, at which time it becomes law.

♦ **Veto** the legislation, whereby the bill dies if a two-thirds majority of Congress cannot overturn the veto.

♦ Neither sign nor otherwise act on the legislation, and it either

— automatically becomes law after 21 days if Congress is in session during that time or

— results in a "pocket veto" if fewer than 21 days remain in the congressional session.

House and Senate Committees

At least 14 committees and subcommittees in the House of Representatives, 24 committees and subcommittees in the Senate, and more than 60 legislative panels directly influence legislation (Falcone and Hartwig 1991). Some implications of this fragmentation are discussed later in the chapter.

ADDITIONAL RESOURCES
Congressional Committees Involved in Health-Related Legislation

The House *Committee on Ways and Means* (http://waysandmeans.house.gov) has sole jurisdiction over Medicare Part A, Social Security, unemployment compensation, public welfare, and healthcare reform.

The House *Energy and Commerce Committee* oversees legislation relating to telecommunications, consumer protection, food and drug safety, public health, air quality and environmental health, the supply and delivery of energy, and interstate and foreign commerce in general. This committee has jurisdiction over Medicaid, Medicare Part B (shared with Ways and Means), and matters of public health.

The House *Committee on Appropriations* (http://appropriations.house.gov) and its Labor, Health and Human Services, Education, and Related Agencies subcommittee are responsible for allocating and distributing federal funds for individual health programs (except those for Medicare and Social Security, which are funded through the Social Security Trust Fund).

The Senate *Committee on Health, Education, Labor and Pensions* (http://help.senate.gov) focuses on health, education, and workplace issues by proposing changes to the healthcare system, the minimum wage, working conditions and compensation, and welfare and labor laws.

The Senate *Committee on Finance* (http://finance.senate.gov) and its Subcommittee on Health, similar to the Ways and Means Committee in the House, have jurisdiction over taxes and revenues, including matters related to Social Security, Medicare, Medicaid, and Maternal and Child Health (Title V of the Social Security Act).

POLICY IMPLEMENTATION

Once legislation has been signed into law, it is forwarded to the appropriate agency for implementation. The US government's principal agency for implementing many of the health laws is the US Department of Health and Human Services (HHS), whose mission is to protect the health of all Americans and provide essential human services, especially for those who are least able to help themselves (HHS 2011). The following operating divisions within HHS focus on specific areas of health concern:

◆   Administration for Children and Families

◆   Administration on Aging

◆ Agency for Healthcare Research and Quality

◆ Agency for Toxic Substances and Disease Registry

◆ Centers for Disease Control and Prevention

◆ Centers for Medicare & Medicaid Services

◆ Food and Drug Administration

◆ Health Resources and Services Administration

◆ Indian Health Service

◆ National Institutes of Health

◆ Office of Inspector General

◆ Substance Abuse and Mental Health Services Administration

The assigned agency develops rules and regulations (the rule-making component), and the proposed rules and regulations are published in the *Federal Register* for public comment and reaction before they are finalized.

Federal Register
A public-access source that publishes presidential and federal agency documents; a daily publication of the US federal government.

Rule Making

Rule making refers to the process by which implementation agencies set detailed rules and regulations for the application of laws. In this process, experts from different disciplines and backgrounds, such as science, economics, and industry, are brought together to agree on the rules by which the new law will be enforced. During the preliminary stage of information collection and as part of the comment or negotiation period, the public—individuals and groups—may also have the opportunity to provide input on the terms of the proposed rule. Once the rules or regulations are finalized, they become the guidelines for operationalizing the law.

Operation

Legislation is operationalized by the HHS agency assigned to develop the regulations to implement or enforce it. This portion of the implementation process focuses on carrying out the rules or regulations in an *efficient* and *effective* manner: The program must meet economic constraints while delivering concrete services to the target population. The ability to attain the policy objective depends on the presence of a host of requirements, including the following:

◆ The logic of the potential solution is sound.

◆ The structure is in place.

◆ Program activities are designed to reflect the policy intent and logic model (see Shi, Oliver, and Huang [2000] for a discussion of logic models).

◆ Program activities are carried out effectively and efficiently.

◆ Unintended outcomes will not jeopardize the continuation of the program.

◆ External factors will not jeopardize the impact of the program.

Factors other than these requirements may also emerge in the operational stage of policy implementation, such as unexpected events or influence from additional determinants (see Chapter 1) that may compromise policy success. An example of uncontrolled determinants is the current prevalence of diabetes and obesity. Since the 1970s, the rate of diabetes, and its main contributing factor, obesity, has steadily increased, triggering major—albeit largely failed—policy initiatives to combat this health problem. One reason these initiatives have failed is that they focus on changing behaviors (e.g., exercise, diet) but do not address other, larger environmental and social determinants that contribute to unhealthy behaviors. Examples of these determinants include a sedentary and stressful work or living environment; easy and cheap access to unhealthy food; limited access to safe, open space; and lack of facilities for exercise.

POLICY MODIFICATION

Policy modification refers to revisions to the rules or regulations pertaining to a piece of original legislation to enhance its benefits to the targeted population, reduce its negative consequences, refine its policy objectives, or address other issues related to the policy. Policy modification typically takes place after the policy has been implemented and incorporates lessons learned from the implementation. It also may occur during agenda setting, where existing similar policies inform the formulation of the new policy; legislation development, where the new development, any budgetary changes, or beneficiary demands dictate the adjustment of policy; rule making, where the nature of the bureaucracy prompts the operationalizing of policy into regulations and where interest groups use their resources to maximize the benefits or minimize the negative consequences; and operation, where administrative structure and budgetary constraints often determine the scope of the enacted program (Longest 2010).

Why Policy Modification?

The need to modify a policy can arise for a number of reasons, including the following.

Change in the logic model. In the course of implementing the policy, new evidence or a new theory comes to light that indicates the logic behind the policy may not be strong. When the logic itself is flawed, it must be adjusted or corrected by modifying the logic model (Shi, Oliver, and Huang 2000). The revision of the logic model often necessitates revision of the policy itself.

Consequences of implementation. Although policymakers try to anticipate potential consequences, not all consequences can be foreseen, particularly if new events take place in the course of policy implementation or if the consequences are determined to be negative for the policy beneficiaries or other stakeholders.

Policy analysis and evaluation. Results of policy evaluation often provide important input into the modification of an existing policy. The Congressional Research Service is a legislative agency within the Library of Congress that provides Congress with information and analyses on implemented policy.

Resource constraints. The economic climate may decline following a policy's implementation, and a particular issue may no longer be a priority in the face of an economic downturn and budget cuts.

Changing goals. The policy goals of one administration may differ from those of the next. As the administration of the US government changes every four years (in addition to the more frequent changes in Congress), many policy priorities change accordingly.

Interest group involvement. In the American democracy, interest groups influence policies at the modification stage as well as at the formulation and implementation stages. Interest groups that are adversely affected by a policy are likely to expend extra effort to overturn or modify the enacted policy.

Oversight. The executive, legislative, and judicial branches each have **oversight** responsibility for enacted legislation. The following are examples for each branch:

- *Executive branch*: In addition to the agencies assigned to a particular piece of legislation, the **Office of Management and Budget** plays a critical role in supervising, assessing, and ensuring the successful implementation of a policy.

- *Legislative branch*: Any congressional committee with **jurisdiction** over a particular policy can hold oversight hearings to review progress and assess modification needs.

- *Judicial branch*: The courts may become involved in policy modification by ruling on how laws are interpreted and enforced, especially in cases of disputes over the interpretation, application, and constitutionality of laws.

Incremental nature of policy development. In the American political landscape, radical policy is rarely enacted; most policies are incremental and evolve over time. In fact, the

---

Oversight
Activities to review, monitor, or supervise the process of formulating, implementing, and modifying public policy.

Office of Management and Budget
The largest component of the Executive Office; implements and enforces the commitments and priorities of the president and assists executive departments and agencies across the federal government.

Jurisdiction
The authority to interpret and apply the law.

basic nature of policy development dictates modification of existing policies. Revisions to the 1935 Social Security Act have spanned decades, serving as a prime example.

ATTRIBUTES OF HEALTH POLICYMAKING IN THE UNITED STATES

US health policymaking is shaped by several important characteristics, as described in this section.

GOVERNMENT IN SUBORDINATE ROLE TO THE PRIVATE SECTOR

Because the federal government takes a subordinate role to the private sector in providing healthcare services and private insurance plans, policymaking by government is limited to addressing market failures or deficiencies. For example, left alone, the healthcare market could not ensure adequate insurance coverage for the elderly (who tend to be sicker) or the poor (who typically cannot afford the premiums). Therefore, government intervened and created health insurance plans for the elderly (Medicare) and the poor (Medicaid). One consequence

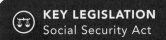

KEY LEGISLATION
Social Security Act

The 1935 Social Security Act is a landmark policy that established the Social Security program for the elderly. Since its enactment, a number of health-related modifications have been made.

- Kerr-Mills Act (1960): established a program of medical assistance for the medically indigent elderly
- Medicare and Medicaid (1965): created as insurance programs for the elderly and the poor, respectively
- Expansion of public coverage (1967): expanded Medicaid to cover eligible children up to age 21 and mandated improvement in the quality of care provided in nursing homes
- Professional standards review organizations (1972): created to monitor the quality and medical necessity of services provided to Medicare recipients
- Block grant program (1974): consolidated federal–state social services programs, placing a ceiling on federal matching funds while giving states more flexibility in prioritizing services than they had prior to the program's implementation
- Prospective payment system (1983): instituted predetermined payments set by diagnosis-related groups

of government intervention is that policies tend to be implemented piecemeal, addressing one market deficiency at a time rather than in a comprehensive and coordinated manner.

FRAGMENTED GOVERNMENT AND PROGRAMS

The fragmentation of the American political institution is reflected in the development of health policy legislation.

Healthcare programs are similarly fragmented among federal, state, and local governments, which pursue their own policies with limited coordination. Exhibit 2.4 provides an example of the variability in healthcare insurance that has emerged.

INCREMENTAL APPROACH TO REFORM

Such fragmentation inevitably leads to incremental change rather than systematic reform. Compromises struck in the resolution of issues also contribute to the piecemeal nature of healthcare reform. Consider the broadening of the Medicaid program since its start in 1965. Rather than adopt a single, comprehensive initiative, Medicaid underwent numerous disjointed expansion efforts in the 1980s and 1990s (see the Key Legislation box on page 43).

IMPORTANCE OF CONGRESSIONAL SUPPORT

As Exhibit 2.5 shows, most of the important US health legislation has been passed when both congressional chambers are controlled by the same party. When the president is of the same party affiliation, chances of success are even greater.

EXHIBIT 2.4 Example of Fragmented Healthcare Programs: Funding of Health Insurance	
The employed	Predominantly covered by voluntary private insurance to which they and their employers make contributions
The elderly	Funded by Social Security tax revenues (Medicare Part A) and government-subsidized voluntary insurance for physician, supplementary, and prescription drug coverage (Medicare Parts B and D)
The poor	Covered by Medicaid, which is financed with federal, state, and local revenues
Special population groups (e.g., veterans; American Indians; members of the armed forces, Congress, and the executive branch of government)	Covered by the federal government directly

For example, President Lyndon B. Johnson achieved passage of Medicare and Medicaid in 1965 not only by virtue of his leadership skills but also because he was operating in an unusually favorable political environment in which to advance legislation. Johnson was a Democrat serving at a time when Congress was also dominated by the Democrats. Johnson mobilized the public and Congress behind the bill and efficiently shepherded it through the legislative process. As a result, the Social Security Amendments of 1965 were signed into law, setting the stage for creating Medicare and Medicaid.

EXHIBIT 2.5
Relationship Between Health Legislation and Party Affiliation

Date	Legislation	President	Senate	Congress
1921	Maternity and Infancy Act	**Republican**	**Republican**	**Republican**
1935	Social Security Act	**Democrat**	**Democrat**	**Democrat**
1937	National Cancer Institute Act	**Democrat**	**Democrat**	**Democrat**
1944	Public Health Service Act	**Democrat**	**Democrat**	**Democrat**
1946	National Mental Health Act	**Democrat**	**Democrat**	**Democrat**
1946	Hospital Survey and Construction Act	**Democrat**	**Democrat**	**Democrat**
1952	Immigration and Nationality Act	**Democrat**	**Democrat**	**Democrat**
1956	Dependents Medical Care Act	Republican	*Democrat*	*Democrat*
1963	Health Professions Educational Assistance Act	**Democrat**	**Democrat**	**Democrat**
1963	Clean Air Act	**Democrat**	**Democrat**	**Democrat**
1965	Social Security Amendments	**Democrat**	**Democrat**	**Democrat**
1971	Comprehensive Health Manpower Training Act	Republican	*Democrat*	*Democrat*
1972	Consumer Product Safety Act	Republican	*Democrat*	*Democrat*
1973	Health Maintenance Organization Act	Republican	*Democrat*	*Democrat*
1974	Employee Retirement Income Security Act	Republican	*Democrat*	*Democrat*
1983	Social Security Amendments	Republican	Republican	Democrat
1990	Americans with Disabilities Act	Republican	*Democrat*	*Democrat*
1990	Ryan White Comprehensive AIDS Resources Emergency Act	Republican	*Democrat*	*Democrat*

(continued)

Exhibit 2.5 Relationship Between Health Legislation and Party Affiliation *(continued)*	1996	Health Insurance Portability and Accountability Act	Democrat	*Republican*	*Republican*
	1997	State Children's Health Insurance Program	Democrat	*Republican*	*Republican*
	2000	Minority Health and Health Disparities Research and Education Act	Democrat	*Republican*	*Republican*
	2002	Health Care Safety Net Amendments	Republican	Democrat	Republican
	2005	Patient Safety and Quality Improvement Act	**Republican**	**Republican**	**Republican**
	2008	Health Care Safety Net Act	Republican	*Democrat*	*Democrat*
	2009	American Recovery and Reinvestment Act	**Democrat**	**Democrat**	**Democrat**
	2010	Patient Protection and Affordable Care Act	**Democrat**	**Democrat**	**Democrat**

NOTE: **Bold** indicates both houses of Congress are controlled by the same party and the president is affiliated with that party. *Italics* indicate both houses of Congress are controlled by the same party and the president is affiliated with a different party.

ROLE OF INTEREST GROUPS IN US HEALTH POLICYMAKING

Interest groups' efforts to promote their positions affect health policy just as they do any other policy debate in American politics. Each group aims to protect its own best interests, and although most groups are satisfied with the benefits they receive, the result for any single group may be less than optimal.

Organizations tend to be effective at demanding health policy. They usually have the resources necessary to advance their interests, and those interests tend to be more focused than the diverse interests of individuals. Well-organized interest groups

- ◆ combine and concentrate their members' resources;

- ◆ pursue an active agenda to influence all phases of policymaking, from formulation to implementation to modification; and

- ◆ represent a variety of individuals and entities.

Here we discuss the traditional types of interest groups involved in health policymaking in the United States.

PHYSICIANS

Physicians as a group have difficulty lobbying for their interests because they represent many specialties. The American Medical Association (http://ama-assn.org) now represents

ADDITIONAL RESOURCES
Interest Groups New to Healthcare Policymaking

Two relatively new types of interest groups have emerged in the health policymaking paradigm: corporate America and healthcare consumers.

Corporate America

Business has emerged as a singular interest group, albeit one with two prongs: large employers and small employers. American employers' health policy concerns often are shaped by the extent to which they are expected to provide health insurance benefits to their employees, their employees' dependents, and their retirees. In general, they are likely to pay attention to health policies that affect worker health or labor–management relations.

Healthcare Consumers

The health policy spectrum has expanded to include consumer interests. Among the most vocal voters on this issue are members of the Tea Party movement (http://theteaparty .net), although their influence has begun to wane as of this writing. This uniquely American populist political movement represents conservative and libertarian interests as demonstrated by the following stances:

- It endorses reductions in government spending.
- It seeks reduction of the national debt and federal budget deficit.
- It opposes taxation.
- It opposes the expansion of insurance coverage to those who are currently uninsured.

The Tea Party movement is known for its demonstrations in Washington, D.C., and around the United States prior to and during the passage of the Affordable Care Act of 2010.

only 17 percent of US physicians, down from its peak of 70 percent in the 1960s. Other medical groups include the American Academy of Pediatrics (www.aap.org), Physicians for a National Health Program (www.pnhp.org), the American Society of Anesthesiologists (www.asahq.org), and the Society of Thoracic Surgeons (www.sts.org). These groups come together on issues that pose a potential threat to the interests of physicians as a whole, as in 1992, when the Health Care Financing Administration (now the Centers for Medicare & Medicaid Services) changed the reimbursement system from fee-for-service to the Resource-Based Relative Value Scale (the physicians did not prevail in their efforts to overturn the policy). Other issues of interest to some physician groups are income maintenance, professional autonomy, and malpractice reform.

SENIOR CITIZENS

AARP (www.aarp.org) assists people age 50 or older by providing them with information, advocating for fulfillment of their needs, and offering certain services. It advocates expansion of financing the public benefits for the elderly covering housing, food, income, and health. AARP supported the Medicare Prescription Drug Improvement and Modernization Act of 2003, but it did not oppose the proposed Medicare cuts in the Affordable Care Act, perhaps because AARP's interests related to the funding of Medicare were outweighed by its support of a national healthcare system.

HOSPITALS

The American Hospital Association (AHA) (www.aha.org) represents approximately 5,000 hospitals, health systems, health networks, and other providers of care in issues of national health policy development, legislation, regulation, and legal concerns. The implications of **administrative simplification**, the reduction of bad debt write-offs, and profitability are among the current topics of interest to hospitals in general.

Administrative simplification
Provision in the Health Insurance Portability and Accountability Act and the Affordable Care Act that aims to reduce administrative costs through the adoption of electronic transactions and standardization of operating rules.

INSURANCE COMPANIES

America's Health Insurance Plans (www.ahip.org) represents nearly 1,300 health insurance companies. The organization supports health insurers in their efforts to ensure that affordable healthcare coverage is expanded to include all Americans. Among the issues holding insurers' interest are the elimination of cost shifting and the implications of administrative simplification.

PHARMACEUTICAL RESEARCH AND MANUFACTURING

The Pharmaceutical Research and Manufacturers of America (PhRMA) (www.phrma.org) represents US pharmaceutical research and biotechnology companies by supporting their efforts to discover new medicines. PhRMA also alerts its members to changes in health policy and attempts to influence policy formulation related to the approval and monitoring of drugs and pharmaceutical devices.

KEY POINTS

➤ The major stages of policymaking are policy formulation, policy implementation, and policy modification.

➤ Characteristics of US health policymaking include a fragmented governing system, a heavy influence of public opinion, and incremental (rather than radical) changes.

➤ Interest groups have become increasingly influential in the policymaking processes, representing a wide variety of healthcare stakeholders.

CASE STUDY QUESTIONS

On the basis of your research of the events leading to the enactment of Medicare and Medicaid legislation and your knowledge of these programs, answer the following questions:

1. Why did the United States forgo attempts to achieve universal health insurance in favor of focusing on insurance for the elderly and the poor?
2. What are the major similarities of and differences between Medicare and Medicaid?

FOR DISCUSSION

Find examples of policymaking in the health sector at the US federal level and answer the following questions:

1. How is the policymaking process demonstrated in your examples?
2. Which components of policymaking are evident in each stage of the process?

3. How do the different stages influence each other?
4. Which characteristics of health policymaking do the examples illustrate?
5. What interest groups were involved in your examples of policymaking? What were their roles in the making of that policy?
6. What policymaking successes and failures can you identify in the example?

REFERENCES

Bogdanich, W. 1987. "False Negative." *Wall Street Journal*, February 2.

Centers for Disease Control and Prevention (CDC). 2007. "Bioterrorism Overview." Updated February 12. www.bt.cdc.gov/bioterrorism/overview.asp.

Falcone, D., and L. C. Hartwig. 1991. "Congressional Process and Health Policy: Reform and Retrenchment." In *Health Politics and Policy*, 2nd ed., edited by T. Litman and L. Robins, 126–44. New York: Wiley.

Longest, B. 2010. *Health Policymaking in the United States*, 5th ed. Chicago: Health Administration Press.

Otten, A. 1992. "The Influence of the Mass Media on Health Policy." *Health Affairs* 11 (4): 111–18.

Shi, L., T. R. Oliver, and V. Huang. 2000. "The Children's Health Insurance Program: Expanding the Framework to Evaluate State Goals and Performance." *Milbank Quarterly* 78 (3): 403–46.

Shi, L., and D. A. Singh. 2011. *Delivering Health Care in America*, 5th ed. Burlington, MA: Jones & Bartlett.

US Department of Health and Human Services (HHS). 2011. "About HHS." Accessed April 22. www.hhs.gov/about/.

ADDITIONAL RESOURCES

Administration on Aging (AoA). 2011. "About AoA." Accessed April 22. www.aoa.gov/AoA-Root/About/index.aspx.

Administration for Children and Families (ACF). 2011. "ACF Services." National Resource Center, Office of Community Services. Accessed April 22. www.acf.hhs.gov/index.html.

Agency for Healthcare Research and Quality (AHRQ). 2011. "AHRQ at a Glance." Accessed April 22. www.ahrq.gov/about/ataglance.htm.

Agency for Toxic Substances and Disease Registry (ATSDR). 2011. "About ATSDR." Accessed April 22. www.atsdr.cdc.gov/.

Alford, R. R. 1975. *Health Care Politics: Ideology and Interest Group Barriers to Reform.* Chicago: University of Chicago Press.

Centers for Disease Control and Prevention (CDC). 2011. "Budget Information." Financial Management Office, CDC. Published in 2011. www.cdc.gov/fmo/topic/Budget%20Information/index.html.

Centers for Medicare & Medicaid Services (CMS). 2011. "About CMS." Accessed April 22. www.cms.gov/home/aboutcms.asp.

Health Resources and Services Administration (HRSA). 2011. "About HRSA." Accessed April 22. www.hrsa.gov/about/index.html.

Kingdon, J. 1995. *Agendas, Alternatives, and Public Policies,* 2nd ed. New York: HarperCollins College.

National Institutes of Health (NIH). 2011. "About NIH." Accessed April 22. www.nih.gov/about/.

Office of Inspector General (OIG). 2011. "About OIG." Accessed April 22. http://oig.hhs
.gov/organization.asp.

Substance Abuse and Mental Health Services Administration (SAMHSA). 2011. "About the
Agency (SAMHSA)." Accessed April 22. www.samhsa.gov/about/.

United States Code. 2010 Edition. "Purpose; State child health plans." Title 42—The Public
Health and Welfare, Chapter 7—Social Security, Subchapter XXI—State Children's Health
Insurance Program, Sec. 1397aa. US Government Printing Office. www.gpo.gov/fdsys/
pkg/USCODE-2010-title42/html/USCODE-2010-title42-chap7-subchapXXI-sec1397aa
.htm.

US Department of Health and Human Services (HHS). 2011. *Healthy People 2020*. Accessed
April 25. www.healthypeople.gov/2020/about/default.aspx.

———. 2010. *Health, United States, 2010*. Washington, DC: HHS.

———. 2002. *Health, United States, 2002*. Washington, DC: HHS.

US Food and Drug Administration (FDA). 2011. "About FDA." Accessed April 22. www.fda
.gov/AboutFDA/WhatWeDo/default.htm.

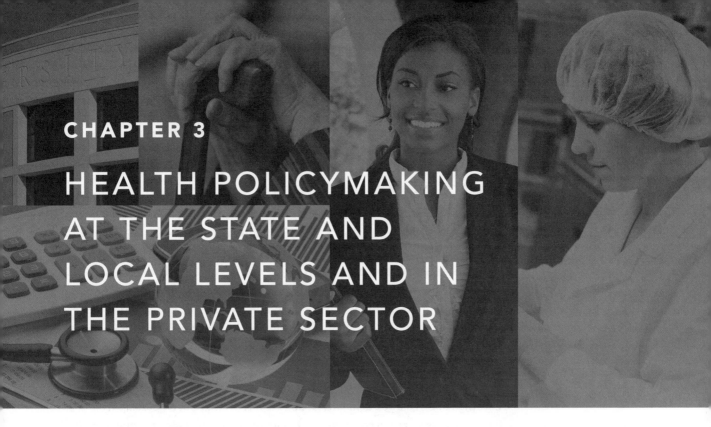

CHAPTER 3

HEALTH POLICYMAKING AT THE STATE AND LOCAL LEVELS AND IN THE PRIVATE SECTOR

A policy is a temporary creed liable to be changed, but while it holds good it has got to be pursued with apostolic zeal.

— Mohandas Gandhi

LEARNING OBJECTIVES

Studying this chapter will help you to

➤ describe features of the US state-level policymaking process and political system and provide examples of state healthcare legislation,

➤ discuss features of the US local government policymaking process and local political system and provide examples of local healthcare legislation,

➤ address the health policy–related activities of private health research institutes and foundations,

➤ understand the implications for the US healthcare system of policies created and practices followed by private industry, and

➤ appreciate the attributes of health policy development at the US state and local levels and in the private sector.

CASE STUDY

MASSACHUSETTS HEALTHCARE REFORM

In 2006, Massachusetts enacted landmark legislation to provide health insurance coverage to nearly all state residents (Kaiser Family Foundation 2012). The legislation led to
the creation of the Commonwealth Care health insurance program to provide subsidized
coverage for individuals whose income is below 300 percent of the federal poverty level.
It also developed a health insurance exchange for individuals and small businesses to
purchase insurance at more affordable rates than could be obtained on the open market.
The state's Medicaid program was expanded and merged with the Children's Health Insurance Program to form MassHealth. Children whose family's income is up to 300 percent of
the federal poverty level are covered by this program.

As part of that legislation, Massachusetts mandated that residents purchase health
insurance coverage or be charged a penalty of up to $912. In addition, employers with 11 or
more employees were required to contribute to health insurance coverage for their employees or pay an annual fair-share contribution of up to $295 per employee.

As of 2012, Massachusetts percentage of residents without insurance had declined to
6.3 percent, in comparison to the 2006 level of 10.9 percent uninsured. Additionally, unin-
surance in Massachusetts is about one-third that of the rest of the United States (18.4
percent). Employer health coverage remains the most common type of insurance, but the
MassHealth public insurance plan and Commonwealth Care (which provides subsidies for
families and individuals to purchase private coverage) have grown substantially (Kaiser
Family Foundation 2012).

Community health centers and safety net hospitals play a dominant role in caring for
those Massachusetts residents who now have health insurance as a result of the state
healthcare reform legislation. In addition, they continue to provide care for those who
remain uninsured.

Massachusetts' experience with healthcare reform legislation provides a real-world case
study demonstrating the potential to significantly reduce the number of uninsured through
an individual mandate combined with affordable health coverage options.

Although US health policies are developed primarily at the federal level, state and
local governments and industries in the private sector (nonfederal arenas) also
engage in health policymaking. This chapter focuses on health policymaking in
these arenas. First, state-level health policymaking is presented; that discussion is followed
by sections covering local government and private-sector health-related policy influencers.
The attributes of health policymaking in these sectors are also summarized.

STATE GOVERNMENTAL STRUCTURE

The federal and state sectors share a common government structure composed of the legislative, executive, and judiciary branches. However, each state has its own constitution and bill of rights, which together define the structure and function of the state government and of the local governments within the state's boundary (Longest 2010). Following is a brief discussion of the typical state political system.

POLITICAL SYSTEM

State governments are modeled after the US federal government in that each is composed of an executive, legislative, and judicial branch (Exhibit 3.1). States are bound by the US (federal) Constitution to maintain a **republican** form of government, although they are not specifically required to adhere to the three-branch system. The executive branch of the state government is headed by the governor and other **state executives**, such as the attorney general, the lieutenant governor, the secretary of state, auditors, and commissioners. All states' governors are directly elected by the people, as are most other positions in their executive branch. The exact structure of the executive branch varies from state to state.

The state legislative branch is the main lawmaking body of the government; it also approves the state's budget and fulfills other functions of government. As in the federal government, the **state legislature** consists of a house of representatives—known in some states as the assembly or house of delegates—and a senate chamber. (Nebraska has only one chamber in its legislature.) In most states, senators are elected by the state's voters to four-year terms, and members of the house are elected to two-year terms.

Republican

A type of democratic government in which the head of state is not a monarch; governmental activities and affairs are open to all interested citizens.

State executives

Officials in the executive branch of state government. Examples include the governor, who is chief executive of a state or territory, and the attorney general, who serves as the main legal adviser to the state government and has executive responsibility for law enforcement.

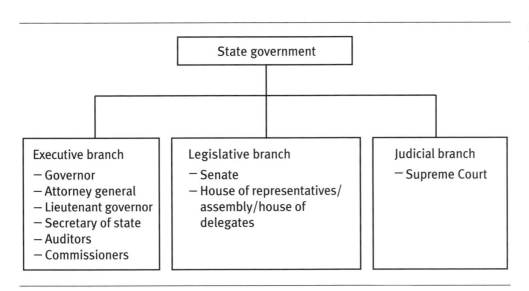

EXHIBIT 3.1

The US State Political System

State legislature
A generic term refer-
ring to the legislative
body of a US state. It
may also be called the
Legislature, General As-
sembly, or Legislative
Assembly.

A state's judiciary is generally headed by its version of the Supreme Court (with some exceptions; for example, New York's Supreme Court is the trial-level court, whereas the state's highest court is referred to as the Court of Appeals). This court hears appeal cases from lower-level state courts; no trials are held in state supreme courts. Decisions made by a state's supreme court are binding unless they do not adhere to the US Constitution, in which case, decisions may be appealed in the US Supreme Court.

The exact structure of the courts and the rules governing judicial appointments and elections are determined on a state-by-state basis, either through state legislation or by the state's constitution.

POLICYMAKING PROCESS AT THE STATE LEVEL

The policymaking process at the state level can vary substantially from state to state. In general, however, states apply the same legislative system as does the federal government (see, e.g., Alabama State Legislature 2011; Maryland General Assembly 2006; Oregon State Legislature 2011; State Legislature of Alaska 2011; West Virginia Legislature 2011). The idea for a new law can come from an elected representative, a group of elected representatives, the governor, or any other concerned citizen or interest group. The proposed law is drafted into a bill, which is then sponsored by an elected member of either the state's senate chamber or its lower chamber (house of representatives, general assembly, etc.). Although a bill must be introduced into the legislature by a representative or senator, both legislators and interest groups draft significant amounts of legislation.

Bills can be introduced in either chamber of the legislature, where they are reviewed by committees. Many states require that the bill also be accompanied by a financial projection showing the budgetary impact of the potential law. The bill goes through three readings before being voted on by the elected representatives. Often, amendments are made after each reading, and the merits of the bill are debated among the members.

Once it passes one chamber, the bill proceeds to three readings in the other chamber. The same process of debates and amendments is followed. After both houses have agreed on and passed a final version of the bill, it goes to the governor to be signed into law. In many states, the governor has the ability to veto a bill that is passed by both chambers. In other states, such as Oregon, the governor's veto can be overridden by a favorable vote of two-thirds or more of the members in both houses.

EXAMPLES OF STATE HEALTHCARE LEGISLATION

The power and responsibility of states to establish laws that protect the public's health and welfare derive from the US Constitution. The focus of healthcare legislation can range from promoting health, including environmental protection, occupational health, safe food services, and injury prevention, to providing health services, such as public health nursing, communicable disease control, family planning and prenatal care, and nutritional counseling. (See Exhibit 3.2 for examples of state health policies, and review the Learning Point box titled "Illustrations of States' Involvement in Health Policy Development" for a description of health policy activity in Oregon and Connecticut.)

LOCAL GOVERNMENT STRUCTURE

Local US governments typically fall into one of two levels: county or municipality (e.g., cities, towns, villages). Counties—called *boroughs* in Alaska and *parishes* in Louisiana— may be further divided into townships. Service districts, such as school districts and police and fire protection districts, may be congruent with county or municipal boundaries or set their own borders.

The structures of county and municipal governments vary greatly, but they all follow the **democratic** model. States assign powers to the local governments rather than to individuals; however, mayors, city council members, and members of other governing bodies are usually elected directly by the local residents. Laws are typically passed by majority votes at local council sessions.

The powers granted to a given municipality or county often depend on the size of its population. New York City, for example, has millions of residents and controls its own fire, police, and emergency medical services as well as its own libraries, parks and recre-

Democratic
The term *democratic* ("small-d") refers to processes carried out in the democratic, representative tradition. It is not the same as *Democratic* ("big-D"), which often refers to the Democratic political party in the United States.

EXHIBIT 3.2
Examples of States' Responsibilities Through Health Policy

- Serve as a major payer of healthcare services—an average of 22.3 percent of all state expenditures were Medicaid-related in 2010 (Miller 2012)

- Fund the Children's Health Insurance Program, health insurance benefits for state employees and other public-sector workers, and stand-alone state programs that provide health services to the uninsured

- Regulate the state's healthcare system (e.g., licensing and monitoring health professionals and health-related organizations, regulating states' private health insurance industry)

- Establish and monitor compliance with quality standards for environmental protection

- Provide safety net facilities through support of local health departments and community-based healthcare organizations and through programs that provide charity care to low-income populations

- Provide subsidies for graduate medical education and support large-scale educational campaigns

---

LEARNING POINT
Illustrations of States' Involvement in Health Policy Development

Oregon

Known as a leader in state healthcare reform (Oregon.gov 2011; Oregon Health Authority 2011; Health Care for All Oregon 2011), in 2009, Oregon's Legislative Assembly passed House Bill 2009, which established the Oregon Health Authority. The legislation created an insurance exchange—a federal subsidy–eligible set of standardized healthcare plans regulated by the state from which individuals may purchase health insurance—through the Oregon Health Authority for individuals and small businesses that do not have group health insurance.

The law also expanded the Oregon Health Plan, the state's Medicaid program, to cover low-income working families, and it allocated $5 billion in additional funds to the Medicaid plan over the following ten years. Other provisions contained in House Bill 2009 called for expanding the use of electronic health records through the Oregon Health Authority, establishing quality standards for hospitals and healthcare providers, and mandating that health insurance companies disclose their administrative costs and executive salaries to maintain transparency and accountability. As with the federal reforms included in the Affordable Care Act (ACA) of 2010, lifetime maximum limits on health benefits will be eliminated, insurers will be prohibited from dropping health coverage to those already enrolled in a plan, and children who are unmarried will be able to stay on their parents' health insurance plan until age 26.

The ACA is expected to provide some financial support for the reforms contained in Oregon's House Bill 2009. Once all the health reforms are implemented, an estimated 90 percent or more of Oregon residents will have health insurance coverage, with the aim to ensure coverage for all Oregon residents by 2015.

(continued)

ation, public transportation, and public works services. Smaller communities, on the other hand, may rely on county or state governments to provide these services.

POLICYMAKING PROCESS AT THE LOCAL GOVERNMENT LEVEL

As with state policymaking, the legislative process can vary significantly between counties and cities or towns (see, e.g., Erie County Legislature 2011; Monroe County 2011; Met-

LEARNING POINT
Illustrations of States' Involvement in Health Policy Development

(continued from previous page)

Connecticut

Connecticut, another of the first states to embrace national healthcare reform efforts (Johnson 2009; House Democrats of Connecticut 2011a, 2011b; State of Connecticut 2011), created Sustinet through legislation passed in May 2009 by the Connecticut General Assembly. Sustinet is a public healthcare plan to provide coverage for 98 percent of Connecticut residents by 2014. Governor M. Jodie Rell initially vetoed the law, but her veto was overridden by more than 67 percent majorities in both the state's House of Representatives and Senate.

Sustinet functions as an insurance pool. State employees, retirees, the uninsured and underinsured, residents receiving public assistance, and small business employers were the first groups to be eligible for the plan. In June 2011, the state legislature voted to extend Sustinet coverage to nonprofit organization and local government employees. Large employers will soon have an opportunity to buy into the Sustinet plan on behalf of their employees.

Sustinet's focus is on preventive care and the management of chronic illnesses. The law creating Sustinet also established task forces to address the problems of obesity, tobacco use, and the healthcare workforce shortage.

ropolitan Government of Nashville and Davidson County 2011). However, in general, these local government structures follow the same democratic process to make laws as federal and state legislatures. The exception is that local legislatures and councils typically have only one chamber, unlike the federal and state legislatures, which also have an upper chamber. Proposals for new laws are written into resolutions, also referred to as referrals, ordinances, or bills. They are brought in front of the county legislature, city council, or other local governing body to be considered.

Resolutions can be introduced by the local government or elected representatives. In some counties, concerned citizens can write a resolution for presentation at the local government meeting. Resolutions are usually reviewed by committees in larger counties or cities and by the entire council or legislature in smaller local governments. The resolution then proceeds through multiple readings—amendments to the legislation are often introduced after each reading—and its merits debated before being voted on by the elected representatives. Some types of resolutions, such as tax laws, may require a greater than 50 percent majority vote to pass.

After the resolution has passed, it may need to be signed into law by the mayor or council executive. Once they become law, resolutions may continue to be called resolutions or become known as bylaws, local laws, or ordinances.

EXAMPLES OF LOCAL HEALTHCARE LEGISLATION

The public health departments of county and city governments enforce laws that complement state-level healthcare legislation. One of the most common areas for health legislation at the local level is the regulation of tobacco products and smoking in public environments. In Monroe County, New York, for example, the local government has instituted a general smoking code and a law intended to prevent adolescent tobacco use (Monroe County Department of Public Health 2011; Monroe County 2005). Monroe County's smoking laws are part of a wider public health campaign in the state of New York to curb tobacco use and reduce nonsmokers' exposure to second-hand and environmental smoke.

Public health campaigns in many US municipalities have also begun to urge adults and children to be more active and engage in outdoor activities to curb obesity. Examples of recent measures include offering healthy lunches and limiting soft drinks in schools and providing portion-control and nutrition information in restaurants (mandatory in some states).

PRIVATE HEALTH RESEARCH INSTITUTES

As with federal, state, and local government, the private sector has contributed to health policy development. Here, the role of private research institutes—also known as think tanks—in influencing health policy is demonstrated through the work of the RAND Corporation.

RAND CORPORATION

The RAND Corporation conducts research and analysis to improve and inform policymaking in the areas of health, education, and national security. RAND, located in Santa Monica, California, strives to provide objective analysis and operates independently of commercial or partisan ties (RAND 2011).

The RAND Health division conducts studies on public policy issues related to healthcare reform, health insurance coverage, and the use of information technology in healthcare. Obesity, post-traumatic stress disorder, and complementary and alternative medicine are RAND's public health focus areas. As a well-regarded participant in policymaking circles, RAND is highly influential through its studies and reports. See the Research from the Field box for an example of health policy research conducted by RAND.

PRIVATE HEALTH FOUNDATIONS

In addition to conducting health policy research, private health foundations work to advance policy through grant programs that fund promising social experiments. The Pew Charitable Trusts comprise one such foundation.

RESEARCH FROM THE FIELD
RAND Health Policy Research:
An Assessment of High-Deductible Health Plans

High-deductible health plans (HDHPs), also known as consumer-directed health plans (CDHPs), have increased in popularity in recent years as methods for controlling healthcare costs. By shifting a larger portion of the cost to the patient through increased deductibles, some believe, consumers will use less care, especially unnecessary care. Approximately 20 percent of Americans covered under employer-sponsored health plans were enrolled in an HDHP or a CDHP in 2009, and more than 54 percent of employers offered at least one such plan in 2010.

In 2011, researchers at RAND Corporation conducted a cost-related assessment of HDHPs (Beeuwkes Buntin et al. 2011). The researchers for this retrospective study looked at data previously collected from the healthcare plan claims and enrollment information reported for 808,707 households by 53 major employers in the United States. Of these employers, 28 offered HDHPs or CDHPs to their employees. The increase in healthcare costs for those who enrolled in one of these types of plans for the first time from 2004 to 2005 was compared to the cost increases for those enrolled in traditional healthcare plans during the same period. Similar comparisons were made for the rates of use of preventive care services between the two groups.

Overall, through the duration of the study, the RAND researchers found that healthcare costs increased for both those with high-deductible plans and those with traditional plans. However, costs grew at a lower rate for those in the HDHP group. Similarly, expenditures for those families with HDHPs were lower for inpatient and outpatient care and for prescription drugs than for those enrolled in traditional health plans; spending on urgent care did not differ between the two groups.

(continued)

RESEARCH FROM THE FIELD
RAND Health Policy Research:
An Assessment of High-Deductible Health Plans

(continued from previous page)

The RAND study also found that families who enrolled in HDHPs reduced their use of preventive care services. These included childhood immunizations, the rates of which increased among traditional plan users; mammography; cervical cancer screening; and colorectal cancer screening.

The popularity of HDHPs is expected to increase further with the advent of healthcare reform in the United States. They will be among the featured health plans offered by the insurance exchanges being established in many states to assist those without health coverage to find insurance. Studies such as that conducted by RAND can guide policymakers when assessing the effectiveness of government health programs. Under the Affordable Care Act (ACA), for example, deductibles must be waived for preventive healthcare services. Thus, one implication of the RAND study is that clearly communicating information to families enrolled in HDHPs and the employers that offer these plans about this provision of the ACA must be a priority if the goal of increasing preventive care is to be met.

SOURCE: Beeuwkes Buntin et al. (2011).

PEW CHARITABLE TRUSTS

The Pew Charitable Trusts conduct research and public policy work to address the challenges facing the United States and global community. Areas of study include the environment, early education, and public health. The trusts also conduct public opinion polls to study trends in specific issues relevant to Americans. Pew's mission is to advance solutions to these issues (Pew Charitable Trusts 2011).

The Pew trusts support health research in four policy areas: consumer product safety, emerging science, food and health, and medical safety. Within these four topics, the Pew Health group focuses on identifying and reducing potential risks and hazards with everyday items such as foodstuffs, financial products, household items, and prescription drugs. Solutions are policy oriented, such as supporting mandatory food safety standards and organizing informational campaigns to curb the overuse of antibiotics in livestock (Pew Charitable Trusts 2011). The Research from the Field box presents an example of Pew Charitable Trusts' work to ensure that children have access to safe and nutritious food.

RESEARCH FROM THE FIELD
An Example of Pew Health Policy Research:
The Kids' Safe and Healthful Foods Project

The Kids' Safe and Healthful Foods Project, funded by the Pew Health Group in partnership with other private foundations, aims to improve the food choices available in schools to curb the rate of childhood obesity and to reform food safety policies in schools to stop the spread of foodborne illnesses. As part of the project, the Pew Health Group works with the US Department of Agriculture (USDA) by providing the agency with evidence-based analysis and policy recommendations.

The three major goals of the Kids' Safe and Healthful Foods Project are to (1) ensure that the nutrition standards established by the USDA for foods and beverages available in schools are based on scientific evidence, (2) make sure schools have sufficient resources to properly train cafeteria employees and keep cafeteria equipment in good working order, and (3) help the USDA to establish and enforce stringent food safety policies for use in schools. (Prior to the launch of the Kids' Safe and Healthful Foods Project, the USDA nutritional standards for school meals had not been updated in more than 15 years.)

As a result of the project, which also is closely aligned with the White House Task Force on Childhood Obesity, food safety has improved. Under the new school food safety policies, which arose from the Healthy, Hunger-Free Kids Act and was guided by the Kids' Safe and Healthful Foods Project, the USDA is required to enhance its communication with other government agencies, including its hold and recall procedures, so that notifications of food recalls are disseminated to schools in a timely manner. The agency must also ensure that food served outside the cafeteria—in classrooms or elsewhere—meets the same safety standards. These additional requirements will help schools to avoid outbreaks of foodborne illness, such as in 2009 when schools may have served students peanut products contaminated with Salmonella because they did not receive the recall notices in time (Kids' Safe and Healthful Foods Project 2013).

SOURCE: Kids' Safe and Healthful Foods Project (2011).

PRIVATE INDUSTRY

Corporate America influences health and health policy primarily through the services or products it provides and through its lobbying activities. The fast-food and tobacco industries, for example, have extensive business interests in the United States and around the world, and their products are key influencers of the population's health status.

Corporate America
An informal term referring to the corporations based and operating in the United States; they are not under direct governmental control.

FAST-FOOD INDUSTRY

Fast food
Refers to the ready-
to-eat, often portable
and inexpensive foods
available through many
outlets in the United
States. This type of
food tends to be less
healthy than home-
made food and has
been criticized for con-
tributing to the obesity
epidemic in the United
States.

More than 25 percent of American adults eat **fast food** every day. In 2000, Americans spent approximately $110 billion on fast food, whereas in 1970, they spent only $6 billion. In addition to those with drive-through access, fast-food restaurants can be found in airports, hospitals, schools and universities, stadiums, cruise ships, and many other locations where people gather (CBS News 2009; Schlosser 2001; Walker 2001).

In general, fast food is inexpensive, convenient, filling, and prepared quickly for the consumer. The food does not require dishes or utensils for eating, is mostly deep-fat fried, and comes in large portions with uniform specifications. Few vegetables are used because they are difficult to store long term.

The fast-food industry consists mainly of multimillion-dollar national restaurant chains. McDonald's Corporation alone franchised 32,737 restaurants worldwide in 2010 and continues to expand each year (*NASDAQ.com News* 2011). It hires more people per year than does any other American organization and is the country's largest purchaser of beef, pork, and potatoes. McDonald's is also the largest owner of retail property in the world and spends the most money of any brand on marketing (Schlosser 2001).

In addition to its vast marketing campaigns, the fast-food industry and its suppliers spend large sums lobbying the US government to promote or oppose legislation according to their interests. Worker safety, food safety, and minimum wage laws have historically been opposed by the fast-food industry.

The consumption of fast food contributes to obesity among American adults and children (CBS News 2009; WHO 2011a). In addition to the commonly cited factors linking fast-food consumption to obesity (e.g., large amounts of fat, highly processed ingredients), studies have shown that proximity to fast-food outlets is a factor (e.g., Currie et al. 2009; Rabin 2009). Currie and colleagues (2009) found that when a fast-food restaurant was located within a tenth of a mile of a school, the obesity rates for children attending the school increased 5.2 percent more than for children who attended a school with a fast-food restaurant a quarter of a mile or farther away.

In 2002, a group of obese and overweight children filed a class-action lawsuit against McDonald's, asking the court to award compensation for their obesity-related health problems and requesting that it force McDonald's to improve its nutritional labeling and provide funding for a health education campaign on the dangers of fast food. The lawsuit was dismissed a year later, but it raised important questions about legal accountability for the poor nutritional standards of most fast-food menu items. Mello, Rimm, and Studdert (2003) draw parallels between the fast-food industry's intention to process and manufacture food to be addictive and the tobacco industry's aim to manufacture addictive cigarettes. However, observers generally agree that eating fast food is a consumer choice.

CIGARETTE AND TOBACCO INDUSTRY

The tobacco industry is composed mainly of large, multinational corporate tobacco growers and cigarette manufacturers. The industry represents historical significance in the United States, as it was an important commodity in colonial times. Tobacco is the seventh largest cash crop in the country; in 2009, the industry reported $614 billion in revenue (American Lung Association in Washington 2011; IRS 2011; Lepore 2011).

Tobacco products are the most heavily taxed consumer product in the United States when measured by percentage of retail price. The industry is also highly regulated, with quotas set for each farmer's land and the end product graded by US Department of Agriculture (USDA) inspectors. The sale of tobacco to dealers and warehouses is monitored by the USDA's Agricultural Stabilization and Conservation Service.

The five largest cigarette manufacturers in the country spent a total of $12.5 billion on advertising in 2006, the last year in which data were available. Most promotional efforts came in the form of price discounts to wholesalers and retailers (American Lung Association 2011b). It has been shown that lowering the price of cigarettes increases youth consumption; conversely, with each 10 percent increase in the price of cigarettes, youth consumption drops by 6 to 7 percent (Boonn 2012).

According to the American Lung Association (2011a), smoking cigarettes is the number one preventable cause of morbidity and mortality worldwide. Nearly 450,000 Americans die from tobacco smoking–related diseases annually (CDC 2011; Cummings, Morley, and Hyland 2002; WHO 2011b). The smoke from one cigarette contains more than 4,800 different chemicals—69 of which are known to be carcinogenic (cancer causing). Chronic lung disease, including lung cancer and chronic obstructive pulmonary disease, accounts for about three-quarters of smoking-related morbidity in current smokers and half of smoking-related morbidity in former smokers.

In 2004, smoking-related deaths and diseases cost the United States $193 billion, including $96 billion from direct healthcare expenditures and $97 billion from lost productivity.

ATTRIBUTES OF HEALTH POLICY DEVELOPMENT IN NONFEDERAL SECTORS

Health policymaking in nonfederal sectors—state and local governments and the private sector—is characterized by several factors:

◆ The constraints imposed by the broader policy landscape

◆ The relationship between politics and policy

+ The level of public health funding

+ The ways in which the private sector shapes policy direction

+ Policy entrepreneurship at the grassroots level

+ The lack of integration and coordination among policymaking groups in creating policy initiatives

CONSTRAINTS UNDER FEDERAL POLICY

Policymaking at the state and local levels is limited by broader federal policy. Although regulation is primarily the states' responsibility, federal laws can preempt state legislation. For example, states cannot require firms to offer insurance to their employees because federal law, in the form of the Employee Retirement Income Security Act, would override any attempt by the state to do so.

The private sector is also influenced and constrained by federal regulations, in areas such as practitioner licensing, security and privacy of patient information, and reimbursement. For example, the Medicare and Medicaid programs periodically adjust their reimbursement methodologies—the methods by which they calculate how much money to pay providers for services rendered—which prompts healthcare organizations to make changes in the way services are delivered.

FOR YOUR CONSIDERATION
Traditional Republican and Democratic Stances

The 2012 election cycle highlighted a number of policy positions (known as planks in their platform) favored by each major party. While Republicans traditionally have sought small government (government that practices limited use of regulation, as opposed to "big," centralized government) and limited taxation and supported business interests, Democrats have historically favored social programs, assistance for vulnerable populations, and a larger tax share from the wealthy than from the middle and lower classes.

How do you view these positions in light of comments made by party leaders during the 2012 presidential and congressional elections as reported by the mainstream media? Do the comments consistently reflect these traditional stances? Why or why not?

RELATIONSHIP BETWEEN POLITICS AND POLICY

Legislation is most likely to pass if the governor and the majority of the legislature carry the same political party affiliation. Similarly, legislation often is stalled or diluted when the policymakers considering it represent different parties.

Another link between politics and policy, which applies to all sectors involved in policymaking, is the election cycle. In the time preceding an election, politicians running for reelection often emphasize legislation that is expected to garner immediate results, thus benefiting their reelection bids. Difficult problems that take a long time to solve are frequently left for future congressional sessions. As a result, many problems facing US residents are cumulative, but the policies meant to address those problems are symptomatic—not addressing the root cause but rather its symptoms—and piecemeal. The underlying problems, left unresolved, tend to worsen over time and exact an even heavier toll on all those affected than an earlier, more comprehensive solution would have.

LEVEL OF PUBLIC FUNDING

The market-oriented economy in the United States attracts private entrepreneurs to carry out key healthcare delivery functions at a profit, leaving the public sector to assume a secondary role when the market alone cannot address all healthcare needs (particularly for members of vulnerable populations who cannot afford expensive care). The resulting healthcare system is functionally fragmented, with little standardization, resulting in duplication of certain services and inadequacy of others.

Funding for public health in the United States is relatively low, at less than $150 per capita, or less than 2.5 percent of the overall healthcare spending (Salinsky and Gursky 2006), compared to that in Canada, which spent 5.5 percent of its total health expenditure on public health (Canadian Institute for Health Information 2005). Little public investment is made in health technology, workforce training and recruitment, or facility construction or renovation. In addition, the fact that spending on public health varies widely across communities raises concerns about whether and how these differences might affect the availability of essential public health services.

SHAPING POLICY DIRECTION

The private sector shapes policy direction more than state and local governments do. As described earlier in this chapter, the research topics addressed by private research institutes and the projects funded by private foundations lead to findings that contribute to better understanding of the health problems studied, their underlying causes, and potential solutions to them, thus paving the way for policy development. Another way private research institutes and foundations drive policy is in their evaluations of existing policies, the results of which are often incorporated in policy modifications or new policies.

POLICY ENTREPRENEURSHIP AT THE GRASSROOTS LEVEL

Grassroots efforts by **policy entrepreneurs** involve community stakeholders and may be funded by private foundations. Such efforts are critical to adapting successful experiences to other environments and identfying innovative approaches to solving health-related issues.

Typically, community-based projects stress participation and empowerment; deeply involving community members leads to acceptance of the initiative and helps promote sustainability of the intervention. Community members plan and manage initiatives, and

Policy entrepreneur
Public innovator who, from outside the formal positions of government, introduces, translates, and implements new ideas into public practice.

through community mobilization, skill building, and resource sharing, communities are empowered to identify and meet their own needs, making them stronger advocates for the vulnerable populations within and across their community boundaries.

KEY POINTS

➤ Although the policymaking process can vary substantially from state to state, states generally apply the same legislative system as the federal government does.

➤ Local government structures follow the same democratic process for making laws as federal and state legislatures do, with the exception that local legislatures and councils typically have only one legislative chamber.

➤ The private sector, including private research institutes, foundations, and industry, contributes to health policy development.

➤ The major attributes of health policymaking in the public nonfederal sector include the constraints imposed by the broader federal policy landscape, influence of politics, availability of funding, level of entrepreneurship at the local level, and lack of integration and coordination among policymaking groups.

CASE STUDY QUESTIONS

Research the events leading to and following the enactment of the Massachusetts healthcare reform legislation introduced in the case study, and answer the following questions:

1. Why was Massachusetts able to enact state-level healthcare reform whereas most other states were not?

2. What are the positive and negative consequences of Massachusetts' healthcare reform?

3. What consequences do you anticipate when similar reform is enacted nationally?

FOR DISCUSSION

1. Describe, and provide an example of, the policymaking process at the US state level.

2. Describe, and provide an example of, the policymaking process at the US local level.

3. What are the health policy–related activities of private health research institutes? Of private health foundations?
4. What kinds of public health information and initiatives are contributed by private industry?
5. List three characteristics of health policy development in the US state government, local government, and private sectors.

REFERENCES

Alabama State Legislature. 2011. "Alabama's Legislative Process." Accessed July 23, 2012. www.legislature.state.al.us/misc/legislativeprocess/legislativeprocess_ml.html.

American Lung Association. 2011a. "Smoking." Accessed July 21, 2012. www.lungusa.org/stop-smoking/about-smoking/health-effects/smoking.html.

———. 2011b. "Tobacco Industry Marketing." Accessed July 21, 2012. www.lungusa.org/stop-smoking/about-smoking/facts-figures/tobacco-industry-marketing.html.

American Lung Association in Washington. 2011. "Facts About Tobacco." Accessed July 21, 2012. www.alaw.org/tobacco_control/facts_about_tobacco/index.html.

Beeuwkes Buntin, M., A. M. Haviland, R. McDevitt, and N. Sood. 2011. "Healthcare Spending and Preventive Care in High-Deductible and Consumer-Directed Health Plans." *American Journal of Managed Care* 17 (3): 222–30.

Boonn, A. 2012. "Raising Cigarette Taxes Reduces Smoking, Especially Among Kids (and the Cigarette Companies Know It)." Campaign for Tobacco-Free Kids. Published October 11. www.tobaccofreekids.org/research/factsheets/pdf/0146.pdf.

Canadian Institute for Health Information. 2005. *National Health Expenditure Trends 1975–2005*, Table C.1.2.7. Ottawa, Ontario: Canadian Institute for Health Information.

CBS News. 2009. "Americans Are Obsessed with Fast Food: The Dark Side of the All-American Meal." Published February 11. www.cbsnews.com/stories/2002/01/31/health/main326858.shtml.

Centers for Disease Control and Prevention (CDC). 2011. "Health Effects of Cigarette Smoking." Accessed July 21, 2012. www.cdc.gov/tobacco/data_statistics/fact_sheets/health_effects/effects_cig_smoking/.

Cummings, K. M., C. P. Morley, and A. Hyland. 2002. "Failed Promises of the Cigarette Industry and Its Effect on Consumer Misperceptions About the Health Risks of Smoking." *Tobacco Control* 11 (Suppl. 1): 110–17.

Currie, J., S. Della Vigna, E. Moretti, and V. Pathania. 2009. "The Effect of Fast Food Restaurants on Obesity." Published in April. http://elsa.berkeley.edu/~sdellavi/wp/fastfoodApr09.pdf.

Erie County (New York) Legislature. 2011. "How the Legislature Takes Action." Accessed July 29, 2012. www2.erie.gov/legislature/index.php?q=how-legislature-takes-action.

Health Care for All Oregon. 2011. "Oregon Legislation." Accessed July 24, 2012. www.healthcareforalloregon.org/oregon/.

House Democrats of Connecticut. 2011a. "House Passes Healthcare Pooling, Sustinet." Published May 27. www.housedems.ct.gov/healthcare/PR11.asp#a052711.

———. 2011b. "Speaker Donovan Statement on Senate Passage of Health Care Reforms." Published June 6. www.housedems.ct.gov/healthcare/PR11.asp#a060611.

Internal Revenue Service (IRS). 2011. "Market Segment Specialization Program: Tobacco Industry." Accessed July 21, 2012. www.irs.gov/pub/irs-mssp/tobacco.pdf.

Johnson, A. 2009. "Connecticut Pushes Ahead on Health Care." *Wall Street Journal*. Published July 22. http://online.wsj.com/article/SB124822088310970327.html.

Kaiser Family Foundation. 2012. "Massachusetts Health Care Reform: Six Years Later." Focus on Health Reform. Published in May. www.kff.org/healthreform/upload/8311.pdf.

Kids' Safe and Healthful Foods Project. 2013. "School Food Safety." Accessed February 6. www.healthyschoolfoodsnow.org/policy/improving-school-food-safety/.

———. 2011. Home page. Accessed January 3 2013. www.healthyschoolfoodsnow.org.

Lepore, M. 2011. "15 Facts About the Cigarette Industry That Will Blow Your Mind." *Business Insider*. Published April 8. www.businessinsider.com/facts-about-tobacco-industry-2011-4.

Longest, B. 2010. *Health Policymaking in the United States*, 5th ed. Chicago: Health Administration Press.

Maryland General Assembly. 2006. "The Legislative Process: How a Bill Becomes a Law." Published in June. www.msa.md.gov/msa/mdmanual/07leg/html/proc.html.

Mello, M., E. B. Rimm, and D. M. Studdert. 2003. "The McLawsuit: The Fast-Food Industry and Legal Accountability for Obesity." *Health Affairs* 22 (6): 207–16.

Metropolitan Government of Nashville and Davidson County, Tennessee. 2011. "Overview of Metropolitan Council." Accessed July 29, 2012. www.nashville.gov/mc/council/legislative_process.htm.

Miller, D. 2012. "Medicaid Spending." Council of State Governments. Accessed February 6, 2013. http://knowledgecenter.csg.org/drupal/content/medicaid-spending.

Monroe County, New York. 2011. "Legislature." Accessed January 3, 2013. www2.monroecounty.gov/legislature-index.php.

———. 2005. "Public Health Law—Article 13-F: Regulation of Tobacco Products and Herbal Cigarettes; Distribution to Minors." Published December 1. www.monroecounty.gov/File/Health/ATUPA/13F_05.pdf.

Monroe County, New York, Department of Public Health. 2011. "Smoking Code/Adolescent Tobacco Use Prevention Act." Accessed July 30, 2012. www.monroecounty.gov/eh-smoking.php.

NASDAQ.com News. 2011. "Subway Tops McDonald's for Number of Stores in World." Published March 21. www.nasdaq.com/article/subway-tops-mcdonalds-for-number-of-stores-in-world-cm63138#.URIvUlrFT_l.

Oregon Health Authority. 2011. "U.S. House Health Reform Vote." Accessed February 6, 2013. www.oregon.gov/oha/pages/features/feature_federal_intersect_ore.aspx.

Oregon State Legislature. 2011. "Citizen's Guide to the Oregon Legislative Process." Accessed July 23. www.leg.state.or.us/citizenguide/.

Oregon.gov. 2011. Press Release: June 30, 2011. Accessed July 24, 2012. www.oregon.gov/gov/media_room/pages/press_releasesp2011/press_063011.aspx.

Pew Charitable Trusts. 2011. Home page. Accessed January 3, 2013. www.pewtrusts.org.

Rabin, R. C. 2009. "Proximity to Fast Food a Factor in Student Obesity." *New York Times*. Published March 25. www.nytimes.com/2009/03/26/health/nutrition/26obese.html.

RAND Corporation. 2011. "History and Mission." Accessed June 29, 2012. www.rand.org/about/history.html.

Salinsky, E., and E. A. Gursky. 2006. "The Case for Transforming Governmental Public Health." *Health Affairs* 25: 1017–28.

Schlosser, E. 2001. "Fast Food Nation: The Dark Side of the All-American Meal" [book review]. *New York Times*. Published January 21. www.nytimes.com/books/first/s/schlosser-fast.html.

State of Connecticut. 2011. "Sustinet: About Us." Published April 8. www.ct.gov/sustinet/cwp/ view.asp?a=3826&q=450132.

State Legislature of Alaska. 2011. "Legislative Process in Alaska." Accessed July 23, 2012. http://w3.legis.state.ak.us/docs/pdf/legprocess.pdf.

Walker, R. 2001. "No Accounting for Mouthfeel." *New York Times*. Published January 21. www.nytimes.com/books/01/01/21/reviews/010121.21walkert.html.

West Virginia Legislature. 2011. "How a Bill Becomes Law." Accessed July 23, 2012. www.legis.state.wv.us/Educational/Bill_Becomes_Law/Bill_Becomes_Law.cfm.

World Health Organization (WHO). 2011a. "Obesity and Overweight." Published in March. www.who.int/mediacentre/factsheets/fs311/en/index.html.

———. 2011b. "Tobacco." Published in July. www.who.int/mediacentre/factsheets/fs339/en/index.html.

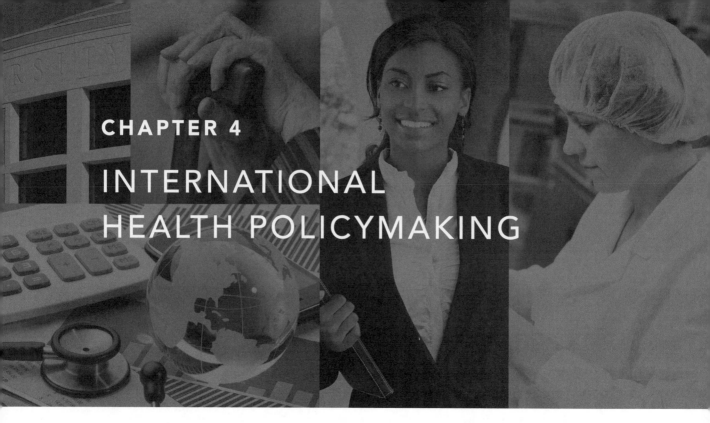

CHAPTER 4

INTERNATIONAL HEALTH POLICYMAKING

The one who adapts his policy to the times prospers, and likewise the one whose policy clashes with the demands of the times does not.

—Nicolo Machiavelli

LEARNING OBJECTIVES

Studying this chapter will help you to

➤ provide examples of health policymaking at the international level;

➤ describe the functions and policy-related activities of the World Health Organization; and

➤ become familiar with health-related policymaking in Canada, Sweden, and China.

CASE STUDY

CHINA'S HEALTHCARE REFORM

China's latest healthcare reform effort began in July 2005 and took four years to complete, from agenda setting to final policy formulation. The initiative culminated in the publication of the policy document "Opinions on Deepening the Reform of the Health Care System" in April 2009. Following is a timeline of the five main stages of this reform process.

STAGE 1, JULY 2005–OCTOBER 2006: ISSUE RAISING AND AGENDA SETTING

In July 2005, the Development Research Center of the Chinese government's State Council and the World Health Organization completed a study entitled "The Evaluation and Recommendations of China's Health System Reform," which concluded that a market-oriented approach to healthcare reform, the model often used in democratic societies, would not be effective for China. This report triggered broad discussion among the general public and attracted attention from high-level government officials. In June 2006, the government State Council established a department, the Health Reform Inter-ministerial Coordination Group—later named the Health Reform Coordination Group—marking the start of agenda setting on health reform policy. Thereafter, policy experts and research institutions throughout the country were provided the opportunity to participate in raising policy concerns and helping establish the direction healthcare reform would take.

STAGE 2, OCTOBER 2006–FEBRUARY 2008: DESIGNING AND SELECTING POLICY OPTIONS

The Health Reform Coordination Group conducted in-depth research, which lasted for more than a year. The process included soliciting opinions from all policy stakeholders and healthcare experts and studying various policy options. On September 28, 2007, the Group drafted the health reform program. On February 29, 2008, a State Council executive meeting was held to accomplish two tasks: modifying the initial version of the program on the basis of inputs gathered and formulating the first draft of its "Opinions" report.

STAGE 3, FEBRUARY 2008–SEPTEMBER 2008: DELIBERATING THE FINAL HEALTHCARE REFORM PROGRAM

The central decision makers from the government State Council deliberated over the proposed reform program and consulted with other ministries, provinces, and municipalities.

On September 10, 2008, another State Council executive meeting was held to consider and adopt the revised draft of the report, which laid the blueprint for implementing the healthcare reform package.

STAGE 4, OCTOBER 2008–NOVEMBER 2008: CONSULTING THE PUBLIC

The period for public consultation began on October 14, 2008, and lasted one month. The public submitted letters and messages via post, fax, e-mail, and online messaging to express their opinions on the revised policy document. At the same time, pilot projects were carried out by designated local governments. By November 14, 2008, the Health Reform Coordination Group had received nearly 36,000 suggestions and comments from the public. On the basis of these opinions, the Group included ten amendments in the reform document.

STAGE 5, DECEMBER 2008–MARCH 2009: UNVEILING THE FORMAL HEALTHCARE REFORM POLICY

In March 2009, the policy documents "Opinions on Deepening the Reform of the Health Care System" and "The Plan for Recent Focus of Health System Reform (2009–2011)" were issued. The policies proposed the future establishment of a basic healthcare system for all urban and rural residents and outlined five major aspects of the reform plan to be implemented in the near future. These components included the development of a medical insurance system, an essential drug system, a basic medical service system, a public health system, and the reform of public hospitals.

SOURCE: Freeman and Boynton (2011).

This chapter focuses on health-related policymaking in the international arena. The World Health Organization (WHO), recognized as the leading international health authority, is described, and examples from three countries—Canada, Sweden, and China—illustrate diverse policymaking processes in different geographic regions.

World Health Assembly

The decision-making and policymaking body of WHO, composed of delegations from all WHO member states.

WORLD HEALTH ORGANIZATION

WHO is composed of the **World Health Assembly**, the Assembly's executive board, and the WHO's Secretariat (WHO 2011a). Delegations from WHO's 193 member countries make up the World Health Assembly, which is the decision-making and policymaking body of the organization (WHO 2011b). The executive board facilitates the work of the World Health Assembly and advises on technical issues related to health. The Secretariat is the main implementation body of WHO's policymaking work and includes approximately 8,000 health experts and support staff.

WHO's FUNCTIONS

WHO has six core functions, which are outlined in its 11th General Programme of Work for the years 2006–2015 (WHO 2013):

◆ Act as a leader and partner on health issues worldwide.

◆ Set research priorities and encourage the sharing of health-related knowledge.

◆ Establish standards of practice and support and monitor their adoption.

◆ Advance policy options founded on ethical and evidence-based principles.

◆ Lend technical support to health initiatives and contribute to capacity building.

◆ Monitor health issues around the world and identify patterns and trends.

In practice, WHO not only sets international health policy but also coordinates population health programs, such as mass immunization campaigns, emergency response efforts to natural disasters and disease outbreaks, and statistical monitoring of disease prevalence.

THE WHO POLICYMAKING PROCESS

Proposals for new WHO resolutions or motions can be submitted by any World Health Assembly member. With the exception of sessions convened in times of emergency and other administrative considerations, proposals for new projects and initiatives can be included on the supplementary agenda of any session of the Assembly. Following a preliminary impact analysis conducted by WHO's director-general, a proposal is referred to the appropriate committee, which examines the proposal and related report at plenary meetings. Once the proposal or resolution passes through the committee, it is considered for adoption by a vote in the World Health Assembly. Those of particular importance, such as the appointment of the director-general and proposals that involve other United Nations agencies, require a two-thirds majority vote to be adopted. Most policy implementation is carried out through WHO's Secretariat, which oversees specific aspects of program design and the logistics involved in launching programs.

WHO Health Programs

WHO currently operates more than 150 programs and projects (WHO 2013). They range from monitoring chronic diseases such as diabetes, to conducting eradication efforts for diseases such as leprosy, to operating initiatives to prevent disease by ensuring access to clean water.

One example is the WHO Global Task Force on Cholera, which was established in 1992 to decrease the incidence of the disease and the social and economic consequences associated with it. The task force provides training on combating endemic or epidemic cholera to health professionals in the countries in which it operates and distributes information about cholera prevention to the public in at-risk areas (WHO 2007). WHO also plays an instrumental role in containing disease outbreaks. For example, it helped to coordinate the response to the outbreak of SARS (severe acute respiratory syndrome) in 2003 and is currently monitoring the incidence of **avian influenza** around the world. Perhaps the most well-known WHO program was the campaign to eradicate smallpox, which came to a successful conclusion in 1979. This effort represents the first and only time thus far that the eradication of a major infectious disease has been achieved (WHO 2007).

WHO's Involvement in Health Policy

WHO is the global leader in formulating health policy. For example, WHO writes and distributes regular policy reports on major diseases, such as HIV/AIDS, tuberculosis, and malaria. It also issues policy statements in response to disease outbreaks and natural disasters.

WHO and its policies and actions have often drawn criticism from various groups (Stein 2010; Peabody 1995). While WHO has increasingly focused its efforts on disease surveillance, many observers believe that the bureaucratic nature of the organization and its perceived slow reaction time undermine WHO's ability to respond in urgent situations.

For example, an independent assessment of WHO's response to the **H1N1 (swine) flu** pandemic in 2009 conducted by the Institute of Medicine concluded that WHO needed improvement in a number of areas (Cohen 2011), including the following points of criticism:

- ◆ WHO does not have a standard way to measure the severity of an outbreak.

- ◆ WHO was not transparent about the members who served on the Emergency Committee, which led to speculation that they had ties to influenza vaccine–producing pharmaceutical companies.

- ◆ WHO had difficulty distributing the vaccines in developing countries.

The report recommended that WHO establish an emergency fund for disease outbreaks, have advance agreements in place with pharmaceutical companies to supply vac-

Avian influenza
A type-A influenza viral infection in wild or domestic birds. The avian flu virus can become a public health danger if a change (mutation) allows it to more easily infect humans, and it can potentially start a worldwide epidemic.

H1N1 (swine) flu
A respiratory disease caused by influenza type-A viruses first detected in 2009. The new strain of influenza A (H1N1) virus is a mix of swine, human, and/or avian influenza viruses that is contagious and can cause seasonal flu.

cines on an as-needed basis, and set up a health emergency corps of personnel to mobilize in the event of an outbreak.

HEALTH POLICYMAKING FROM SELECTED COUNTRIES

Although WHO conducts high-level research, policy analysis, and emergency response, the vast majority of health policy in a country is made at the national level. This section provides examples from Canada, Sweden, and China to illustrate the diverse political and healthcare systems, health challenges, and policymaking processes.

CANADA

Canada is a parliamentary democracy founded on the British system of government. The king or queen of England is Canada's head of state and is represented by the governor general in Canada, who carries out the British monarch's formal duties.

The House of Commons is the main legislative body. It is composed of elected local representatives called Members of Parliament (MPs), who typically belong to one of Canada's five major political parties:

◆   Conservative Party

◆   Liberal Party

◆   New Democratic Party

◆   Bloc Québécois

◆   Green Party

Canada is divided into electoral districts, or *ridings*, on the basis of population, with one MP elected per riding.

The Senate acts as a review board for legislation introduced by the House of Commons, and senators are chosen for appointments by the prime minister. The government is formed by the party with the most elected representatives; the leader of this party becomes prime minister. Elected officials who are not members of the ruling party become the official opposition (Atlantic Canada Opportunities Agency 2011; Settlement Ontario 2011).

Elected members of the federal and provincial governments can introduce legislation, which is voted on in the Parliament or, for regional legislative issues, in the province's Legislative Assembly. The prime minister selects MPs from within his or her party to form a cabinet. Cabinet ministers take on special responsibility for one or more federal platform issues (e.g., defense, finance, foreign affairs) in addition to representing the members of their electoral riding.

Canada is made up of ten provinces and three territories. Responsibility for such areas as national defense, foreign policy, and international trade rests with the federal government, while healthcare and education are provincial or territorial responsibilities. Large towns and cities also have their own local government, which is responsible for providing services such as police and fire departments and trash collection. See the International Policymaking box for a summary of Canada's policymaking process.

INTERNATIONAL POLICYMAKING
Policymaking in Canada

- The Canadian legislative process is based on the British model (Parliament of Canada 2011a, 2011b). Proposals for new laws or changes to existing laws are referred to as *bills*.
- Bills are usually introduced in the House of Commons; they may also be introduced in the Senate.
- Once a bill is introduced, it must go through three rounds of readings and reviews, first by the House of Commons and later by the Senate (Government of Canada Publications 2012).
- The bill is also sent to a committee to be examined clause by clause before the third and final reading. The committee may bring in experts to testify on the contents of the bill before the first parliamentary chamber passes, amends, delays, or defeats the bill.
- If a bill is accepted and passed by both chambers, it is submitted for Royal Assent. In Canada, this approval is given by the governor general on behalf of the queen of England. After receiving Royal Assent, a bill becomes law.

The Healthcare System

An overview of key statistics related to Canada's healthcare system is shown in Exhibit 4.1. The Canadian healthcare system is administered by the provincial and territorial governments and is taxpayer funded, mainly on the provincial level but also through federal taxation by way of the Canada Health Transfer. The 13 provinces and territories must meet the national standards outlined in the Canada Health Act to receive the full amount of federal funding available (Health Canada 2013).

The act stipulates that provinces and territories insure residents for all medically necessary primary and tertiary care provided by physicians and hospitals. Some provinces may provide additional benefits, such as coverage for dental or chiropractic care. Most physicians work in for-profit private practices; however, they bill and are paid through the public insurance system of their respective province or territory on a fee-for-service basis. Many large hospitals are not-for-profit and are associated with a religious group or university.

Health Policymaking

The Canada Health Act, the primary piece of health-related legislation at the federal level, was signed into law in 1984 (Health Canada 2013). The law ensures that all eligible Canadian citizens and residents have access to

Population	34,173,900	
GDP per capita (in PPP)	$38,841	
% of GDP spent on healthcare	11%	
Healthcare spending per capita (in PPP)	$4,196	
Life expectancy, male/female	79/84	
Infant mortality rate	5 per 1,000 live births	
No. of hospital beds per 1,000 people	3	

EXHIBIT 4.1
Canadian
Healthcare System
Key Statistics
(2009–10 data)

NOTE: GDP = gross domestic product; PPP = purchasing power parity.
SOURCES: OECD iLibrary (2010); World Bank (2011a).

prepaid health insurance and services. It also provides the legal framework for provincial healthcare plans receiving federal funding.

Specifically, the Canada Health Act sets forth the following tenets:

1. The healthcare system must be administered publicly and as a not-for-profit operation.

2. The system must provide insurance for all necessary health services.

3. All residents have the right to the same level of care.

4. Insurance must be portable from one province or territory to another.

5. All insured residents should have reasonable access to healthcare services.

Key Health Policy Stakeholders

Key stakeholders include the federal government; Health Canada, the federal health department; the provincial governments, which administer the insurance plans; physicians' and nurses' associations and the Canadian Medical Association; industry and trade groups, such as the pharmaceutical industry; and the Canadian public (CBC 2006, 2005; Canadian Doctors for Medicare 2011; Health Canada 2013).

None of the political parties of Canada seek to dismantle the universal healthcare system; however, they have differing views on the degree to which it should be privatized. The Conservatives are generally in favor of more **privatization**, whereas Liberal, New Democrat, Bloc Québécois, and Green Party members generally favor less. Some politi-

Privatization
The movement of an industry in a country from the public to the private sphere.

cians advocate for a two-tier health system, in which consumers can choose between public and private care. The implementation of this framework has become increasingly likely since June 2005, when the Canadian Supreme Court struck down a Quebec law prohibiting residents from buying private insurance that covered services already covered by the public system.

Many doctors' and nurses' associations favor the public healthcare system and do not support privatization of clinics and hospitals. Some, however, feel they would be paid more for their services if they worked in a private system than they are currently paid by the public insurance. The Canadian public is generally in favor of the universal healthcare system, but similar to the disagreements between the political parties that represent them, opinions vary on whether the system should remain public or the degree to which the system should become privatized.

Major Health Issues

When prioritizing current health issues, the Public Health Agency of Canada, Health Canada, and the Ministry of Health rely on public policy documents and analytical reports, such as the *Report on the Health of Canadians* (Parliament of Canada 2002), which are developed on the basis of national health surveys conducted by Statistics Canada.

Those conditions and diseases noted in the report as causing the greatest amount of mortality or morbidity in the population as a whole, in certain geographic areas, or within specific demographic groups are considered high priority in terms of intervention. In addition, the report addresses determinants of health in targeted interventions in the most at-risk communities. This aspect of the reporting reflects the Canadian government's overall focus on preventive health.

Other major areas of focus include the health of the elderly and access to healthcare in rural and remote areas. These priorities directly address two key demographic challenges in Canada: the aging population and the low population density outside of major urban areas. Specific health concerns include chronic diseases, such as arthritis and diabetes, and mental health concerns, such as depression, which affect a significant portion of the population.

SWEDEN

Sweden is a constitutional monarchy and parliamentary democracy. Citizens elect members to represent them in the Riksdag, Sweden's legislative assembly. Elections are held every four years. The political party whose members win the most seats in the Riksdag forms the government, which is led by the prime minister. The prime minister selects 21 other representatives to become ministers and form the cabinet. The Swedish head of state is the reigning monarch; he or she has no political powers (US Department of State 2011; Government Offices of Sweden 2013; *The Economist* 2009).

The Swedish Constitution is made up of four fundamental laws:

◆ The Institute of Government (outlines the functioning of Sweden's government and elections)

◆ The Act of Succession (regulates who inherits the throne of the Swedish monarchy)

◆ The Freedom of the Press Act (guarantees the people's right to disseminate information)

◆ The Fundamental Law on Freedom of Expression (gives citizens the right to access government documents)

Sweden is also subject to the legislation of the European Union (EU). Some EU laws are automatically adopted by Sweden, and some must pass through a vote in the Riksdag to be formally incorporated. See the International Policymaking box for a summary of Sweden's policymaking process.

Healthcare System

Exhibit 4.2 provides key statistics related to the Swedish healthcare system. Healthcare in Sweden is primarily financed through a county council income tax paid by individuals (Sweden .se 2011). Patients are charged a small fee for services, and the county council pays the remaining costs. The national government sets an annual out-of-pocket ceiling for individuals. Less than 3 percent of the population has private insurance because of the comprehensiveness of the public healthcare system.

The national government is responsible for healthcare regulation but plays no role in healthcare delivery; this responsibility lies with

INTERNATIONAL POLICYMAKING
Health Policymaking in Sweden

- The Swedish government is responsible for proposing new laws (Government Offices of Sweden 2013). It must appoint a committee of inquiry to study the feasibility of a proposed initiative.
- The committee writes a report that is circulated to relevant agencies and the Council on Legislation for consideration.
- Once the committee has gauged the feasibility of the proposed law, the government presents a bill to the parliament, known as the Riksdag. The Riksdag then votes on the bill. If it passes, the bill becomes a new law and is published in the *Swedish Code of Statutes*.
- Sweden is also subject to the legislation of the European Union (EU). Some EU laws are automatically adopted by Sweden, and some must pass through a vote in the Riksdag to be formally incorporated.

EXHIBIT 4.2

Swedish
Healthcare System
Key Statistics
(2009–10 data)

Population	9,394,130
GDP per capita (in PPP)	$38,885
% of GDP spent on healthcare	10%
Healthcare spending per capita (in PPP)	$3,690
Life expectancy, male/female	79/83
Infant mortality rate	2 per 1,000 live births
No. of hospital beds per 1,000 people	no data

NOTE: GDP = gross domestic product; PPP = purchasing power parity.
SOURCE: World Bank (2011c).

county councils and municipal governments. County councils deliver most primary and tertiary care, while municipal governments arrange for elderly care, including basic healthcare delivered in the patient's home or in a nursing home.

Residents with nonurgent conditions first seek healthcare services from general practitioners (GPs) at primary healthcare centers. The GPs refer patients to a specialized care provider if needed. Primary healthcare centers offer basic medical and public health services. County and district hospitals provide specialized care, such as dermatology and ophthalmology. Regional hospitals provide highly specialized healthcare services, such as organ transplants and heart surgery. Sweden's healthcare system also includes centers of teaching and research.

Health Policymaking and Key Health Policy Stakeholders

The national, county, and municipal levels of government in Sweden collectively wield influence on healthcare and health policy (Sweden.se 2011). As such, they are the primary stakeholders in health policymaking. The various levels of government provide services for the vast majority of the population's healthcare needs. As mentioned, private health insurers cover less than 3 percent of the population, and they enjoy less popularity in Sweden than in many other countries with universal healthcare systems.

The public is also a major stakeholder in Sweden's healthcare system, because it can indirectly influence health policy on the national level and health priorities on the county level through the voting process.

Major Health Issues

Healthcare priorities in Sweden are established by the National Board of Health and Welfare's Health Reports (see, e.g., National Board of Health and Welfare 2009). These reports are based on data collected from a variety of sources: government healthcare inquiries; patient data from public hospitals; literature reviews and existing studies; and national surveys, including interviews with and questionnaires administered to target populations. Data sets include the Living Conditions Survey, Household Finances Survey, National Public Health Survey, National Database on Waiting Lists and Wait Times, and Health Care Barometer.

Progress is primarily measured against the goals of the National Public Health Strategy of 2003. The 11 target areas set forth in the strategy were developed from an earlier Health Report, which identified the most pressing issues facing Sweden in terms of mortality and morbidity in the coming decade. The 2003 goals fall into the following general areas:

◆ Safe reproduction and expression of sexuality

◆ Decreased alcohol and tobacco use

◆ Safe working conditions

◆ Prevention of communicable diseases

In these assessments, public health researchers consider not only the direct causes of mortality and morbidity when setting priorities but also the determinants of health and the social and economic conditions that may indirectly contribute to an increased disease burden in certain populations.

Over the past decade, Sweden targeted reduction of tobacco use and coronary heart disease, achieving improvement against the 2003 goals in these areas. The government continually monitors access to healthcare and healthcare effectiveness to identify additional areas for improvement.

CHINA

Key statistics for China and its healthcare system are shown in Exhibit 4.3. The People's Republic of China operates under a single-party socialist system of government (Congressional Research Service 2010). The Communist Party of China (CPC) manages the national government through the National People's Congress (NPC), which is the main legislative body in China, and the State Council, which is the executive body of the Chinese government. The president, elected by the NPC, leads the government and appoints a premier to lead the State Council, who in turn nominates individuals for vice premier and other ministerial posts. Local people's congresses are also in place throughout China.

Although elections are held to select representatives to the NPC and local people's congresses, each candidate for office is affiliated with the CPC.

China is governed by a written constitution. In part, it stipulates that the CPC is the sole political party in power, that China will remain a socialist society, and that all power belongs to the people. See the International Policymaking box for a summary of China's policymaking process.

Healthcare System

The laws governing the healthcare system in China are the Fundamental Health Law and the Hygienic Common Law. In 2009, China introduced a universal healthcare system intended to cover 90 percent of the population by 2010 (China Daily 2011). This target was met, but the level of coverage varies by type of insurance scheme. This reform effort resulted largely from the expansion of the four government insurance schemes: the basic scheme, for urban workers; the urban-resident scheme, for other urban residents, such as children and students; the rural cooperative system, for the rural population; and the medical assistance program, for the poor. These insurance schemes work by collecting funds from all insured persons, the local government, and employers; pooling the funds; and dispensing them according to health need. The Learning Point box describes the schemes in more detail.

Healthcare is primarily delivered by local governments. In some communities, large employers, such as mining companies, may also set up health clinics. Primary care is deliv-

EXHIBIT 4.3 Chinese Healthcare System Key Statistics (2009–10 data)	
Population	1,338,300,000
GDP per capita (in PPP)	$7,536
% of GDP spent on healthcare	5%
Healthcare spending per capita (in PPP)	$309
No. of doctors per 1,000 people	1
Life expectancy, male/female	72/75
Infant mortality rate	17 per 1,000 live births
No. of hospital beds per 1,000 people	4

NOTE: GDP = gross domestic product; PPP = purchasing power parity.
SOURCE: World Bank (2011b).

> **⊕ INTERNATIONAL POLICYMAKING**
> Health Policymaking in China
>
> - The National People's Congress (NPC) and its Standing Committee are the main legislative bodies in China (China Internet Information Center 2013). Local people's congresses also draw up legislation on a regional level.
> - The Political Bureau of the Central Committee of the Communist Party of China plans legislation in five-year periods.
> - On the basis of the preparations made in this planning stage, bills are introduced to the NPC or Standing Committee. Most bills are introduced by the State Council. Important bills are published for public feedback before being submitted to the NPC.
> - After bills are submitted for consideration, the president of the NPC and the Council of Chairmen of the Standing Committee decide whether to add the bill to the agenda or to discard it. Bills submitted by the president are automatically considered. The remaining bills on the agenda are debated by the delegates. The Law Committee may make amendments to a bill before a final vote.
> - The bill becomes formal law after it passes a majority vote and is signed by the president. The president may not veto a bill once it is passed.

ered through local health clinics and small hospitals. Specialized care is provided at regional borough hospitals or larger teaching and research hospitals in urban areas.

Health Policymaking

The healthcare reform package of 2009 serves as an example of China's legislative process; refer to the case study at the beginning of this chapter for a detailed discussion of the initiative. China's State Department sets regulations for the healthcare system, and other governmental departments, such as the State Food and Drug Administration and the Quarantine Bureau, can institute Department Rules concerning public health.

Key Health Policy Stakeholders

China's national government, including the Ministry of Health (renamed the Commission of Public Health and Family Planning), plays an enormous role in the healthcare system, but it is not the only stakeholder (Ministry of Health, Government of China 2009).

> **✳ LEARNING POINT**
> **China's Four Insurance Programs**
>
> **Basic insurance scheme:** Designed for urban employees, with relatively generous and comprehensive benefit packages. Employees pay premiums and copayments and receive comprehensive care at designated hospitals and providers.
>
> **Urban-resident scheme:** Implemented in 2007 to cover primary and secondary school students who are not covered by the urban employee medical insurance system. Higher premiums are assessed than those for basic insurance.
>
> **Rural cooperative system:** Covers rural residents. Government and local subsidies are typically provided to operate facilities. Benefits are generally low and may only cover catastrophic illness. Not considered a viable insurance scheme by most policy analysts.
>
> **Medical assistance program:** Aims to cover those who are designated by the government as poor, but eligibility varies widely across regions. Less than 10 percent of the population is eligible for medical assistance coverage.

Exhibit 4.4 summarizes the responsibilities and roles, resources, and functions of the following stakeholders:

- The central government
- Relevant ministries
- Local governments
- Hospitals and medical institutions
- Medical staffs
- The pharmaceutical industry
- The public
- Think tanks
- The media

Stakeholders		Resources and roles	Interests	Functions
Government	Central government	The main body in policymaking, plays a leadership role	Represents social interests and political interests	Directly responsible for decisions at the national level, overall economic and social policy formulation
	Relevant ministries	The main body in policymaking within jurisdiction	Tend to focus on the interests of own department	Directly responsible for policymaking within jurisdictions
	Local governments	Policy interpretation and implementation	Focuses on local interests	Directly responsible for the interpretation of central policy, local policymaking; expresses local opinion to central government
The supply side of healthcare	Hospitals and medical institutions	Market power, have influence and ability to evade administrative power	Secure government funding, hospital ratings, and market share	Have influence on policymaking by relationship with decision makers and own market reputation
	Medical staff	Have the right to prescribe, hold information superiority	Personal development, income, and professional reputation	Use information superiority and right of prescription
	Pharmaceutical industry	Market power	Maximize profits	Provides funding to research institutions, hires experts and scholars as consultants, forms coalitions of interest with media and local government
The demand side of healthcare	The public	Has the right to choose medical services	Healthcare quality, fairness and access to healthcare	Uses media to form public opinion, expresses opinion to decision makers or experts in the research process
Think tanks	Government-affiliated policy advisory body	Provide policy advisory services	Consistent with the interests of their respective ministries	Directly involved in the policymaking process or provide policy advice to decision makers
	Independent research institutions	Provide policy advisory services	Social interests	Provide policy advisory support, submit report to government and releases to the media
Media		Influence public opinion, support different stakeholders	Diverse interests according to policy preferences	Guide public opinion, help form public agenda, join in different policy networks

EXHIBIT 4.4
Major Stakeholders in China's Health Policymaking Process

Major Health Issues

China's size and its geographic and socioeconomic variability can stymie efforts to collect comprehensive data about all populations and in all regions. The Chinese Ministry of Health sets health priorities by collecting and analyzing data on the conditions that contribute most to morbidity and mortality in the entire country or in specific regions or populations (WHO 2005; Zheng et al. 1998). Some analysis is carried out in conjunction with WHO and other United Nations agencies, such as UNAIDS.

China also has a number of health surveillance systems in place to collect data, such as the Ministry of Health's National Nutritional Surveillance System and the National Disease Reporting System (Zhang et al. 2007). The latter, established in 1959, reports on 37 infectious diseases.

Other areas on which Chinese health policymakers focus are the prevention of infectious disease outbreaks, diabetes, hypertension, cardiovascular disease, and cancers. More than half of all men in China smoke, which is another long-term public health concern. The size of China's population also fuels government concern over family planning measures (e.g., the "one child" policy, free contraceptives, educational subsidies for the single child) and care for the elderly (e.g., mandatory support for elderly by adult family members; subsidies for elderly without children; development of "respect the elderly" housing, similar to the nursing home model in the United States).

KEY POINTS

➤ As the world's health authority, the World Health Organization acts as a leader and partner on health issues worldwide, sets research priorities and encourages the sharing of health-related knowledge, establishes standards of practice and supports and monitors their adoption, advances policy options founded on ethical and evidence-based principles, lends technical support to health initiatives and contributes to capacity building, and monitors health issues around the world and identifies patterns and trends.

➤ The Canada Health Act is the primary piece of health legislation in Canada. It ensures that all eligible Canadian citizens and residents have access to prepaid health insurance and services. It also provides the legal framework for provincial healthcare plans receiving federal funding.

➤ The national, county, and municipal levels of government in Sweden collectively wield influence on healthcare and health policy, and they provide services for the vast majority of the population's healthcare needs.

➤ China's State Council sets regulations for the healthcare system. Other governmental departments, such as the Ministry of Health, State Food and Drug Administration, and Quarantine Bureau, can institute department rules concerning healthcare delivery and public health.

CASE STUDY QUESTIONS

Considering China's recent health reform policymaking process and on the basis of your own research of the events surrounding this round of healthcare reform, answer the following questions:

1. Why did China embark on healthcare reform?
2. What are the similarities and differences in health policymaking between China and the United States?
3. How would you assess the current state of healthcare reform in China?

FOR DISCUSSION

1. What are the functions of WHO?
2. How are health policies made at WHO?
3. Cite examples of WHO-sponsored health programs.
4. Answer the following questions for each country profiled in this chapter:
   a. How are health policies made in the country?
   b. What is the primary legislation related to healthcare policy in the country, and what are its main features?
   c. What are the top health issues in the country?
5. Using examples from Canada, Sweden, and China, identify stakeholders and describe their interests in and influence on health policymaking.

REFERENCES

Atlantic Canada Opportunities Agency. 2011. "Political System." Accessed May 7. www.acoa .ca/English/investment/About%20Atlantic%20Canada/Pages/PoliticalSystem.aspx.

Canadian Broadcasting Corporation (CBC). 2006. "In Depth—Health Care: Introduction." Published August 22. www.cbc.ca/news/background/healthcare/.

———. 2005. "In Depth—Health Care: Studied to Death?" Published June 10. www.cbc.ca/news/background/healthcare/ studiedtodeath.html#rr.

Canadian Doctors for Medicare. 2011. "Background." Accessed May 15. www.canadiandoctorsformedicare.ca/background.html.

China Daily. 2011. "China's Medical Care System Leaps Forward." Published May 30. www.chinadaily.com.cn/china/2011-05/30/content_12601168.htm.

China Internet Information Center. 2013. "The Legislative System of China." Accessed March 20. www.china.org.cn/english/features/legislative/75857.htm.

Cohen, J. 2011. "Committee Sharply Critiques WHO's Pandemic Response." Published March 11. http://news.sciencemag.org/scienceinsider/2011/03/committee-sharply-critiques-whos.html.

Congressional Research Service. 2010. "Understanding China's Political System." Published April 14. www.fas.org/sgp/crs/row/R41007.pdf.

The Economist. (2009). "Sweden: Political Structure." Published August 5. www.economist.com/node/14155425.

Freeman III, C. W., and X. L. Boynton (eds.). 2011. *Implementing Health Care Reform Policies in China*. Published in December. http://csis.org/files/publication/111202_Freeman_ImplementingChinaHealthReform_Web.pdf.

Government of Canada Publications. 2012. "About the Depository Services Program." Updated February 2. http://publications.gc.ca/site/eng/programs/aboutDsp.html.

Government Offices of Sweden. 2013. "The Government." Accessed January 22. www.sweden.gov.se/sb/d.

Health Canada. 2013. "Health Care System." Accessed May 15, 2011. www.hc-sc.gc.ca/hcs-sss/index-eng.php.

Ministry of Health, Government of China. 2009. "Ministry of Health." Updated December 22. www.gov.cn/english/2005-10/09/content_75326.htm.

National Board of Health and Welfare. 2009. "The 2009 Swedish Health Care Report." Published September 18. www.socialstyrelsen.se/Lists/Artikelkatalog/Attachments/17742/2009-9-18.pdf.

OECD iLibrary. 2010. "Country Statistical Profile: Canada 2010." Updated May 2010. www.oecd-ilibrary.org/sites/20752288-2010-table-can/index.html;jsessionid=mbq9yj6u9pbd.epsilon?contentType=/ns/Statistical Publication,/ns/KeyTable&itemId=/content/table/20752288-table-can&containerItemId=/content/tablecollection/20752288&accessItemIds=&mimeType=text/html.

Parliament of Canada. 2011a. "Legislative Process." Accessed May 7. www.parl.gc.ca/About/House/compendium/web-content/c_g_legislativeprocess-e.htm.

———. 2011b. "The Senate Today: Making Canada's Laws." Accessed May 7. www.parl.gc.ca/About/Senate/Today/laws-e.html.

———. 2002. *The Health of Canadians—The Federal Role: Final Report*. Published in October. Accessed May 15, 2011. www.parl.gc.ca/Content/SEN/Committee/372/soci/rep/repocto2vol6-e.htm.

Peabody, J. W. 1995. "An Organizational Analysis of the World Health Organization: Narrowing the Gap Between Promise and Performance." Published in March. www.sciencedirect.com/science/article/pii/027795369400300I.

Settlement Ontario. 2011. "What Is Canada's Political System?" Accessed May 7. www.settlement.org/sys/faqs_detail.asp?k=GOVT_GOVT&faq_id=4000074.

Stein, R. 2010. "Reports Accuse WHO of Exaggerating H1N1 Threat, Possible Ties to Drug Makers." *Washington Post*. Published June 4. www.washingtonpost.com/wp-dyn/content/article/2010/06/04/AR2010060403034.html.

Sweden.se. 2011. "Swedish Health Care." Accessed June 18. www.sweden.se/eng/Home/Society/Health-care/.

US Department of State. 2011. "Background Note: Sweden." Accessed June 16. www.state.gov/r/pa/ei/bgn/2880.htm.

World Bank. 2011a. "World Databank: Canada." Accessed August 10. http://databank.worldbank.org/ddp/home.do.

———. 2011b. "World Databank: China." Accessed August 10. http://databank.worldbank.org/ddp/home.do.

———. 2011c. "World Databank: Sweden." Accessed August 10. http://databank.worldbank.org/ddp/home.do.

World Health Organization (WHO). 2013. "Programmes and Projects." Accessed February 4. www.who.int/entity/en/.

———. 2011a. "Constitution." Accessed July 31. http://apps.who.int/gb/bd/PDF/bd47/EN/constitution-en.pdf.

———. 2011b. "Rules of Procedure of the World Health Assembly." Accessed July 31. http://apps.who.int/gb/bd/PDF/bd47/EN/rules-of-procedure-en.pdf.

———. 2007. "Working for Health: An Introduction to the World Health Organization." Accessed February 4, 2013. www.who.int/about/brochure_en.pdf.

———. 2005. "China: Health, Poverty, and Economic Development." Published in December. www.who.int/macrohealth/action/CMH_China.pdf.

Zhang, X., Y. Ding, Z. Chen, and C. Schable. 2007. "Development of an Integrated Surveillance System for Beijing." *Advances in Disease Surveillance* 2: 127.

Zheng, G., J. K. Zhang, K. M. Rou, C. Xu, Y. K. Cheng, and G. M. Qi. 1998. "Infectious Disease Reporting in China." *Journal of Biomedical Environmental Science* 11 (1): 31–37.

ADDITIONAL RESOURCES

Canadian Institutes of Health Research. 2011. "Building a Strong Foundation for Rural and Remote Health Research in Canada." Accessed May 16. www.cihr-irsc.gc.ca/e/27498.html.

China View. 2009. "Backgrounder: Chronology of China's Health-Care Reform." Published April 6. http://news.xinhuanet.com/english/2009-04/06/content_11139417.htm.

Embassy of the People's Republic of China in the Republic of Malta. 2011. "China's Medical Care System Covers 96 Percent of Rural Residents." Published June 13. http://mt.china-embassy.org/eng/zyxwdt/t830041.htm.

Hu, S., S. Tang, L. Yuanli, Z. Yuxin, M.-L. Escobar, and D. de Ferranti. 2008. "Reform of How Health Care Is Paid for in China: Challenges and Opportunities." *The Lancet* 372: 9652.

Public Health Agency of Canada. 2011. "Toward a Healthy Future: Second Report on the Health of Canadians." Accessed August 12. www.phac-aspc.gc.ca/ph-sp/report-rapport/toward/over-eng.php.

Swedish National Institute of Public Health. 2011a. "The National Public Health Strategy for Sweden in Brief." Accessed June 18. www.fhi.se/PageFiles/4411/public%20health%20strat(1).pdf.

———. 2011b. "Public Health in Sweden." Accessed June 18. www.fhi.se/en/Public-Health-in-Sweden/.

WHO Framework Convention on Tobacco Control. 2009. "History of the WHO Framework Convention on Tobacco Control." Accessed August 1, 2011. http://whqlibdoc.who.int/publications/2009/9789241563925_eng.pdf.

World Health Organization. 2013. "The Role of WHO in Public Health." Accessed February 4. www.who.int/about/role/en/index.html.

———. 2011. "Rules of Procedure of the Executive Board of the World Health Organization." Accessed July 31. http://apps.who.int/gb/bd/PDF/bd47/EN/new-rules-of-procedure-of-the-eb-en.pdf.

Yamey, G. 2002. "WHO's Management: Struggling to Transform a 'Fossilised Bureaucracy.'" *British Medical Journal.* Published November 16. www.bmj.com/content/325/7373/1170.short.

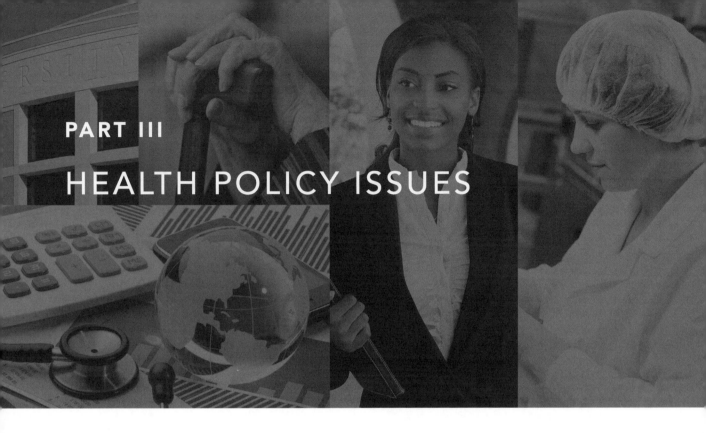

PART III

HEALTH POLICY ISSUES

P art III consists of three chapters that provide examples of a variety of health policy issues. Chapter 5 focuses on health policies related to US healthcare delivery and financing. Chapter 6 discusses health policy concerns for people with special needs and for
vulnerable populations. And Chapter 7 illustrates health policy concerns in the international
community, including both industrialized and developing countries.

The broad health policy issues presented in this part of the book should help students
understand how health policy is applied in the context of healthcare delivery and in terms of
other determinants of health. Knowledge of policy applications prepares readers to examine how
health policies are studied and evaluated—the focus of Part IV.

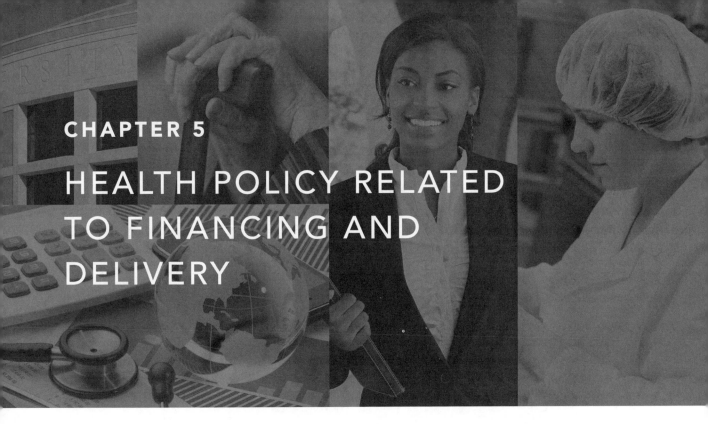

CHAPTER 5

HEALTH POLICY RELATED TO FINANCING AND DELIVERY

Nearly a century after Teddy Roosevelt first called for reform, the cost of our health care has weighed down our economy and the conscience of our nation long enough. So let there be no doubt: health care reform cannot wait, it must not wait, and it will not wait another year.

— Barack Obama

LEARNING OBJECTIVES

Studying this chapter will help you to

➤ describe how healthcare is financed and delivered in the United States and

➤ provide examples of and discuss health policy issues related to financing and delivery.

CASE STUDY

THE FEDERALLY FUNDED HEALTH CENTER PROGRAM: PROVIDING ACCESS, OVERCOMING DISPARITIES

The Health Resources and Services Administration (HRSA), a government agency within the US Department of Health and Human Services, supports access to care for US residents through community-based, patient-directed (i.e., at least 51 percent of the governing board's members must be patients of the health center), federally funded health centers (HCs) (HRSA 2011). The HCs have been providing accessible and affordable healthcare services to individuals in the most resource-deprived communities since the 1960s. To be designated as an HC, healthcare organizations must meet the following criteria:

1. Be located in or provide services to high-need communities—those designated by the government as medically underserved areas or populations

2. Provide primary care services and promote access to care that exceeds access previously offered through supportive services (e.g., translation, transportation)

3. Provide services with fees charged on the basis of ability to pay

The scope of HC services includes primary care, dental care, mental health, and substance abuse services (HRSA 2009, 2011).

Although HCs do not specifically target minority populations or the uninsured, a disproportionate number of their patients are from racial or ethnic minorities and are uninsured patients from low-income, underserved communities: 36 are of a racial or ethnic minority background, and about 40 percent are uninsured (NACHC 2012).

In 2010, HRSA granted HC status to 1,124 organizations nationally, serving more than 19.5 million patients (NACHC 2012). HCs fill a critical healthcare access gap for people who lack insurance by providing good-quality primary care services; delivering cost-effective care; and offering catalysts for local economic development, particularly in underserved communities.

This chapter highlights examples of healthcare policies in the United States that affect the financing and delivery of healthcare. To help you begin to appreciate the underlying rationales for healthcare policy, this chapter begins with a summary of the current methods of financing and delivering healthcare in the United States.

FINANCING US HEALTHCARE

Healthcare spending is often described in terms of a country's *national health expenditure*. The United States, for example, leads the world in national health expenditure: In 2009, national health spending accounted for 17.6 percent of the *gross domestic product* (GDP)—more than a threefold increase from its 1960 level of 5.2 percent (NCHS 2011).

Another way to quantify healthcare spending is by average per capita (per person) spending. This measure adjusts the percentage according to population size. In the United States, the amount spent on healthcare per capita increased from $147 in 1960 to $8,680 in 2011 (CMS 2011a).

In 2006, of the healthcare dollars being spent in the United States, costs for physician and other professional services (31 percent), hospital care (31 percent), and prescription drugs and medical products (13 percent) accounted for 75 percent of the total national healthcare expenditures; the remaining expenditures went to nursing home and home healthcare (8 percent); research, structures, and equipment (7 percent); administrative operations (7 percent); and public health (3 percent). The distribution of spending was similar in 2011 (see Exhibit 5.1).

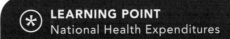

LEARNING POINT
National Health Expenditures

National health expenditures, also referred to as national health spending or national healthcare costs, are estimates of annual spending on health services, healthcare supplies, and research and construction activities related to health.

Total healthcare expenditures are often compared with total economic consumption, represented by the gross domestic product, which measures the total value of goods and services produced and consumed during a calendar year.

Hospitals are the largest source of healthcare spending among institutions. Exhibit 5.2 profiles US hospitals by size and type.

Multiple factors have contributed to the dramatic increases in US healthcare costs, including the following:

◆ An emphasis on curing disease rather than maintaining wellness

◆ Advances in and extensive use of technology in delivering healthcare

◆ The inefficiency of a multiple third-party payer system

◆ An increase in the elderly population and accompanying chronic illness

◆ Waste and abuse within the system, resulting in part from practice variations across geographic areas

◆ General inflation

EXHIBIT 5.1
The Nation's
Health Dollar,
Calendar Year
2010

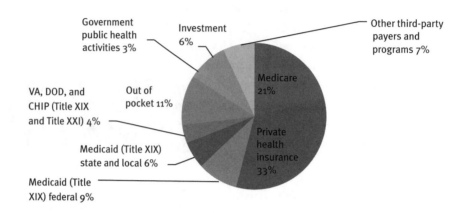

Where it came from

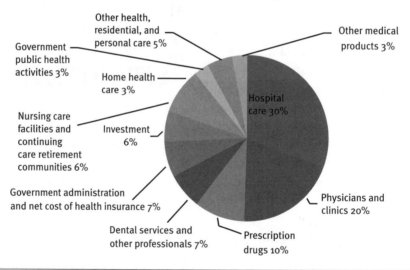

Where it went

SOURCE: Information from Longest (2010).

Defensive medicine
The practice of
medicine in which the
main goal is to avoid
malpractice claims,
not to ensure good
health for the patient
or maximum medical
efficiency.

◆   The recent economic recession and continuing recovery

◆   The practice of **defensive medicine**

Several forms of health insurance have been developed to help patients pay—and allow providers to be paid—for healthcare. These mechanisms fall under two general types: private health insurance and public health insurance.

Total number of US hospitals	**5,724**
Number of US community hospitals	4,973
Number of federal government hospitals	208
Number of nonfederal psychiatric hospitals	421
Number of nonfederal long-term care hospitals	112
Number of hospital units of institutions (prison hospitals, college infirmaries, etc.)	10
Total number of beds in US hospitals	**924,333**
Beds in community hospitals	797,403

SOURCE: Data from AHA (2013).

EXHIBIT 5.2
A Profile of US Hospitals, 2011

PRIVATE HEALTH INSURANCE

Private health insurance is offered by commercial insurance companies, such as Aetna and Metropolitan Life; nonprofit organizations, such as Blue Cross and Blue Shield associations; self-insured employers; and **managed care organizations (MCOs)**, which pay a large portion of the healthcare expenses that subscribers incur. Together, they account for about 33 percent of the funding sources for medical expenditures (see Exhibit 5.1).

Private insurance is an important source of healthcare coverage for most Americans. Among the private insurance options, **managed care** predominates. *Managed care plans* are available through MCOs, such as health maintenance organizations (HMOs), which tend to be large, integrated companies that employ doctors on salary and have their own network of providers and sometimes hospitals, and preferred provider organizations (PPOs), which contract with doctors and hospitals to offer their patients a preferred provider network for care). In exchange for an insurance **premium** and **deductible** from their enrollees, MCOs assume the financial risk, as well as the responsibility, for delivering care to enrollees through networks of providers.

PUBLIC HEALTH INSURANCE

Public insurance programs are health plans financed by the government. Together, these programs account for about 52 percent of the funding sources for medical expenditures (see Exhibit 5.1).

In this system, the government provides benefits to certain categories of individuals who meet eligibility criteria by reimbursing providers in the private sector for care given to beneficiaries. The Medicare and Medicaid programs were created in 1965 under the

Managed care organizations (MCOs)
Organizations that seek to apply the components of managed care to a population in the hope of providing high-quality care at a lower cost than that incurred by the provision of fee-for-service care.

Managed care
A care model characterized by a designated provider network, standardized review and quality improvement measures, an emphasis on preventive rather than acute care, and financial incentives for doctors and patients to reduce unnecessary medical care use.

Premium
The amount an enrollee must pay to join the managed care plan. It serves as a membership fee and is typically adjusted annually.

Deductible

The amount an insured patient must pay out-of-pocket for his medical care per year before the insurance plan covers the costs.

Social Security Amendments of 1965 and are administered by the Centers for Medicare & Medicaid Services (CMS) under the US Department of Health and Human Services. These and other public insurance programs are described in more detail next.

Medicare

The Medicare program provides coverage to (1) individuals aged 65 or older, (2) people of any age with disabilities who are entitled for Social Security benefits, and (3) individuals who have end-stage renal (kidney) disease. The number of Medicare beneficiaries has increased substantially, from 19.1 million in 1966 to 44.1 million (36.9 million elderly and 7.2 million nonelderly) in 2007 and is expected to reach 61 million by 2020 with the aging of the baby boomers.

Medicare is a four-part program. *Medicare Part A* covers healthcare services received in hospitals, at nursing facilities, through hospice care, and from some home healthcare programs. Subscribers do not pay a monthly premium. Part A is financed by mandatory payroll taxes paid by all working individuals.

Medicare beneficiaries willing to pay a monthly premium—determined on the basis of income—may also enroll in *Medicare Part B*. This supplemental insurance pays for physicians' services and outpatient care not covered by Part A. Neither Part A nor Part B covers some services and devices, such as vision care, eyeglasses, dentures, and hearing aids. However, Pap smears; mammography; screening for colorectal cancer, prostate cancer, and glaucoma; and vaccinations against flu and pneumonia are covered by Medicare Part B.

Medicare Part C, known as Medicare Advantage, is an optional, private plan that contracts with Medicare and provides all Part A and Part B services, plus additional services as specified by the individual plan. The insurance plan pays participating private health insurers for services received by beneficiaries in exchange for a monthly insurance premium. *Medicare Part D*, which provides coverage for prescription drugs, offers two types of private insurance plans that help pay for brand-name and generic prescription drugs purchased at pharmacies listed in the Medicare program.

Medicaid

Medicaid provides healthcare benefits to eligible low-income elderly and nonelderly individuals, with separate programs for low-income women and children and for individuals with disabilities. In this joint federal–state program, the federal government provides financial support to states by matching the funding that each state allocates for its program. The federal funding is calculated on the basis of the state's per capita income.

Each state sets its own eligibility criteria and covered services—which must meet a minimum threshold of services required by the federal government—as well as amounts of payments made to providers. It also has the discretion to establish and define other medically needy categories for coverage; these often include individuals living in institutions (e.g., nursing homes, psychiatric facilities) and those who receive care in community-based settings.

Children's Health Insurance Program

Children in uninsured families whose income falls within 200 percent of the **federal poverty level (FPL)** are eligible to enroll in the Children's Health Insurance Program (CHIP). This federal program allows states to expand Medicaid eligibility and establish a special child health assistance program by providing additional funds to states' Medicaid coffers. States can expand the eligibility criteria to cover children younger than 19 years of age in families with incomes exceeding the FPL established for Medicaid eligibility, pregnant women, parents of CHIP children, and caretaker relatives.

IMPACT OF HEALTHCARE REFORM

The Affordable Care Act of 2010 (ACA) is being implemented over the course of several years and will likely introduce new funding mechanisms in both public and private health insurance. For example, the ACA is expected to provide financing to increase the proportion of legal, nonelderly residents with insurance from about 83 percent to about 94 percent, resulting in a reduction of 32 million nonelderly individuals without insurance by 2019 (CBO 2010).

The law will also require individuals to maintain a minimum level of essential coverage for themselves and their dependents, with some exceptions. These individuals, as well as small businesses, will have access to qualified, affordable health plans through state health insurance exchanges. Additional features of the ACA will affect funding as well. (See the Learning Point box for more detailed discussion of the healthcare reform law and its funding implications.)

> *Federal poverty level (FPL)*
>
> A calculation reflecting a set of federal government guidelines related to income that is based on the cost of living (the amount of income needed by families of different sizes to be self-supportive). Many federal assistance programs use a percentage of FPL as part of their eligibility criteria.

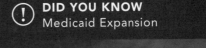

① DID YOU KNOW
Medicaid Expansion

The Affordable Care Act of 2010 expands Medicaid to cover all non-Medicare-eligible individuals under age 65 (i.e., children, pregnant women, parents, and adults without dependent children) whose incomes fall within 133 percent of the federal poverty level.

US HEALTHCARE DELIVERY

The United States does not have a single, coherent healthcare system. In its place are multiple subsystems of healthcare delivery. Access to care through these subsystems—managed care plans, safety net providers, public health programs, long-term care services, and military-operated healthcare—depends on the eligibility factors, as explained below, for each subsystem.

LEARNING POINT
Covering the Uninsured

The ACA aims to reduce the number of uninsured Americans by expanding eligibility for Medicaid and offering tax credits for the purchase of private insurance. Much of the funding for these initiatives comes from the public sector. For example, the ACA includes funding for creating health insurance exchanges; expanding the healthcare workforce, especially primary care; and adding community health centers. The mechanisms of funding include tax credits (e.g., for private insurance and increasing eligibility for Medicaid), grants (e.g., community-based prevention, health centers, long-term care, market reform), special programs (e.g., health workforce, maternal and child health, Medicaid and CHIP expansion, Medicare innovation), and taxes (e.g., penalty on individuals and corporations, certain medical services deemed luxuries).

MANAGED CARE PLANS

Managed care is currently the most prevalent method of healthcare delivery in the United States. In this system, employers and the government purchase health plans for their employees through contracts with MCOs, which offer HMO, PPO, point-of-service (POS) plans, and, more recently, high-deductible health plans (HDHPs).

Managed care expanded rapidly over conventional health insurance from 1981 (covering about 5 percent of health insurance subscribers, primarily through HMOs) to 1996 (covering 73 percent of subscribers, through a mix of HMOs, PPOs, and POSs) and then to 2010 (covering 99 percent of subscribers, through a mix of HMOs, PPOs, POSs, and HDHPs) (KFF and HRET 2010).

Managed care plans provide specific healthcare services depending on the type of plan, paying providers through **capitation**, which is a fixed fee for each patient; a **discounted fee-for-service** scheme, whereby providers accept discounted fees in exchange for a guaranteed pool of patients; or salary, such as that paid in some Kaiser HMO plans. Enrollees choose their providers from within a set network, and primary care providers function as **gatekeepers**, who manage routine services and referrals for higher-level care or specialty services.

Capitation
A fixed fee for each patient.

SAFETY NET PROVIDERS

Healthcare services for vulnerable populations are unique in that they seek to provide medical care and **enabling services** to the poor, the uninsured, and those of minority or immigrant status. These services are provided by **safety net providers**, which include federally funded health centers (see the case study at the beginning of this chapter), physicians' offices, and hospital outpatient and emergency departments. Health policy related to diverse populations is discussed in detail in Chapter 6.

Discounted fee-for-service
A fee agreed on between an insurance plan and physicians to provide medical services at a lower cost than is common for the area in exchange for access to the insurance plan's pool of patients.

PUBLIC HEALTH PROGRAMS

State public health agencies operate numerous programs and services. The five most common are the following:

- ◆ Preparedness (100 percent of state health departments offer such a program)

- ◆ Vital statistics (98 percent)

- ◆ Tobacco prevention and control (96 percent)

- ◆ Public health laboratories (96 percent)

- ◆ Women, infants, and children (WIC) programs (96 percent)

Local public health agencies also operate programs, generally at the county level.

LONG-TERM CARE SERVICES

Long-term care (LTC) is healthcare provided in nursing homes; in skilled nursing, subacute care, and specialized care facilities; by respite care, restorative care, and hospice care agencies; and by noninstitutional, community-based programs, such as home healthcare and adult foster care (Shi and Singh 2009). Most clients of LTC services are elderly, and because aging increases the probability of developing chronic illnesses and functional limitations, they typically suffer from chronic conditions. Functional limitations are measured by **activities of daily living (ADLs)** and **instrumental activities of daily living (IADLs)**. A growing elderly population and rising prevalence of obesity and diabetes are expected to result in increased utilization of LTC services. The Learning Point box summarizes the key features of LTC.

Most nursing home services are paid by Medicaid; Medicare Part A covers a limited amount of services. Private insurance is the least popular funding source for LTC because of the high cost of premiums and its limited coverage.

Gatekeeper

A qualified health professional, usually a primary care physician, who must approve specialist visits before they are covered by an insurance program.

Enabling services

Services (e.g., transportation, interpretation, education, community outreach) that enhance access to medical care.

FOR YOUR CONSIDERATION
Health Services Provision for Diverse Populations

Despite the public insurance options mentioned here, members of vulnerable populations often lack access to safety net providers. One factor is the variation from region to region in the type and level of healthcare services available from providers who offer such care. Another is the mounting pressure being placed on safety net providers from increasing numbers of poor and uninsured people seeking care. The situation is further complicated by the fact that the costs for providing uncompensated care—care that is provided to patients but for which no one pays—cannot be transferred to private insurance (e.g., by charging higher fees for privately insured patients to cover anticipated uncompensated care).

What do you think? Are safety net providers available in your region? How might they provide better care and access to people from diverse populations?

Safety net providers
As defined by the Institute of Medicine, "providers that by mandate or mission organize and deliver a significant level of health care and other health-related services to the uninsured, Medicaid, and other vulnerable patients" (IOM 2006).

LEARNING POINT
Key Features of Long-Term Care

Individualized, coordinated services

Appropriate services are provided according to individualized plans. These plans are determined by assessing various factors, such as physical, mental, and emotional conditions; medical and social history; former occupation; and cultural factors. As the patient's needs change, such as when an acute episode (e.g., stroke, bone fracture, pneumonia) occurs, the LTC provider coordinates care with outpatient settings or hospital inpatient settings, occasionally followed by intensive rehabilitation at a hospital-based transitional care unit or the LTC facility.

Maximized functional independence

LTC aims to enable patients to maintain maximum possible functional independence and prevent further decline of patients' current abilities by motivating them to perform as many activities as possible by themselves.

Holistic approach, quality of life

Holistic healthcare emphasizes taking physical and mental needs, as well as social and spiritual preferences, of patients into consideration when designing delivery of care and the living environment. Lifestyle pursuits (personal enrichment through enjoyable activities), living environment (hygiene, furnishings, aesthetic features), clinical palliation (relief from unpleasant symptoms), and human factors (caregiver attitudes and practices, latitude for independency, adequate privacy) are the four factors of quality of life.

Activities of daily living (ADLs)
Measure of functioning that includes six basic activities: eating; bathing; dressing; using a toilet; maintaining bowel and bladder control; and transferring, such as getting out of bed or moving into a chair.

Instrumental activities of daily living (IADLs)
Measure of an individual's ability to perform activities that are necessary to live independently in non-institutional settings, such as driving a car, shopping, preparing meals, and performing light housework.

Because of the substantial growth in recent years of community-based LTC (e.g., home healthcare, adult day care and foster care, senior centers, home-delivered meals, homemaker and handyman services) institution-based facilities (i.e., nursing homes) have experienced a slight decline in the number of residents (Kahn 2012). However, the growing elderly population will eventually increase the demand for institutional LTC.

CARE DELIVERY FOR MEMBERS OF THE MILITARY AND THEIR FAMILIES

The military medical care system offers ambulatory care and hospital care services free of charge to active-duty military personnel of the US Army, Navy, Air Force, Coast Guard, and certain uniformed nonmilitary services (e.g., Public Health Service, National Oceanographic and Atmospheric Association). It operates through base dispensaries and hospitals, sick bays, first-aid stations, medical stations, and regional military hospitals.

Families and dependents of active-duty or retired military personnel are covered through the military-financed TRICARE program. Retired veterans receive healthcare services through the Veterans Administration healthcare system, which provides care to more than 5.5 million people at over 1,100 sites across the nation, including hospitals, ambulatory and community-based clinics, nursing homes, counseling centers, residential care facilities, and home healthcare programs.

POLICY ISSUES RELATED TO HEALTHCARE FINANCING AND DELIVERY

Exhibit 5.3 illustrates the intersection of medical expenditures and health outcomes in the United States. It reveals a relationship between financing and health status that is seen by many observers as counterintuitive. First, we address the finance policy issues at play in this relationship; later, we discuss delivery issues.

FINANCE

As shown in the exhibit, costs incurred while delivering services such as preventive health and primary care (the intersection at point A) lead to improved health, whereas expendi-

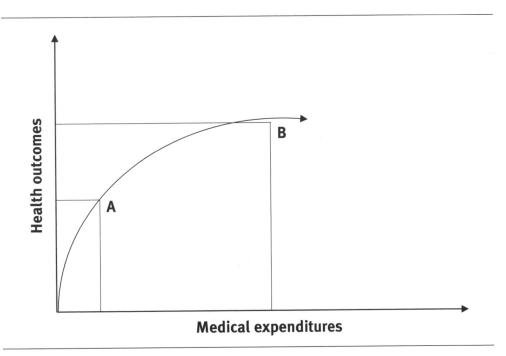

EXHIBIT 5.3
Effect of Increased Medical Expenditures on Health Outcomes

tures made while delivering disease-focused medical care, such as secondary and tertiary care (the intersection at point B) do not proportionally improve health status. And at a certain point (beyond point B, say, delivering high-tech treatment for terminal patients), medical care brings minimal health benefits while potentially prolonging suffering and incurring costs.

Because of this disproportionate relationship, cost containment has become a major policy priority in the United States.

Regulatory Approaches

Regulation-based cost containment is typically achieved through control of supply (how many providers are available), price (fees charged for services), and utilization (extent to which services are provided). Countries that operate a national healthcare system are in a favorable position to achieve simultaneous and comprehensive cost containment by tightly controlling supply and using global budgets to limit payments to providers. In contrast, the US multipayer system requires cost control to be undertaken sector by sector. Various attempts to contain health expenditures through regulation have been undertaken in the United States; the following are just two examples (IOM 2006):

◆ *Health planning*—An example is the implementation of certificate-of-need (CON) statutes at the state level, whereby approval from a state government agency is required for construction or expansion of healthcare facilities. (CON did not appear to reduce hospital expenditures on a per patient, per day basis or affect reimbursement rates, offering no incentive for providers and patients to change utilization behavior.)

◆ *Price controls*—A recent example is pay for performance (P4P), a Medicare initiative that reimburses providers on a scale according to the quality of care they achieve. (Although a study by the Institute of Medicine [IOM] showed that P4P could result in decreased access to and increased disparities in care, IOM advised Medicare to launch a phased implementation with careful monitoring.)

DELIVERY

Policy related to healthcare delivery has focused on both the provider and the patient. Provider-related policies target the healthcare workforce, accreditation, and antitrust regulations; patient-side policy areas include access issues and patient rights concerns.

Workforce

Donelan and colleagues (2010) conducted a survey among leadership representatives of key stakeholder groups about health workforce policies to examine their perceptions on nurse workforce issues. Because nurses are critical to the quality and safety of healthcare and considering current shortages of nurses will likely intensify following the passage of healthcare reform, Donelan and colleagues determined that stakeholders should focus on the current lack of effective policy advocacy and leadership to advance nurse workforce issues on the national health agenda and in the media (Donelan et al. 2010). (The Critical Concept box describes workforce shortages of another kind: rural health professionals.)

Accreditation

To participate in the Medicare or Medicaid programs, healthcare organizations—hospitals and healthcare systems, critical access hospitals, skilled nursing facilities, portable X-ray service providers, ambulatory surgery centers, and others, as well as suppliers to these organizations—must meet eligibility requirements set forth in federal regulations, including a certification of compliance with **Conditions of Participation** (CMS 2011b).

Healthcare organizations have the option of being accredited by a private accrediting organization, such as The Joint Commission, that has developed standards that meet or exceed Medicare's Conditions of Participation. CMS grants *deeming authority* to accreditors that it considers an appropriate proxy (AHRQ 2011).

Antitrust

Anticompetitive activities that lead to higher healthcare costs and a substantial reduction of competition without expanding access to care are scrutinized by the Federal Trade Commission (FTC 2010). Such activities include the following:

Conditions of Participation
Health and safety standards defined by CMS as the minimum requirements that hospitals and medical centers must meet to be eligible to serve publicly insured patients.

- ◆ Mergers and acquisitions involving hospitals, clinics, and pharmaceutical companies that will reduce competition and patients' access to care

- ◆ Price fixing and boycott agreements among healthcare providers to increase the fees they charge healthcare plans without improving quality of care

- ◆ "Pay for delay" drug patent settlements, whereby a drug company that has a brand-name pharmaceutical on the market pays a competitor intending to sell a generic version of the drug to delay bringing the lower-cost drug to market

The FTC and the US Department of Justice Antitrust Division provide antitrust guidance related to various types of healthcare arrangements.

> **⚠ CRITICAL CONCEPTS**
> Rural Health Professional Shortage
>
> MacDowell and colleagues conducted a nationwide survey of rural hospital CEOs in the United States while studying shortages of health professionals in rural areas. According to their analyses from 335 respondents (34.4 percent), 75.4 percent of rural CEOs reported physician shortages, where shortages in family medicine (FM), general internal medicine (IM), and psychiatric physicians were identified as the top three specialty shortages. Seventy percent of rural CEOs reported shortages of two or more primary care specialties (FM, IM, or pediatrics). The four most commonly needed allied health professionals were registered nurses, physical therapists, pharmacists, and occupational therapists. Among US regions, rural hospital CEOs located in states in the New England through Virginia region reported the highest shortages in all health professions. Their findings are consistent with results from related literature in concluding that (1) the physician supply in most rural areas in the United States is less than adequate; and (2) there is a shortage of specialty physicians, especially psychiatrists and general surgeons. Similarities in shortages and attributes influencing recruitment across regions indicate the need for substantial and targeted policy and program interventions to develop a rural health professions workforce that can meet increased demand resulting from the recent health reform.
>
> The study also identified four recruitment and retention factors significantly correlated with the reported primary care physician shortage: "(1) healthcare is a major part of the local economy; (2) community is a good place for family; (3) doctors are well-respected and supported; and (4) people in the community are friendly and supportive of each other." The authors suggest that rural hospital CEOs seeking to improve the recruiting situation work with community leaders to build stronger public education systems and economy and to improve overall quality of life.
>
> *SOURCE:* MacDowell et al. (2010).

Access to Care

The primary goal of health policy concerning access to care is to serve the most needy and underserved populations. Categories of healthcare services to be included in the basic level of care, however, are always up for debate. Elsewhere in this chapter and throughout the book, we discuss the various aspects of access to care as it relates to health policy.

Patients' Rights

Patients' rights consist of issues such as informed consent, adherence to the Health Insurance Portability and Accountability Act of 1996 (HIPAA), and emergency medical treatment.

Informed Consent

The aims of informed consent are to (1) respect and promote the autonomy of patients and research participants and (2) protect patients and research participants from potential harm (Jefford and Moore 2008). The ability to fulfill these aims depends on the presence of three basic components: *prerequisites*, including competence (being able to understand and make decisions) and voluntariness; clear and truthful *information*; and free and voluntary *enrollment*, including the opportunity to withdraw consent without any impact on the quality of treatment received by the patient (Petrini 2010).

HIPAA

HIPAA helps protect patients in the following ways:

- ◆ It prohibits insurers from discriminating against their subscribers through enrollment restrictions or prohibitively expensive premiums assessed on the basis of health factors, including prior medical conditions, previous claims, and genetic information (Department of Labor 2011).

- ◆ It allows certain individuals to enroll in group or individual health plans following the loss of their employment-based coverage.

- ◆ It mandated the development of personal health records to increase patients' access to their healthcare information and their sense of ownership over the information by putting in place data-breach notification laws and other privacy protection mechanisms.

EMTALA

The Emergency Medical Treatment and Labor Act (EMTALA) was passed in 1986 to eliminate discriminatory practices by providers and consequently increase access to healthcare for the indigent and uninsured. Under the law, all Medicare-participating hospitals with emergency departments must provide a medical screening examination, stabilization, and further care or a transfer as needed to all patients, regardless of the patient's ability to pay. The law also requires hospitals to maintain a list of on-call physicians and prohibits hospitals with specialized capabilities or facilities from refusing an appropriate transfer if the hospital has the ability to treat the individual (CMS 2010).

KEY POINTS

➤ Multiple factors have contributed to the dramatic increases in US healthcare costs, including an emphasis on curing disease rather than maintaining wellness, the inefficiency of a multiple third-party payer system, and an increase in the elderly population and accompanying chronic illness.

➤ The United States does not have a single, coherent healthcare system; rather, multiple subsystems of healthcare delivery exist. These include managed care plans, safety net providers, public health programs, long-term care services, and military-operated healthcare.

➤ Triggered by high healthcare costs, cost containment has become a major policy priority for US policymakers through both regulatory (e.g., price controls) and delivery (e.g., promoting accountable and integrated care) approaches.

CASE STUDY QUESTIONS

On the basis of your research of the federally funded health center program and its achievements, answer the following questions:

1. Provide examples of recent studies that demonstrate the value of the HC program.
2. Are HCs sufficient to address the lack of access of diverse and vulnerable populations?
3. How can HCs prepare for future challenges?

FOR DISCUSSION

1. Describe healthcare financing in the United States, and list some reasons for the country's high healthcare expenditures.
2. What are the major types of private health insurance in the United States? Who are the beneficiaries of these programs?
3. What are the major types of public health insurance in the United States? Who are the beneficiaries of these programs?
4. What are the major subsystems of healthcare delivery in the United States? Why were they developed?
5. What important policy issues are related to healthcare financing in the United States?

6. Cite examples of price control in healthcare.
7. What are the important policy issues related to healthcare delivery in the United States?
8. What kinds of current healthcare issues involve patients' rights?

REFERENCES

Agency for Healthcare Research and Quality (AHRQ). 2011. "Hospital Preparedness Exercises Guidebook—Chapter 2. Accreditation Requirements." Accessed February 8, 2013. http://archive.ahrq.gov/prep/hospexguide/hospex2.htm.

American Hospital Association (AHA). 2013. "Fast Facts on US Hospitals." Updated January 3. www.aha.org/research/rc/stat-studies/fast-facts.shtml.

Centers for Medicare & Medicaid Services (CMS). 2011a. "National Health Expenditures Tables: Selected Calendar Years 1960–2011." Accessed February 19, 2013. www.cms .gov/Research-Statistics-Data-and-Systems/Statistics-Trends-and-Reports/National-HealthExpendData/Downloads/tables.pdf.

———. 2011b. "State Operations Manual: Chapter 2—The Certification Process." Accessed February 8, 2013. www.cms.gov/manuals/downloads/som107c02.pdf.

———. 2010. "CMS Advanced Notice of Proposed Rulemaking; Emergency Medical Treatment and Labor Act (EMTALA): Applicability to Hospital and Critical Access Hospital Inpatients and Hospitals with Specialized Capabilities." Published December 23. http://edocket.access.gpo.gov/2010/pdf/2010-32267.pdf.

Congressional Budget Office (CBO). 2010. Letter to the Honorable Nancy Pelosi providing an analysis of the amended reconciliation proposal, March 20. Accessed February 8, 2013. www.cbo.gov/ftpdocs/113xx/doc11379/AmendReconProp.pdf.

Donelan, K., P. I. Buerhaus, C. DesRoches, and S. P. Burke. 2010. "Health Policy Thought Leaders' Views of the Health Workforce in an Era of Health Reform." *Nursing Outlook* 58 (4): 175–80.

Health Resources and Services Administration (HRSA). 2011. "Operating a Health Center. Legislation and Regulations. Authorizing Legislation." Accessed June 7. http://bphc.hrsa .gov/policiesregulations/legislation/index.html.

———. 2009. *Health Center Data. 2009 National Data*. Accessed June 8, 2011. http://bphc .hrsa.gov/healthcenterdatastatistics/nationaldata/2009/2009nattotsumdata.html.

Institute of Medicine (IOM). 2006. "Rewarding Provider Performance: Aligning Incentives in Medicare." [Report brief.] Published in September. www.iom.edu/~/media/Files/ Report%20Files/2006/Rewarding-Provider-Performance-Aligning-Incentives-in-Medi-care/ReportBriefRewardingProviderPerformanceAligningIncentivesinMedicare.pdf.

Jefford, M., and R. Moore. 2008. "Improvement of Informed Consent and the Quality of Consent Documents." *Lancet Oncology* 9: 485–93.

Kahn, K. 2012. "Assisted Living Options Grow, Nursing Home Occupancy Declines." Center for Advancing Health. Published May 23. www.cfah.org/hbns/2012/assisted-living-options-grow-nursing-home-occupancy-declines#.USNNdlpTL_k.

Kaiser Family Foundation (KFF) and Health Research & Educational Trust (HRET). 2010. *Employer Health Benefits: 2010 Annual Survey*. Published September 2. http://ehbs.kff .org/2010.html.

Longest, B. 2010. *Health Policymaking in the United States*, 5th ed. Chicago: Health Administration Press.

MacDowell, M., M. Glasser, M. Fitts, K. Nielsen, and M. Hunsaker. 2010. "A National View of Rural Health Workforce Issues in the USA." *Rural and Remote Health* 10: 1531.

National Association of Community Health Centers (NACHC). 2012. *A Sketch of Community Health Centers: Chart Book 2012*. Accessed February 19, 2013. www.nachc.com/client// Chartbook%202012.pdf.

National Center for Health Statistics (NCHS). 2011. *Health, United States, 2010*. Hyattsville, MD: US Department of Health and Human Services.

Petrini, C. 2010. "Informed Consent in Experimentation Involving Mentally Impaired Persons: Ethical Issues." *Annali dell' Istituto Superiore di Sanita* 46 (4): 411–21.

Shi, L., and D. A. Singh. 2009. *Essentials in Health Care Delivery*, 2nd ed. Sudbury, MA: Jones and Bartlett.

US Department of Labor. 2011. "FAQs About the HIPAA Nondiscrimination Requirements." Accessed February 8, 2013. www.dol.gov/ebsa/faqs/faq_hipaa_ND.html.

US Federal Trade Commission (FTC). 2010. "Prepared Statement of the Federal Trade Commission on Antitrust Enforcement in the Health Care Industry." Published December 1. www.ftc.gov/os/testimony/101201antitrusthealthcare.pdf.

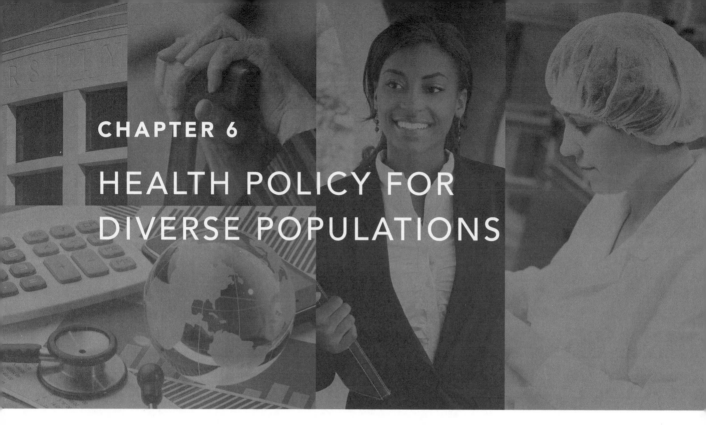

CHAPTER 6

HEALTH POLICY FOR DIVERSE POPULATIONS

The moral test of government is how it treats those who are in the dawn of life . . . the children; those who are in the twilight of life . . . the elderly; and those who are in the shadow of life . . . the sick . . . the needy . . . and the disabled.

—Hubert Humphrey

LEARNING OBJECTIVES

Studying this chapter will help you to

➤ define vulnerable populations;

➤ identify policy issues for racial and ethnic minorities;

➤ describe policy issues for those with low income;

➤ highlight policy issues for the uninsured; and

➤ discuss policy issues for vulnerable subpopulations, such as the elderly, the chronically ill, the mentally ill, women and children, the disabled, the homeless, and people with HIV/AIDS.

CASE STUDY

THE HEALTH CENTER PROGRAM

For more than four decades, health centers (HCs)—not-for-profit, community-directed healthcare providers also known as federally qualified health centers—have provided primary and preventive care to predominantly low-income, racial or ethnic minority patients in medically underserved urban and rural areas. In addition to clinical care, HCs provide enabling services, such as transportation, translation, and health education to facilitate access to care for diverse populations. HCs coordinate with other community services and are governed by boards made up mainly of health center patients.

HCs face significant challenges, including the following:

- The persistent economic slowdown
- Demographic trends
- A shifting disease burden
- The increasing complexity of the healthcare delivery system
- Health and healthcare disparities
- The healthcare workforce shortage
- The rapid rate of technological innovation

HCs are making a difference in underserved communities all across the United States. The National Association of Community Health Centers (2013) has chronicled the stories of how HCs have provided access to affordable primary healthcare and are saving lives and tax-payer dollars. Following are several examples:

- West Cecil Health Center (Cecil County, Maryland) uses the federal stimulus investment to expand services to include more evening hours.
- Westside Healthcare (northern Delaware) built a new site to expand access to more than 5,000 people.
- East Jordan Family Health Center (northern Michigan) has placed computers in every exam room.
- United Neighborhood Health Services (Nashville, Tennessee) serves as a medical home to mothers and children.
- Will County Community Health Center (suburban Chicago) has a new dental van that provides Will County families with healthy smiles.

- Family Health Services (Twin Falls, Idaho) has three expansion projects under way throughout Magic Valley that include medical, behavioral, dental, and pharmacy services.

- Family Practice and Counseling Network (Philadelphia) recruits new dentists and provides many children with regular cleaning before they start school.

- Crescent Community Health Center (Dubuque, Iowa) invests in electronic medical records implementation and patient education.

- La Clinica Health Care (Medford, Oregon) installed a new ultrasound machine to provide better imaging for uninsured and underinsured pregnant women.

- Center for Family Health (Jackson, Michigan) serves as a one-stop center for women's health, pediatrics, and other medical services.

This chapter discusses healthcare policies that focus on diverse populations and on vulnerable subpopulations composed of people with special needs. The populations covered in the chapter include racial or ethnic minorities, the uninsured, and individuals with low incomes. The elderly, the chronically ill, the mentally ill, women and children, the disabled, the homeless, and people with HIV/AIDS comprise the vulnerable subpopulations we discuss.

DEFINING VULNERABILITY

No consensus has been reached on how to define *vulnerability* and *vulnerable populations*. For purposes of our discussion, this chapter defines *vulnerability* as the convergence of health risks. Health risks can be manifested within the following dimensions:

- Physical (as with having a fever or other physical symptoms)

- Mental (as with feeling depressed)

- Social (as with poor school or job performance)

Because poor health along one dimension can be compounded by poor health along one or more of the other dimensions, health needs are considerably greater for those with multiple health problems than for those with a single health problem (Shi and Stevens 2010). Health risks consist of *predisposing*, *enabling*, and *need* characteristics at the individual and ecological levels. (See the Learning Point box for definitions of these characteristics.)

Vulnerable subpopulations such as those presented in this chapter experience a convergence of these health risk factors and, consequently, typically exhibit poorer health status than those who avoid these factors. The For Your Consideration box describes some compelling reasons to focus national attention on their needs to reduce the health and healthcare disparities they experience.

LEARNING POINT
Definitions of Health Risk Characteristics

Predisposing characteristics (those that describe the propensity of individuals to use services):

- Demographic characteristics (e.g., age, sex, family size)
- Social structure variables (e.g., race or ethnicity, education, occupation)
- Health beliefs (e.g., beliefs about health and the value of healthcare)

Enabling characteristics:

- The resources available to individuals and families for the use of services (e.g., income, insurance coverage)
- The attributes of the surrounding community or region that affect the availability of healthcare services

Need factors:

- The specific illnesses or health needs that drive the receipt of healthcare

SOURCE: Andersen (1995).

HEALTH POLICY ISSUES FOR DIVERSE POPULATIONS

RACIAL OR ETHNIC MINORITIES

The US Census Bureau (2010) estimates that more than 34 percent of the country's population is made up of racial or ethnic minorities:

Blacks or African Americans	12.2 percent
Hispanics or Latinos	15.4 percent
Asians	4.4 percent
Native Hawaiian and other Pacific Islanders	0.1 percent
American Indian and Alaska Natives	0.8 percent
Identified as two or more races	1.5 percent

Racial and ethnic minorities experience significant problems in accessing high-quality healthcare, leading to disparities in health status compared to the white, non-Hispanic population.

FOR YOUR CONSIDERATION
Why Should We Care About
Vulnerable Populations?

- Vulnerable populations have greater health needs.
- The prevalence of vulnerability in the United States is increasing.
- Vulnerability is influenced and therefore should be remedied by social forces.
- Vulnerability is fundamentally linked with national resources.
- Vulnerability and equity cannot coexist.

   What do you think? Are these points valid? Explain your answer.

Healthcare Access

The **regular source of care (RSC)** measure is commonly used to assess an individual's access to care. Several research studies indicate that having an RSC increases one's chances of receiving better coordinated care, better treatment for chronic and acute health conditions, fewer delays in care, and access to preventive care. Studies show, however, that compared to whites, racial and ethnic minorities are less likely to have an RSC, even when socioeconomic status (SES), insurance status, and health conditions are controlled for (accounted for in the measure) (Shi and Stevens 2005). Hispanic adults were found to be the least likely to have an RSC, followed by American Indians and Alaska Natives, blacks, and Asians. Whites were shown to be the most likely to have an RSC. Similar trends were seen with children from racial and ethnic minority populations compared to children from the white, non-Hispanic population (HHS 2011).

   Factors contributing to the lack of an RSC include the following:

◆   Absence of health insurance coverage

◆   Low family income

◆   Language other than English spoken in the home

   The inability to afford care was reported as the most common reason for Hispanic adults to lack an RSC (Shi and Stevens 2005). Additional factors that limit access to care, especially for Hispanics and Asians, include English language difficulty, poor geographical proximity to a source of care, and lack of providers that offer **culturally appropriate services**.

Healthcare Quality

Racial and ethnic minority patients are more likely to report dissatisfaction with quality of care and patient–provider interactions than white patients are. One reason is that patients from these groups commonly perceive discrimination in quality of treatment. Just as Eng-

---

*Regular source of
care (RSC)*

A usual place where, or
a usual provider from
whom, an individual
receives healthcare
services.

---

*Culturally appropriate
services*

Efforts by healthcare
organizations and
providers to increase
understanding and
produce effective interventions for patients by
taking into account patients' cultural and linguistic characteristics.

lish language fluency affects access to care for racial or ethnic minorities, it also contributes to whether racial or ethnic groups experience disparities in receiving high-quality preventive care (Ngo-Metzger et al. 2006).

Health Status

Racial and ethnic minorities experience disparities in health status perception, causes of death, and health risk behaviors when compared to non-Hispanic whites. In terms of perception, for example, the 2007 National Children's Health Survey shows that Hispanic and African American children were the least likely to be rated by their parents as in "excellent" or "good" health, even after adjusting for SES and family demographics (CDC 2007). Regarding cause of death, blacks have the highest mortality rates for homicide, breast cancer, and HIV/AIDS (CDC 2011). These causes of death have important implications for healthcare policy because they are preventable through law enforcement, regular screening and early detection, health education, and access to effective medications. As for health risk behaviors, blacks and American Indians/Alaska Natives have the highest smoking prevalence among the populations (Garrett et al. 2011). Additionally, Asians and Hispanics are more likely to live in an area with substandard air quality as measured against the US Environmental Protection Agency standard (Yip et al. 2011).

Programs to Eliminate Racial and Ethnic Disparities

Federal Initiatives

The Office of Minority Health (OMH) and the Indian Health Service (IHS), both of which are part of the US Department of Health and Human Services (HHS), are among the federal agencies that address issues related to the health of racial or ethnic minorities. The OMH (1) provides funds to state minority health agencies and to communities and organizations dedicated to improving minority health, (2) collects data on minority health, (3) increases national attention on health disparities in racial and ethnic minorities, and (4) promotes minority health policy in Congress (OMH 2011). The IHS provides comprehensive health services to federally recognized American Indians and Alaska Natives residing in 12 Indian Health Service Areas across the country.

State and Local Initiatives

State and local programs work independently to meet the specific needs of the minority populations in each state, county, and local community. At the same time, state programs often serve as models for future federal initiatives. Two examples are Minnesota's Eliminating Health Disparities Initiative and the California Department of Public Health Strategic Plan, both released in 2008. They serve large numbers of individuals, and their goals are closely aligned with the determinants of health in *Healthy People 2020* (HHS 2013).

Private Initiatives

One example of private endeavors in this area is the Association of Schools of Public Health, which, with the support of the W.K. Kellogg Foundation, was formed to promote health professionals' involvement in racial and ethnic health disparities research. Another, the California Endowment's Building Healthy Communities Initiative, seeks to promote long-term changes in communities through broad investment in social, environmental, and medical interventions with a primary focus on children and youths.

THE UNINSURED

In 2009, more than 15 percent of the US population did not have health insurance (US Census Bureau 2012). Studies have shown that those without health insurance risk facing barriers to healthcare access, quality of care, and positive health outcomes (Moonesinghe, Zhu, and Truman 2011; Kenney et al. 2012; Garfield and Damico 2012; Weissman et al. 2008). Advocates have urged lawmakers to expand public insurance programs, such as Medicare, Medicaid, and the Children's Health Insurance Program (CHIP), and have called for the improvement of the quality of care received through these programs.

One main goal of the Affordable Care Act of 2010 (ACA) is to reduce the number of uninsured Americans and promote healthcare access. Several provisions within this legislation seek to extend coverage to previously uninsured groups. Examples include the development of health insurance exchanges, which would establish insurance markets for individuals and small business owners, and the expansion of Medicaid, which would provide insurance coverage to all individuals and families whose income is at or below 133 percent of the federal poverty level (FPL) (Redhead et al. 2012).

Healthcare Access

Lack of health insurance increases the likelihood of delayed care because of the increased chances that the uninsured individual does not have an RSC. Uninsured children in particular suffer negative consequences without health coverage. A study on young children aged 0 to 3 showed that uninsured children had a lower chance than insured children of obtaining needed medical care, prescription medications, dental care, and an RSC (Newacheck et al. 2002). Studies have further shown that the type of insurance an individual has affects emergency department (ED) use and the level of preventable hospitalization rates. According to one study, individuals with public insurance were more likely than privately insured individuals to use an ED instead of a physician's office as their primary source of care (Gindi, Cohen, and Kirzinger 2012).

Healthcare Quality

The association between the quality of healthcare and health insurance type has been well documented, as has the impact of insurance status on how much of specific recommended services an individual receives. One study found that, when compared to those who were insured at the time of the study, uninsured individuals experienced deficits in the receipt of preventive care and that the likelihood of receiving care decreased as the length of time without health insurance increased (Moonesinghe, Zhu, and Truman 2011; KFF 2010; Garfield and Damico 2012; Weissman et al. 2008). This pattern was consistent across most preventive services.

Furthermore, poorer access to primary care services among uninsured individuals has been reported to result in preventable hospitalizations, which could have been avoided with timely and high-quality primary care (KFF 2010).

Programs to Eliminate Disparities in Health Insurance

Federal Initiatives

On the forefront of the national drive toward universal and more comprehensive health coverage, government and community organizations have created several programs to increase the number of individuals with health insurance. Federal programs, such as Medicare, Medicaid, and CHIP, cover nearly 40 percent of the US population. The impact of these programs has been especially noticeable in reducing the number of the uninsured among vulnerable populations.

State and Private Initiatives

Many states are expanding the eligibility level for Medicaid or CHIP, and these programs have been credited by several evaluation studies to have improved access to care and health status (Sommers, Baicker, and Epstein 2012; Dubay and Kenney 2009; Holahan and Headen 2010; Howell and Kenney 2012). To assist the remaining uninsured individuals, some states and private organizations have created their own programs for those who cannot afford to purchase health insurance but whose income level makes them ineligible for Medicaid or CHIP.

For example, California Coverage & Health Initiatives (CCHI) is an association of 28 California Children's Health Initiatives (CHIs), which are not-for-profit, county-based private initiatives to connect low-income uninsured or undocumented children to

Medi-Cal, Healthy Families programs, and locally funded health programs (CCHI 2011). CHIs have been credited with improving the health status of undocumented children and reducing preventable hospitalizations. In recent years, however, CCHI has experienced serious financial constraints, and its future is uncertain.

PEOPLE WITH LOW SES

Socioeconomic status is defined by several factors, the most common being income level, educational attainment, and occupational status. Those with lower SES typically face greater barriers in accessing healthcare than those who fall higher on the SES scale. For those in the lower segments of SES who are able to receive care, their overall health status and the quality of care they receive are typically inferior to the healthcare experiences of those with higher SES.

Healthcare Access

SES has been shown to have a greater impact on access to healthcare than race and ethnicity. According to an analysis of the California Health Interview Survey (UCLA Center for Health Policy Research 2007), poor adults are more than twice as likely as nonpoor adults to lack an RSC. Those with higher levels of education were more likely than those with low educational attainment to maintain an RSC and more likely to seek care at a doctor's office than at community clinics and EDs.

Healthcare Quality

Several studies have examined the link between SES and healthcare utilization. For example, women with lower education levels are less likely to report receiving Pap smears and mammograms (NCHS 2009), and women with low household income were found to have lower utilization rates for influenza vaccinations, cervical and colon examinations, and bone densitometry (Earle et al. 2003). Regarding SES and healthcare quality, low income and education levels appear to have a negative impact on physicians' perceptions of patients, which in turn influences physicians' treatment selection and recommendations according to SES (van Ryn and Burke 2000).

Health Status

Low income, education, and occupational status have long been associated with high health risks, poor health status, and high mortality rates (see, e.g., Syme and Berkman 1976). For example, individuals living in poverty were four times more likely to assess their health status as fair or poor than those who were not poor (i.e., above 200 percent

FPL). Furthermore, the percentage of adults aged 55 to 64 with functional limitations also appears to increase as income level decreases, differing by almost six times between the highest and the lowest income levels (Minkler, Fuller-Thomson, and Guralnik 2006).

Analyses conducted by the Centers for Disease Control and Prevention (CDC 2009) on the relationship between SES and mental health status showed that the likelihood of reporting frequent mental distress was two to three times higher in individuals with low income than in those with high income. Prevalence of health risk behaviors (e.g., physical inactivity, smoking, smoking during pregnancy, short breast-feeding period) was also high among low-income adults.

Disparities in mortality rates by SES have also been documented. For example, the Health, United States reports show that infant mortality rates, mortality from communicable diseases, and HIV mortality rates among men are closely associated with education level (NCHS 2003). A 2011 study found that states with the highest proportions of residents under 200 percent of the FPL had twice as high amenable (defined as death "before age 75 from complications of conditions that might be avoided by timely effective care and prevention") mortality rates as states with lower poverty rates (Schoenbaum et al. 2011).

Programs to Eliminate Socioeconomic Disparities

Federal Initiatives

Commonly referred to as the healthcare safety net, federal programs to address SES disparities have focused on increasing access to care for low-income populations. Federal programs targeted to specific low-income subpopulations include the Public Housing Primary Care program; the Health Care for the Homeless program; and Head Start, which helps disadvantaged preschool-aged children attain fundamental math and reading skills. Unlike federal programs that focus on reducing economic and geographical barriers to healthcare, Head Start is the only federal program that invests in increasing the education level of individuals—an often overlooked contributor to SES disparities in healthcare.

State and Local Initiatives

One state program of note is South Carolina's Welvista program, a public–private nonprofit partnership that offers free or low-cost primary care, free prescription services, and free pediatric dental care to low-income people without health insurance. Services are provided by volunteer health professionals, pharmaceutical companies, hospitals, and laboratories, and numerous corporate and community providers are involved in offering resources.

A local initiative targeting those without insurance is TeleKidcare, in Kansas City, Kansas. It was established through a partnership between the Kansas University Medical

Center and a local school district with four elementary schools and later expanded to include middle and high schools. Videoconferencing technology allows providers to conduct physical exams on school children who need medical assistance and to provide acute care and mental healthcare services to those in need.

Private Initiatives

Project HealthDesign, funded by the Robert Wood Johnson Foundation, is one example of privately funded programs addressing SES disparities, through which undergraduate students volunteer in community clinics and connect patients with local health resources. Another, the Health Foundation of Greater Cincinnati, awards grants to improve health in Cincinnati, Ohio, and surrounding counties.

HEALTH POLICY ISSUES FOR VULNERABLE SUBPOPULATIONS

THE ELDERLY

For the elderly, concerns about primary care and health policy broadly revolve around the following:

- Containing costs

- Reforming the health system to better serve a new, large generation of the elderly

- Increasing quality of life as far as possible into old age

Cost Containment

Healthcare costs can be daunting for any American. For the elderly, they are often prohibitive to seeking care. The AARP Public Policy Institute has found that more than 25 percent of American adults aged 50 to 64 (who are not yet eligible for Medicare) spend a significant amount of their disposable income (at least 10 percent) on healthcare; perhaps more surprisingly, nearly two in five older adults covered under a public insurance plan (like Medicare or Medicaid) also spent at least 10 percent of their disposable income on healthcare (Smolka, Purvis, and Figueiredo 2009). This report also determined that costs increase when the patient has at least one chronic disease, and many elderly patients have a considerably higher disease burden (two or more diseases). For example, according to

Bodenheimer, Chen, and Bennett (2009), a Medicare patient living with a single chronic health condition will see, on average, four physicians per year. This increase in numbers of providers appears to be related to the total number of chronic conditions; patients with many chronic conditions (five or more) see, on average, 14 different physicians per year.

Any out-of-pocket healthcare cost for typical elderly individuals is significant, whether they are covered through public insurance, are insured through a private health plan, or pay completely out-of-pocket because they lack insurance. Additionally, care costs for the elderly are on the rise, predominantly due to increases in the number of chronic diseases per patient and the overall aging of the population: "In 2002, beneficiaries with five or more chronic conditions accounted for 76 percent of Medicare expenditures [and] the population over age eighty-five, the group with the highest proportion of people with multiple chronic conditions, is projected to grow from five million in 2005 to twenty-one million in 2050, ensuring a major increase in the number of very-high-cost patients" (Bodenheimer, Chen, and Bennett 2009). Most efforts to rein in these expenditures will require major health system reforms.

Quality of Life

Bodenheimer, Chen, and Bennett (2009) note that the most proactive ways to raise the quality of life for the elderly are to

1. provide effective and low-cost preventive treatments designed to lower risk factors for future adverse health outcomes and

2. provide such treatments throughout the patient's life.

If policies were implemented to help reduce behavioral risk factors, such as smoking, earlier in life, the researchers hypothesize, the increase in chronic disease may slow, and in turn, lower disease prevalence would improve quality of life (Bodenheimer, Chen, and Bennett 2009).

Some evidence does show that the relationship between quality of life and absence of disease is not absolute. Christensen and colleagues (2009) note, "Most evidence for people aged younger than 85 years suggests postponement of limitations and disabilities, despite an increase in chronic diseases and conditions. This apparent contradiction is at least partly accounted for by early diagnosis, improved treatment, and amelioration of prevalent diseases so that they are less disabling." This finding suggests that a highly functioning health services system will be crucial to improving quality of life by its potential to help postpone disability.

Service Availability

The availability of assistive technology, specialized facilities, and customized services may be placing further distance between disease and disability, as do changes in areas that contribute indirectly to health, such as housing, transport, structural improvements to accommodate people with disabilities, gender roles and women's empowerment, and other large-scale social issues (Christensen et al. 2009). Improved funding and coordination of government and private programs addressing these issues within the healthcare system would greatly simplify the process of obtaining necessary care and improving health outcomes for many elderly patients (Reinhard, Kassner, and Houser 2011).

The ACA and the Elderly

Many experts believe that the current system of administering healthcare in the United States is dysfunctional. Issues such as high costs, little emphasis on prevention, recurring medical mistakes, and a general sense of discord among stakeholders now pervade patient care, especially for the elderly. The ACA attempts to address several of these challenges. An analysis in *Health Affairs* found that by changing how healthcare providers are paid by Medicare and Medicaid, the incentives offered to focus on preventive care and coordinate care across different providers and facilities will increase; at the same time, these changes should also reduce the rate at which healthcare spending is currently growing and provide better value for the public payers (Thorpe and Ogden 2010). Specific measures to reduce hospital readmission, improve monitoring of controllable chronic diseases (such as diabetes and hypertension), and help community health teams coordinate care among multiple doctors and organizations will alter the current healthcare delivery system. These changes are expected to result in a system that is less convoluted, more patient centered, and better able to serve the evolving needs of US patients, particularly the elderly (Bodenheimer, Chen, and Bennett 2009; Thorpe and Ogden 2010).

As the US population ages, it faces unique issues, especially in matters of healthcare cost, treatment coordination, and quality of life. As a consequence, these concerns will move to the forefront of the health policy agenda.

THE CHRONICALLY ILL

Chronic illness continues to increase worldwide. In the United States, the primary care system will need to be fundamentally overhauled to accommodate the dramatic increase of chronic disease patients, requiring new ideas on how best to provide high-quality care and meet the needs and expectations of this population (Kimura, DaSilva, and Marshall 2008).

Chronically ill patients in the United States face disorganized care and high costs—$7,000 per capita in 2006 (Schoen et al. 2009; Thorpe and Philyaw 2012). Several programs designed to test alternative approaches to chronic care have already been introduced in the United States, but none has been accepted or implemented on the wide scale that will be required to effect major change (Shortell et al. 2009). New national policies addressing the chronic disease burden should take these experiences into account in attempts to control cost and improve care for the chronically ill.

Uninsured patients with chronic conditions face a double burden. A 2008 study of results from the National Health and Nutrition Examination Survey (conducted by the National Center for Health Statistics, a part of the CDC) found that 11.4 million Americans aged 18 to 65 were living with at least one chronic health condition. These patients faced high barriers to care in that they "were more likely than those with coverage to have not visited a health professional (22.6% vs. 6.2%) and to not have a standard site for care (26.1% vs. 6.2%) but more likely to identify their standard site for care as an emergency department (7.1% vs. 1.1%)" (Wilper et al. 2008). This inability to receive proper and timely primary care leads to more negative health outcomes, which can be especially acute in those patients already suffering from a chronic condition.

The burden of chronic illness is borne both by patients, who experience frustration, high costs, and negative health outcomes, and by the healthcare system, which is often unable to provide appropriate, effective, and efficient care. Policy changes, with a focus on chronic illness, could make a great difference in easing that burden.

THE MENTALLY ILL

Mental health in the United States is an important issue that is only growing in importance. Estimates using the Diagnostic and Statistical Manual of Mental Health Disorders (DSM-IV) classification system found that half of all Americans are affected by at least one mental disorder in their lifetime, and a quarter of Americans meet this criterion in any given year (Kessler and Wang 2008). In addition, mental health disability is on the rise: 2.7 percent of all US adults reported mental health disability in 2009, an increase of 2 million people from 1999 (Mojtabai 2011). In 2005, 27 percent of individuals younger than 65 receiving Medicare coverage were mentally disabled (Goldman, Glied, and Alegria 2008).

These large numbers represent serious health consequences. Poor mental health is associated with increased risk for early mortality, and many mental disorders have an early-age onset (in contrast to most other chronic conditions), which leads to a lifetime of healthcare needs (Goldman, Glied, and Alegria 2008; Kessler et al. 2008). However, as measured over a 12-month period, only 41.1 percent of those Americans identified as having a DSM-IV-recognized mental disorder received any treatment for that disorder (Wang, Lane, and Olfson 2005).

Marginalization

A process in which a person or an idea is pushed aside in favor of another. A marginalized subject typically receives few resources and little attention.

In fact, mental healthcare in the United States has traditionally been **marginalized**. Only fairly recently has focus shifted from specialized, inpatient treatment options to treatment that is integrated within the broader healthcare system; a 2012 study found that the majority of mental health patients are now identified in the primary care system, and because primary care physicians often report difficulties in obtaining mental healthcare referrals for their patients, mental healthcare provided in a primary care setting can improve health outcomes (Kessler 2012).

In the course of this shift, general practitioners have become far more involved in mental healthcare than in the past: 22.8 percent of mental health patients are now treated solely by a general health medical professional, which is higher than the percentage seen by any form of specialist (Wang, Lane, and Olfson 2005).

This trend, while indicative of better integration of mental health services with general medicine, may also reflect a shortage of specialized mental health professionals. A survey of general practitioners found that 66.8 percent had difficulty obtaining a referral to any mental health specialist for their patients (Cunningham 2009), and another analysis detected some level of unmet patient need for mental health professionals in 96 percent of all counties in the United States (Thomas et al. 2009). Evidence also indicates that the mental health services rendered by general practitioners are of lower quality than those provided by mental health professionals, with only 12.7 percent of general practitioner visits resulting in "treatments that exceeded a minimum threshold of adequacy," compared to 48.3 percent of visits to specialists (Wang, Lane, and Olfson 2005).

This need for increased numbers of mental health professionals may be exacerbated by a major legislative development in mental healthcare: the passage of federal and state mental health parity laws. On a national level, the Paul Wellstone and Pete Domenici Mental Health Parity and Addiction Equity Act of 2008 requires equal coverage in group health insurance plans for mental health and physical health benefits (Cunningham 2009). Several states followed with their own similar policies. The impact of these laws is not yet clear, but disparities in care between mental and physical health, and between Americans with mental health disorders and those without, continue.

The ACA is expected to increase access to insurance coverage and thus diminish some barriers to adequate mental healthcare. However, the other issues mentioned, if left unexamined and unaddressed, will continue to prevent progress in mental healthcare delivery in the United States.

WOMEN AND CHILDREN

In 2009, 50.7 percent of the US population was female, and 25 percent of the population was younger than 18 years of age (MCHB 2011, 2010). Both groups face unique health issues that deserve policy attention, and maternity and childbirth present yet another set of concerns.

Women

Women's health is an emerging field centered on health issues and concerns that disproportionately affect women. For instance, women tend to live longer, report more physically and mentally unhealthy days each month, and have higher rates of chronic conditions in old age than men (MCHB 2011; Strobino, Grason, and Minkovitz 2002). Women—especially those who are poor—are less likely to meet minimum physical activity recommendations than men. Women are also more likely to be obese and report activity limitations than men do.

In 2009, 36.6 percent of female-headed households were classified as food-insecure —and 15 percent of all women experienced food insecurity—placing them at increased risk for health problems caused by poor nutrition. Of those adults who receive aid through the Supplemental Nutrition Assistance Program (formerly known as food stamps) benefits, 64.4 percent are women (MCHB 2011; Strobino, Grason, and Minkovitz 2002).

These factors, combined with disparities perpetuated by the limitations of women's traditional roles as caregivers and by economic inequality, call for increased attention to women's health issues.

Children

The health issues faced by children are constantly evolving. For example, chronic conditions in children have increased dramatically in recent years; in 2007, 7 percent of children had a chronic condition that limited their basic daily activities, as opposed to 1.8 percent in 1960 (Perrin, Bloom, and Gortmaker 2007). High-prevalence chronic diseases among children now include obesity (affecting 18 percent of children and adolescents aged 18 to 25, as opposed to 5 percent in the early 1970s), asthma (9 percent of children and adolescents, double the number for the 1980s), and attention deficit hyperactivity disorder (ADHD) (6 percent of school-age children). Poverty is associated with an increased risk for many chronic conditions (Perrin, Bloom, and Gortmaker 2007).

As children become heavier consumers of medical care, the quality of care they receive increases in importance. A medical record analysis conducted by Mangione-Smith, DeCristofaro, and Setodji (2007) shows that, on average, children seeking medical care received only 46.5 percent of the services recommended or prescribed by a healthcare provider, a reminder that simply expanding access to health services, a major policy focus for many years, does "not deliver necessary services [and] will not result in optimal outcomes."

Maternity and Childbirth

Pregnancy and childbirth can lead to both temporary and permanent health conditions, including maternal mortality (Misra and Grason 2006). Receiving proper prenatal care is essential for improving neonatal health in the United States, but preventive care must be obtained early and continued throughout the pregnancy. For example, folate, a substance that helps prevent negative fetal outcomes, such as spina bifida, must be present in adequate levels early on in pregnancy. Thus, women must be able to obtain adequate levels of this nutrient even before conception (Misra and Grason 2006). Considering that 42 percent of the births in the United States in 2008 were reported as unintended, ensuring this level of preventive care is difficult (MCHB 2011).

Women from racial minorities receive prenatal care at lower rates than do non-Hispanic white women, and 7.1 percent of women giving birth in 2007 received no prenatal care at all (MCHB 2011). Pregnant women who had received inadequate prenatal care, and lacked education related to the purpose of that care, experienced an increased risk of providing poor nutrition to the unborn baby; in turn, this practice may increase the risk of the child being diagnosed with obesity, asthma, and ADHD. Maternal cigarette smoking during pregnancy is among the most-documented risks for asthma, obesity, and ADHD in children. And of course, alcohol use during pregnancy introduces risks as well (Perrin, Bloom, and Gortmaker 2007).

While great progress has been made in improving prenatal care, and thus the health of women and children, these gains have not been evenly distributed; health disparities between women and children of different ethnic, racial, and socioeconomic groups still exist, and primary care for these groups has great potential for additional improvement.

THE DISABLED

Disability-adjusted life year (DALY)
A measure of the loss of healthy life. This measurement is intended to capture the economic, social, and functional realities that a person with a disability will face and the corresponding loss in health status and quality of life.

As the US population ages, more people will face disabilities and need specialized care. The Institute of Medicine predicts substantial growth in the disabled elderly population over the next 30 years. On the other side of the spectrum, the number of children and young adults facing disability is increasing as survival odds increase for once-fatal birth and childhood conditions and as chronic conditions in the young become more common (Iezzoni 2011).

Combined, these trends have led to significant and increasing levels of disability in the United States. In 2004, the World Health Organization estimated that the country lost 41.372 million **disability-adjusted life years (DALYs)** that year. The DALY measure has been used since the mid-1990s to capture the true health burden caused by disability, measuring both the years of life lost to disabling conditions and the quality of life lost over the years spent living with a disability (McKenna et al. 2005). While DALYs measure the number of life years lost to disability for the people living with disability, those who care for the disabled, and the country as a whole, feel the effects of disability as well.

In addition to the underlying issues of poor socioeconomic, educational, income, and employment outcomes, disabled people in the United States encounter a health system characterized by difficulty in accessing care and discrimination. Although more than two decades have passed since the Americans with Disabilities Act went into effect, "inaccessible facilities, equipment, and communication systems still compromise healthcare experiences for individuals with disabilities in the United States. . . . The barriers that disabled patients confront represent quality problems and also heighten patients' sense of stigmatization, disenfranchisement, and demoralization" (Kirschner, Breslin, and Iezzoni 2007).

Although little large-scale research has been conducted in this area, studies suggest significantly lower rates of preventive treatments are provided to the disabled. According to Iezzoni (2011), only half of women with a severe disability had received a recommended mammogram or Pap smear, compared to almost three-quarters and more than 80 percent of women, respectively, without any disability. Approximately half of Americans with disabilities are eligible for governmental assistance, such as Medicaid or Medicare, and many more have private coverage. State and federal government spending on the disabled totaled more than $400 billion in 2008, and patients with disabilities account, on average, for almost three times higher healthcare expenditures each year than the nondisabled (Livermore, Stapleton, and O'Toole 2011; Kirschner, Breslin, and Iezzoni 2007). These costs are predicted to rise, especially as the ACA expands Medicaid coverage to more disabled Americans and prohibits refusal of insurance on the basis of preexisting conditions in the private market.

THE HOMELESS

The homeless in the United States are among the most marginalized groups in society; however, their health needs are not marginal. Up to 3.5 million people each year experience homelessness in the United States, and 700,000 people are classified as homeless on any given night. Seven percent of US residents will bear at least one occurrence of homelessness in their lives (Reid, Vittinghoff, and Kushel 2008). Additionally, many more Americans will face housing instability, a precarious position that, while less drastic than homelessness, predisposes individuals to several risk factors that can lead to worse health outcomes (Reid, Vittinghoff, and Kushel 2008).

Homeless and housing-unstable people are subject to much higher resource competition than most of the general population, and health issues that would be considered by others absolutely necessary to resolve may be sidelined by the homeless in favor of basic needs, such as food and shelter (Kidder et al. 2007).

As a result of reduced healthcare, the homeless experience high rates of morbidity and mortality, greatly reduced access to healthcare (especially preventive services), and, therefore, much higher rates of hospitalization and self-reported bad health than the broader population does (Kidder et al. 2007; Baggett et al. 2010).

Up to 75 percent of the homeless population has a chronic mental health disorder or abuses drugs or alcohol (Kushel, Vittinghoff, and Haas 2001). A mid-1990s survey of the homeless reported that only two-thirds of the population had an ambulatory care visit in the previous year, whereas almost one-third had visited an ED and more than 20 percent had been hospitalized. More than 30 percent had been unable to comply with their prescription regimen (Kushel, Vittinghoff, and Haas 2001). Despite having a much poorer health status in general than the broader population, the homeless receive far less care than most groups. For many, by the time they do receive a health intervention, the problem has become so severe that it requires expensive and intensive acute services, such as emergency medicine or hospitalization (Kidder et al. 2007).

Several studies have attempted to identify factors that increase ambulatory and preventive care utilization among the homeless. First and foremost, housing situations with greater stability have been shown to increase the amount of healthcare received, especially ambulatory care (Kushel, Vittinghoff, and Haas 2001). The Housing First program was developed in response to these findings, and it realized positive results in reducing ED visits and hospitalizations among the chronically homeless population in several cities through the provision of basic, no-strings-attached housing (Kertesz and Weiner 2009).

Another factor, the lack of insurance among the homeless population, was analyzed by Reid, Vittinghoff, and Kushel (2008), who suggested that health would improve with better insurance options or options to receive regular care. A different study found that health services utilization by the homeless did not increase greatly with either housing stability or insurance coverage and instead was associated with better community ties and social support. It further indicated that increased community support was, in turn, correlated with housing stability (Stein et al. 2000).

Overall, the plight of the homeless in the United States is complex, distressing, and poorly understood. Many innovative and comprehensive approaches to improving the health outcomes of the homeless are being developed. The Boston Health Care for the Homeless program, a leading outreach program, works to integrate care across the medical spectrum and housing situations to provide continuous services and preventive care (O'Connell et al. 2009).

Such goals are difficult to achieve, and they require significantly more attention than they are given at present. Ignoring the health problems faced by the homeless and housing-insecure will only exacerbate an already desperate situation.

PEOPLE WITH HIV/AIDS

In the relatively short time since the disease was recognized, AIDS has dramatically changed the lives of millions of people, their communities, and the US healthcare system. Although we have seen marked improvements in the prevention and care of HIV and AIDS, approximately 50,000 people contract the virus each year (Hall et al. 2008); in 2010, 47,500 people were newly infected (CDC 2013). A major factor in the continued high number of transmissions is that nearly one in five people infected with HIV do not know they are HIV-positive (KFF 2012a).

Impact on Subpopulations

Current health disparities in the United States are also reflected in the trends in AIDS infection. Men who have sex with other men (a category referred to as MSM) represent only 2 percent of the country's population yet account for 61 percent of new HIV infections. Although the proportion of women who are HIV-positive or have AIDS is significantly lower than that of men, the disease has become more prevalent in the female population over time, and research has shown that more barriers to care exist for women than for men (KFF 2012b). Minorities also carry a disproportionate share of that health burden; for example, blacks, who make up 12 percent of the US population, accounted for 44 percent of new infections and 57 percent of deaths from AIDS. The diagnosis rate for black Americans is nine times higher than the AIDS diagnosis rate for whites (KFF 2013).

As with other health conditions and diseases, socioeconomic factors influence the rate of HIV acquisition. Lower SES is associated with higher AIDS mortality, and infection prevalence is higher among Americans with less education, lower incomes, and higher rates of unemployment (Rubin, Colen, and Link 2010; KFF 2013). Even as the demographic profiles of HIV-infected residents have evolved, those living with AIDS still face discrimination, reduced access to care, and other disparities that greatly affect health outcomes.

> ### ✱ LEARNING POINT
> HIV/AIDS in the United States
>
> HIV is the abbreviation for human immunodeficiency virus; the acronym AIDS stands for acquired immune deficiency syndrome. AIDS is a disease of the human immune system. HIV is a retrovirus that infects the human body and, over time, destroys the immune system, leading to AIDS. A person who has AIDS is typically in the final stages of HIV, after the immune system becomes unable to defend itself. HIV is transmitted by having sex without a condom; by sharing syringes, needles, or drug works; and through pregnancy, childbearing, or breast-feeding.
>
> The CDC identified the first AIDS cases in the United States in 1981. In the following decades, 1.7 million US residents have become infected with HIV, and more than 600,000 have died from AIDS, leaving 1.1 million people in the United States living with HIV/AIDS today (KFF 2012a).

Implications of Advances in Treatment

People infected with HIV/AIDS fare better today than they did ten years ago as a result of the discovery and widespread use of new treatment options, particularly antiretroviral drugs used in combinations of multiple drug classes. These therapies are only effective, however, if administered early and continuously over the course of the infection. For those patients who have access to expert medical care and powerful drug "cocktails," these advances "have transformed HIV/AIDS from a terminal illness to a chronic disease," whereas those with limited means may still face a bleak outcome (Lubinski et al. 2009). The barriers that inhibit HIV-positive people from accessing lifesaving medications are significant; most important among them is the lifetime health costs associated with the diagnosis. In 2006, total costs to treat HIV and AIDS per person were estimated to be more than $385,000, 73 percent of which was spent on antiretroviral medications (Schackman et al. 2006).

Assuming an individual has access to these treatments, the average patients' life expectancy has increased to 24.2 years following diagnosis (as opposed to the average expected 6.8 years in 1998), and this greatly expanded life expectancy accounts for much of the rise in treatment costs (Schackman et al. 2006). As discussed next, the federal government pays a substantial portion of these expenses.

Funding

In fiscal year 2011, the US government spent $14.1 billion on HIV-related care and treatment activities (KFF 2011). Medicare covers about 100,000 people infected with HIV, with the vast majority becoming eligible through disability (KFF 2009b). Medicaid covers even more patients, an estimated 240,000 in 2009, which represents about four out of every ten patients receiving treatment for HIV in the United States (KFF 2009a). The federal government spends $4.1 billion each year for Medicaid HIV activities, which is supplemented by state funding (KFF 2009a).

Additional funding is provided by the Ryan White HIV/AIDS Program, a federal initiative named after a 13-year-old boy who was diagnosed with AIDS in 1984 and fought for the right to attend school. The program aims to assist HIV patients who do not have sufficient means to obtain treatment by disbursing discretionary funds provided by Congress to states, cities, not-for-profit organizations, and healthcare providers.

Policy Initiatives

Two major current initiatives in US healthcare policy are expected to lead to improved health outcomes for people with HIV/AIDS. First, President Barack Obama's 2010 National AIDS Strategy for the United States, hailed as "the most comprehensive federal response to the domestic HIV epidemic to date," sets three targeted goals for the country to achieve in the next ten years (Yehia and Frank 2011):

◆ Reduce new infections

◆ Improve access to care and outcomes

◆ Reduce health disparities

Accompanying this renewed focus on HIV health issues are mandates set forth in the ACA. The act will raise the income level for Medicaid enrollment and outlaw the denial of coverage due to preexisting conditions, both of which should help HIV/AIDS patients continue to receive lifesaving healthcare.

The government's achievements in addressing disparities in HIV/AIDS treatment are making a positive impact on the lives of this subpopulation. However, much progress is yet to be made.

KEY POINTS

➤ Vulnerable subpopulations, such as racial/ethnic minorities, the uninsured, and those with low socioeconomic status, typically experience a convergence of health risk factors and, consequently, exhibit poorer health status than do other subpopulations.

➤ For the elderly, concerns about primary care and health policy broadly revolve around containing costs; reforming the health system to better serve a new, large generation of the elderly; and increasing the quality of life.

➤ The US primary care system will need to be fundamentally overhauled to accommodate the new increase of chronic disease patients, requiring new ideas on how best to provide high-quality care and meet the needs of this population.

➤ Although half of all Americans are affected by at least one mental disorder in their lifetime, mental healthcare in the United States has traditionally been marginalized.

CASE STUDY ASSIGNMENT

On the basis of your own research, provide a summary of the efficacy of health centers, focusing on their roles in improving access, quality, and outcomes for vulnerable populations. In addition, discuss how health centers can cope with the challenges they face.

FOR DISCUSSION

1. Why should health policy focus on vulnerable populations?
2. What health policy issues are racial and ethnic minorities facing?
3. Cite examples of programs to eliminate racial and ethnic disparities in healthcare.
4. What health policy issues are uninsured US residents facing?
5. Cite examples of programs to eliminate insurance disparities.
6. What is socioeconomic status (SES)?
7. What health policy issues are people with low SES facing?
8. Cite examples of programs to eliminate SES disparities.
9. List the health policy issues for each of the following subpopulations:
   a. The elderly
   b. The chronically ill
   c. The mentally ill
   d. Women and children
   e. The disabled
   f. The homeless
   g. People with HIV/AIDS

REFERENCES

Andersen, R. M. 1995. "Revisiting the Behavioral Model and Access to Medical Care: Does It Matter?" *Journal of Health and Social Behavior* 36 (Social Science Module): 1.

Baggett, T. P., J. J. O'Connell, D. E. Singer, and N. A. Rigotti. 2010. "The Unmet Health Care Needs of Homeless Adults: A National Study." *American Journal of Public Health* 100: 1326–33.

Bodenheimer, T., E. Chen, and H. D. Bennett. 2009. "Confronting the Growing Burden of Chronic Disease: Can the U.S. Health Care Workforce Do the Job?" *Health Affairs* 28 (1): 64–74.

California Coverage & Health Initiatives (CCHI). 2011. "Vision, Mission & History." Accessed February 13, 2013. http://cchi4families.org/vision_history.cfm.

Centers for Disease Control and Prevention (CDC). 2013. "HIV/AIDS Statistics and Surveillance: Basic Statistics." Modified February 28. www.cdc.gov/hiv/topics/surveillance/basic.htm#incidence.

———. 2011. "CDC Health Disparities and Inequalities Report—United States, 2011." Published January 14. www.cdc.gov/mmwr/pdf/other/su6001.pdf.

———. 2009. "Minority Health Surveillance—REACH U.S. 2009." Accessed February 13, 2013. www.cdc.gov/Features/dsREACHUS.

———. 2007. "National Survey of Children's Health." Accessed March 20, 2013. www.cdc.gov/nchs/slaits/nsch.htm#2007nsch.

Christensen, K., G. Doblhammer, R. Rau, and J. W. Vaupel. 2009. "Ageing Populations: The Challenges Ahead." *Lancet* 374 (9696): 1196–1208.

Cunningham, P. J. 2009. "Beyond Parity: Primary Care Physicians' Perspectives on Access to Mental Health Care." *Health Affairs* 28 (3): w490–w501.

Dubay, L., and G. Kenney. 2009. "The Impact of CHIP on Children's Insurance Coverage: An Analysis Using the National Survey of America's Families." *Health Services Research* 44 (6): 2040–59.

Earle, C. C., H. J. Burstein, E. P. Winer, and J. C. Weeks. 2003. "Quality of Non-Breast Cancer Health Maintenance Among Elderly Breast Cancer Survivors." *Journal of Clinical Oncology* 21 (8): 1447–51.

Garfield, R., and A. Damico. 2012. "Medicaid Expansion Under Health Reform May Increase Service Use and Improve Access for Low-Income Adults with Diabetes." *Health Affairs* 31 (1): 159–67.

Garrett, B. E., S. R. Dube, A. Trosclair, R. S. Caraballo, T. F. Pechacek, and the National Center for Chronic Disease Prevention and Health Promotion, CDC. 2011. "Cigarette Smoking—United States, 1965–2008." Published January 14. www.cdc.gov/mmwr/preview/mmwrhtml/su6001a24.htm?s_cid=su6001a24_w.

Gindi, R. M., R. A. Cohen, and W. K. Kirzinger. 2012. "Emergency Room Use Among Adults Aged 18–64: Early Release of Estimates from the National Health Interview Survey, January–June 2011." Published in May. www.cdc.gov/nchs/data/nhis/earlyrelease/emergency_room_use_january-june_2011.pdf.

Goldman, H. H., S. A. Glied, and M. Alegria. 2008. "Mental Health in the Mainstream of Public Policy: Research Issues and Opportunities." *American Journal of Psychiatry* 165 (9): 1099–1101.

Hall, H. I., R. Song, P. Rhodes, J. Prejean, Q. An, L. M. Lee, J. Karon, R. Brookmeyer, E. H. Kaplan, M. T. McKenna, and R. S. Janssen. 2008. "Estimation of HIV Incidence in the United States." *Journal of the American Medical Association* 300 (5): 520–29.

Holahan, J., and I. Headen. 2010. *Medicaid Coverage and Spending in Health Reform: National and State-by-State Results for Adults at or Below 133% FPL*. Published in May. www.kff.org/healthreform/upload/medicaid-coverage-and-spending-in-health-reform-national-and-state-by-state-results-for-adults-at-or-below-133-fpl.pdf.

Howell, E. M., and G. M. Kenney. 2012. "The Impact of the Medicaid/CHIP Expansions on Children: A Synthesis of the Evidence." *Medical Care Research and Review* 69 (4): 372–96.

Iezzoni, L. I. 2011. "Eliminating Health and Health Care Disparities Among the Growing Population of People with Disabilities." *Health Affairs* 30 (10): 1947–54.

Kaiser Family Foundation (KFF). 2013. "Fact Sheet: Black Americans and HIV/AIDS." Published February 6. www.kff.org/hivaids/upload/6089-10.pdf.

———. 2012a. "Fact Sheet: The HIV/AIDS Epidemic in the United States." Published December 4. www.kff.org/hivaids/upload/3029-13.pdf.

———. 2012b. "Fact Sheet: Women and HIV/AIDS in the United States." Published December 18. www.kff.org/hivaids/upload/6092-10.pdf.

———. 2011. "Fact Sheet: The Ryan White Program." Published in November. www.kff.org/hivaids/upload/7582-06.pdf.

———. 2010. "The Uninsured: A Primer." Published in December. www.kff.org/uninsured/upload/7451-06.pdf.

———. 2009a. "Fact Sheet: Medicaid and HIV/AIDS." Published in February. www.kff.org/hivaids/upload/7172_04.pdf.

———. 2009b. "Fact Sheet: Medicare and HIV/AIDS." Published in February. www.kff.org/hivaids/upload/7171_04.pdf.

Kenney, G., S. McMorrow, S. Zuckerman, and D. Goin. 2012. "A Decade of Health Care Access Declines for Adults Holds Implications for Changes in the Affordable Care Act." *Health Affairs* 31 (5): 899–908.

Kertesz, S. G., and S. J. Weiner. 2009. "Housing the Chronically Homeless: High Hopes, Complex Realities." *Journal of the American Medical Association* 301 (17): 1822–24.

Kessler, R. 2012. "Mental Health Care Treatment Initiation when Mental Health Services Are Incorporated into Primary Care Practice." *Journal of the American Board of Family Medicine* 25 (2): 255–59.

Kessler, R. C., S. Heeringa, M. D. Lakoma, M. Petukhova, A. E. Rupp, M. Schoenbaum, P. S. Wang, and A. M. Zaslavsky. 2008. "Individual and Societal Effects of Mental Disorders on Earnings in the United States: Results from the National Comorbidity Replication Survey." *American Journal of Psychiatry* 165 (6): 703–11.

Kessler, R. C., and P. S. Wang. 2008. "The Descriptive Epidemiology of Commonly Occurring Mental Disorders in the United States." *Annual Review of Public Health* 29: 115–29.

Kidder, D. P., R. J. Wolitski, M. L. Campsmith, and G. V. Nakamura. 2007. "Health Status, Health Care Use, Medication Use, and Medication Adherence Among Homeless and Housed People Living with HIV/AIDS." *Journal of the American Public Health Association* 97: 2238–45.

Kimura, J., K. DaSilva, and R. Marshall. 2008. "Population Management, Systems-Based Practice, and Planned Chronic Illness Care: Integrating Disease Management Competencies into Primary Care to Improve Composite Diabetes Quality Measures." *Disease Management* 11: 13–22.

Kirschner, K. L., M. L. Breslin, and L. I. Iezzoni. 2007. "Structural Impairments That Limit Access to Health Care for Patients with Disabilities." *Journal of the American Medical Association* 297 (10): 1121–25.

Kushel, M. B., E. Vittinghoff, and J. S. Haas. 2001. "Factors Associated with the Health Care Utilization of Homeless Persons." *Journal of the American Medical Association* 285 (2): 200–206.

Livermore, G., D. C. Stapleton, and M. O'Toole. 2011. "Health Care Costs Are a Key Driver of Growth in Federal and State Assistance to Working-Age People with Disabilities." *Health Affairs* 30 (9): 1664–72.

Lubinski, C., J. Aberg, A. D. Bardeguez, R. Elion, P. Emmanuel, D. Kuritzkes, M. Saag, K. E. Squires, A. Weddle, J. Rainey, M. R. Zerehi, J. F. Ralston, D. A. Fleming, D. Bronson, M. Cooke, C. Cutler, Y. Ejnes, R. Gluckman, M. Liebow, K. Musana, M. E. Mayer, M. W. Purtle, P. P. Reynolds, L. Viswanathan, K. B. Weiss, and B. Yehia. 2009. "HIV Policy: The Path Forward—a Joint Position Paper of the HIV Medicine Association of the Infectious Diseases Society of America and the American College of Physicians." *Clinical Infectious Diseases* 48: 1335–44.

Mangione-Smith, R., A. H. DeCristofaro, and C. M. Setodji. 2007. "The Quality of Ambulatory Care Delivered to Children in the United States." *New England Journal of Medicine* 357 (15): 1515–23.

Maternal and Child Health Bureau (MCHB), Health Resources and Services Administration, US Department of Health and Human Services. 2011. *Women's Health USA 2011*. Rockville, MD: HHS.

———. 2010. *Child Health USA 2010*. Rockville, MD: HHS.

McKenna, M. T., C. M. Michaud, C. J. L. Murray, and J. S. Marks. 2005. "Assessing the Burden of Disease in the United States Using Disability-Adjusted Life Years." *American Journal of Preventive Medicine* 28 (5): 415–23.

Minkler, M., E. Fuller-Thomson, and J. M. Guralnik. 2006. "Gradient of Disability Across the Socioeconomic Spectrum in the United States." *New England Journal of Medicine* 355: 695–703.

Misra, D. P., and H. Grason. 2006. "Achieving Safe Motherhood: Applying a Life Course and Multiple Determinants Perinatal Health Framework in Public Health." *Women's Health Issues* 16: 159–75.

Mojtabai, R. 2011. "National Trends in Mental Health Disability, 1997–2009." *American Journal of Public Health* 101: 2156–63.

Moonesinghe, R., J. Zhu, and B. I. Truman. 2011. "Health Insurance Coverage—United States, 2004 and 2008." Published January 14. www.cdc.gov/mmwr/preview/mmwrhtml/su6001a6.htm?s_cid=su6001a6_w.

National Association of Community Health Centers. 2013. "Community Health Center Stories." Accessed March 20. www.nachc.com/health-center-map.cfm.

National Center for Health Statistics (NCHS). 2009. *Health, United States 2008*. Hyattsville, MD: NCHS.

———. 2003. *Health, United States 2003*. Hyattsville, MD: NCHS.

Newacheck, P. W., Y. Y. Hung, M. Hochstein, and N. Halfon. 2002. "Access to Health Care for Disadvantaged Young Children." *Journal of Early Intervention* 25 (1): 1–11.

Ngo-Metzger, Q., J. Telfair, D. H. Sorkin, B. Weidmer, R. Weech-Maldonado, M. Hurtado, and R. D. Hays. 2006. "Cultural Competency and Quality of Care: Obtaining the Patient's Perspective." The Commonwealth Fund. Published in October. www.commonwealthfund.org/usr_doc/Ngo-Metzger_cultcompqualitycareobtainpatientperspect_963.pdf.

O'Connell, J. J., S. C. Oppenheimer, C. M. Judge, R. L. Taube, B. B. Blanchfield, S. E. Swain, and H. K. Koh. 2009. "The Boston Health Care for the Homeless Program: A Public Health Framework." *American Journal of Public Health* 100: 1400–1408.

Office of Minority Health (OMH), US Department of Health and Human Services. 2011. "About OMH." Updated August 16. http://minorityhealth.hhs.gov/templates/browse .aspx?lvl=1&lvlID=7.

Perrin, J. M., S. R. Bloom, and S. L. Gortmaker. 2007. "The Increase of Childhood Chronic Conditions in the United States." *Journal of the American Medical Association* 297 (24): 2755–59.

Redhead, C. S., H. Chaikind, B. Fernandez, and J. Staman. 2012. "ACA: A Brief Overview of the Law, Implementation, and Legal Challenges." Congressional Research Service. Published July 3. http://fpc.state.gov/documents/organization/195390.pdf.

Reid, K. W., E. Vittinghoff, and M. B. Kushel. 2008. "Association Between the Level of Housing Instability, Economic Standing and Health Care Access: A Meta-Regression." *Journal of Health Care for the Poor and Underserved* 19: 1212–28.

Reinhard, S. C., E. Kassner, and A. Houser. 2011. "How the Affordable Care Act Can Help Move States Toward a High-Performing System of Long-Term Services and Supports." *Health Affairs* 30 (3): 447–53.

Rubin, M. S., C. G. Colen, and B. G. Link. 2010. "Examination of Inequalities in HIV/AIDS Mortality in the United States from a Fundamental Cause Perspective." *American Journal of Public Health* 100: 1053–59.

Schackman, B. R., K. A. Gebo, R. P. Walensky, E. Losina, T. Muccio, P. E. Sax, M. C. Weinstein, G. R. Seage III, R. D. Moore, and K. A. Freedberg. 2006. "The Lifetime Cost of Current Human Immunodeficiency Virus Care in the United States." *Medical Care* 44 (11): 990–97.

Schoen, C., R. Osborn, S. K. H. How, M. M. Doty, and J. Peugh. 2009. "In Chronic Condition: Experiences of Patients with Complex Health Care Needs, in Eight Countries, 2008." *Health Affairs* 28 (1): w1–w16.

Schoenbaum, S. C., C. Schoen, J. L. Nicholson, and J. C. Cantor. 2011. "Mortality Amenable to Health Care in the United States: The Roles of Demographics and Health Systems Performance." *Journal of Public Health Policy* 32: 407–29.

Shi, L., and G. Stevens. 2010. *Vulnerable Populations in the United States*, 2nd ed. San Francisco: Jossey-Bass.

———. 2005. "Vulnerability and Unmet Health Care Needs: The Influence of Multiple Risk Factors." *Journal of General Internal Medicine* 20 (2): 148–54.

Shortell, S. M., R. Gillies, J. Siddique, L. P. Casalino, D. Rittenhouse, J. C. Robinson, and R. K. McCurdy. 2009. "Improving Chronic Illness Care: A Longitudinal Cohort Analysis of Large Physician Organizations." *Medical Care* 47: 932–39.

Smolka, G., L. Purvis, and C. Figueiredo. 2009. "Health Care Reform: What's at Stake for 50- to 64-Year-Olds?" *AARP Public Policy Institute Insight on the Issues,* 1–7.

Sommers, B. D., K. Baicker, and A. M. Epstein. 2012. "Mortality and Access to Care Among Adults After State Medicaid Expansions." *New England Journal of Medicine* 367: 1025–34.

Stein, J. A., R. M. Andersen, P. Koegel, and L. Gelberg. 2000. "Predicting Health Services Utilization Among Homeless Adults: A Prospective Analysis." *Journal of Health Care for the Poor and Underserved* 11 (2): 212–30.

Strobino, D. M., H. Grason, and C. Minkovitz. 2002. "Charting a Course for the Future of Women's Health in the United States: Concepts, Findings and Recommendations." *Social Science and Medicine* 54: 839–48.

Syme, S. L., and L. F. Berkman. 1976. "Social Class, Susceptibility and Sickness." *American Journal of Epidemiology* 104 (1): 1–8.

Thomas, K. C., A. R. Ellis, T. R. Konrad, C. E. Holzer, and J. P. Morrissey. 2009. "County-Level Estimates of Mental Health Professional Shortage in the United States." *Psychiatric Services* 60: 1323–28.

Thorpe, K. E., and L. L. Ogden. 2010. "The Foundation That Health Reform Lays for Improved Payment, Care Coordination, and Prevention." *Health Affairs* 29 (6): 1183–87.

Thorpe, K. E., and M. Philyaw. 2012. "The Medicalization of Chronic Disease and Costs." *Annual Review of Public Health* 33: 409–23.

UCLA Center for Health Policy Research. 2007. "The State of Health Insurance in California: Findings from the 2005 California Health Interview Survey." Published July 1. http://healthpolicy.ucla.edu/publications/search/pages/detail.aspx?PubID=219.

US Census Bureau. 2012. "Table 155. Health Insurance Coverage Status by Selected Characteristics: 2008 and 2009." In *Statistical Abstracts of the United States: 2012*. Accessed February 24, 2013. www.census.gov/compendia/statab/2012/tables/12s0156.pdf.

———. 2010. *Statistical Abstracts of the United States: 2010*. Washington, DC: Government Printing Office.

US Department of Health and Human Services (HHS). 2013. *Healthy People 2020*. Updated February 6. www.healthypeople.gov/2020/default.aspx.

———. 2011. *HHS Action Plan to Reduce Racial and Ethnic Health Disparities: A Nation Free of Disparities in Health and Health Care*. Accessed February 23, 2013. http://minorityhealth.hhs.gov/npa/files/Plans/HHS/HHS_Plan_complete.pdf.

Van Ryn, M., and J. Burke. 2000. "The Effect of Patient Race and Socio-economic Status on Physicians' Perceptions of Patients." *Social Science and Medicine* 50 (6): 813–28.

Wang, P. S., M. Lane, and M. Olfson. 2005. "Twelve-Month Use of Mental Health Services in the United States: Results from the National Comorbidity Survey Replication." *Archive of General Psychiatry* 62: 629–40.

Weissman, J., A. Zaslavsky, R. Wolf, and J. Ayanian. 2008. "State Medicaid Coverage and Access to Care for Low-Income Adults." *Journal of Health Care for the Poor and Underserved* 19 (1): 307–19.

Wilper, A. P., S. Woolhandler, K. E. Lasser, D. McCormick, D. H. Bor, and D. U. Himmelstein. 2008. "A National Study of Chronic Disease Prevalence and Access to Care in Uninsured U.S. Adults." *Annals of Internal Medicine* 149: 170–76.

Yehia, B., and I. Frank. 2011. "Battling AIDS in America: An Evaluation of the National HIV/ AIDS Strategy." *American Journal of Public Health* 101: e4–e8.

Yip, F. Y., J. N. Pearcy, P. L. Garbe, and B. I. Truman. 2011. "Unhealthy Air Quality—United States, 2006–2009." Published January 14. www.cdc.gov/mmwr/preview/mmwrhtml/ su6001a5.htm?s_cid=su6001a5_w.

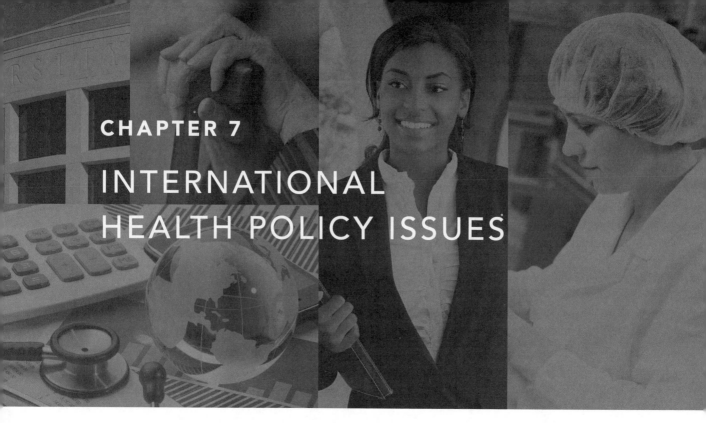

CHAPTER 7

INTERNATIONAL HEALTH POLICY ISSUES

Letting a hundred flowers blossom and a hundred schools of thought contend is the policy for promoting the progress of the arts and the sciences and a flourishing culture in our land.

—Mao Zedong

LEARNING OBJECTIVES

Studying this chapter will help you to

➤ learn about the critical health policy issues in industrialized countries,

➤ discuss the critical health policy issues in developing countries,

➤ understand how various countries address their health challenges,

➤ learn about the common and unique health challenges in an international context, and

➤ explore emerging and intensifying global health issues.

CASE STUDY

CLIMATE CHANGE AND PUBLIC HEALTH

The natural environment has a profound impact on human health, as reflected in the UN Framework Convention on Climate Change (Singh et al. 2011). Climate scientists predict that the world will warm 4° C by 2100, yet the relationship between rising temperatures and human health is not fully understood. Severe weather events, such as heat waves, hurricanes, and cyclones, pose direct threats to human life and health. Some argue that changing weather patterns have already indirectly affected food yields, water flows, patterns of infectious disease (e.g., the increasing reach of tropical diseases beyond the typical geographic areas of occurrence, changes in the seasonality of certain diseases), and population displacement (McMichael et al. 2003).

Public health experts are calling for climate change policy interventions that have an immediate, positive impact on population health. For example, policies to encourage reduced meat consumption mitigate the intake of saturated fats and remove some methane (a greenhouse gas) from cow-producing regions (McMichael and Lindgren 2011). Examples such as these and findings from other emerging research show that a public health discussion must be incorporated into the larger climate change discourse.

Global health
An area of study, research, and practice that focuses on improving health and achieving health equity for all people worldwide (Koplan et al. 2009).

This chapter provides examples of important health policy issues from the international community, using selected countries—both developed and developing—to demonstrate their impact. Students' exposure to these issues not only helps them understand international health policy applications but also introduces them to **global health** as a field and **globalization** as a reality.

The advent of globalization, technological advances, and changing global demographics brings challenges in achieving equitable global health. Although globalization brings conformity in some areas of people's lives, differences in economic policies, political and legal structures, social and cultural norms, and religious beliefs remain from country to country and region to region, creating additional barriers to the equitable delivery of healthcare.

Increased ease of travel and communications not only has diminished some barriers between countries but also has ushered in new concerns of disease transmission and other global health threats. Recently considered a problem predominantly afflicting the developing world, infectious diseases have become a concern for all countries as global trade, tourism, international relations, and migration facilitate the spread of disease. The United Nations (UN) works with several constituent organizations on global health initiatives; in addition, the World Health Organization (WHO) coordinates some health activities between countries and surveillance of global health concerns. These organizations, and

Globalization
Worldwide changes in many aspects of people's lives driven by the exchange of information across borders and characterized by (1) increased production of goods and services by developing countries and (2) the expanded interdependence of developed and emerging economies (Shi and Singh 2011).

policymakers around the world, face varied problems and hard decisions regarding global health.

This chapter begins by discussing issues shared by many industrialized countries. Japan, Denmark, Canada, and South Korea are profiled in terms of their major health issues and the solutions they have proposed to address these issues. Next, the chapter discusses both common and unique challenges faced by developing nations. The variety of unique issues confronted by emerging economies is demonstrated in discussions of China, Ukraine, Nigeria, and Colombia. The chapter also includes several Global Health Impact boxes to illustrate issues that could affect global health in the future, challenging policymakers to rethink their approaches to public health.

GLOBAL HEALTH IMPACT
Noncommunicable Diseases

The global rise in noncommunicable and chronic diseases is one of the greatest current challenges developed, emerging, and developing countries face. In September 2011, WHO Director-General Dr. Margaret Chan discussed noncommunicable disease in an address to the General Assembly (UN Department of Public Information 2010):

The worldwide increase of non-communicable diseases is a slow-motion disaster, as most of these diseases develop over time, but unhealthy lifestyles that feed these diseases are spreading with a stunning speed and sweep. I can understand why some developing countries are being taken by surprise by the onslaught of these diseases. Their initial burden was greatest in affluent societies.

Noncommunicable diseases were once considered to be confined to wealthy people and wealthy nations. That paradigm is shifting as the burden of noncommunicable and chronic diseases, and associated risk factors, is now being felt worldwide. A fundamental shift is also being seen in the United States and other developed countries as community wellness and preventive care are increasingly viewed as vital to the control and reduction of chronic disease prevalence in their populations (Navarro et al. 2007). In general, noncommunicable diseases are quickly becoming the most frequent cause of death worldwide and are associated with nearly two-thirds of all global mortality. Although not currently the largest contributor to mortality in sub-Saharan Africa, projections for the region suggest that deaths from noncommunicable diseases will surpass deaths from maternal, perinatal, and nutrition-related diseases by 2030.

(continued)

GLOBAL HEALTH IMPACT
Noncommunicable Diseases

(continued from previous page)

The risk factors associated with many noncommunicable diseases are well documented in the scientific literature. Behaviors such as tobacco use, alcohol abuse, unhealthy diet habits, and physical inactivity have been linked to cancers, cardiovascular diseases, chronic respiratory diseases, and diabetes. Lifestyles in developing nations are changing to include these behaviors, sometimes as a consequence of development, such as the emergence of supermarkets in low- and middle-income countries (supermarkets are the largest providers of processed foods that are high in fat, sugar, and sodium and low in nutritional value) (Wagner and Brath 2012). The total health-related costs of development are staggering: In 2005, the estimated losses in national income from heart disease, stroke, and diabetes were $18 billion in China, $11 billion in the Russian Federation, $9 billion in India, and $3 billion in Brazil (WHO 2005).

Researchers working in developing countries have produced a robust literature on the epidemiology of noncommunicable diseases in most regions of the world (except for sub-Saharan Africa) (Dalal et al. 2011). They have found that public health policymakers have several tools by which to address noncommunicable diseases and associated risk factors. Yet such health policies have not been well defined at a national or global level, even though science and medicine have made great strides in our understanding of the determinants of chronic disease. Observers note that the most effective policies are long-term, collaborative approaches that engage both the public and private sectors. For example, WHO has deemed "best buy" interventions to be cost-effective in reducing disability-adjusted life years associated with noncommunicable diseases. Examples of such interventions include raising tobacco taxes, restricting access to alcohol, providing primary care diet counseling, promoting healthy living and physical activity in mass media, and offering vaccination programs.

The consequences of failing to stem noncommunicable diseases are enormous. In developed countries, where clinical chronic care is currently available, the increasing burden of disease will place increasingly greater strains on the health financing system. In developing countries, where clinical chronic care is less available and more people go undiagnosed, primary prevention is essential to saving lives and improving life expectancies. Policymakers at all levels, as well as other stakeholders, have the power to reshape this intensifying public health issue.

HEALTH POLICY ISSUES IN DEVELOPED COUNTRIES

Some health policy issues are unique to advanced economies. Most developed nations have controlled the spread of communicable diseases through well-established public health infrastructures and effective sanitation services (although the threat of importation of communicable disease from uncontrolled regions is a concern caused by globalization and increased travel and trade). However, their health systems are strained by an aging population and widespread chronic disease.

COMMON POLICY ISSUES

All industrialized nations with established healthcare systems struggle to adapt these systems to meet changing needs. They must maintain an adequate, well-trained workforce and integrate new technologies while keeping costs at a manageable level.

Researchers first found that healthcare spending was rising among the Organisation for Economic Co-operation and Development (OECD) countries in the 1970s; a 2009 study confirmed the continuation of this trend by showing that OECD countries spent an average of 9.5 percent of their gross domestic product (GDP) on health compared to an average of 5.3 percent in the 1970s (OECD 2011).

Policymakers in industrialized countries constantly seek ways to achieve sustainable growth and allocate adequate funding to ensure fiscal and population health. To meet the challenge of cost control, many countries have experimented with alternative methods of paying for and delivering health services. For example,

- Italy decentralized the authority of the Servizio Sanitaris Nazionale as a way to control federal health spending (Tediosi, Gabriele, and Longo 2009).

- New Zealand replaced its former healthcare model with one called the Primary Health Care Strategy, which increased public funding of preventive and public health activities, encouraged general practitioners to form nongovernmental primary health organizations (PHOs), and changed payments from fee-for-service to capitated fees paid to PHOs (Cumming and Mays 2011).

- Israel placed the health system budget under the jurisdiction of the Ministry of Finance rather than the health ministry as in most other countries. The relationship is intended to help control spending—the Ministry of Finance sets the level at which it will fund the national health insurance after estimating the amount that will be collected from cost-sharing provisions.

- The Danish government consolidated health services administration, decision making, and services provision (Andersen and Jensen 2010).

Each of these countries faced similar problems and shared the goals of providing low-cost healthcare while achieving positive health outcomes. Yet, they developed different solutions, which took into account the country's level of political will and societal values.

In addition to experimenting with health system structure, some countries have developed mechanisms for determining suitable treatment methods in the hope of reducing pharmaceutical expenditures without negatively affecting health outcomes (Clement et al. 2009). Australia, the United Kingdom, Canada, and other countries have governmental agencies that evaluate the cost-effectiveness of certain pharmaceutical products by analyzing cost and comparative effectiveness evidence to make national coverage decisions. Australia has taken this measure a step further by often delaying the recommendation of drugs for use until the price is negotiated to a level low enough to be deemed cost-effective.

Some cost-reduction policies aim to directly improve health outcomes. For example, the United Kingdom has set up a **pay-for-performance** physician payment model, under which physicians treat patients following disease-based **clinical practice guidelines**. The guidelines are drawn from **evidence-based medicine** and are designed to reflect the best path to achieving high-quality healthcare and strong patient outcomes. Not all experts agree that evidence-based care is the best mode of service delivery. Starfield and Mangin (2010), for example, assert that because patients experience diseases differently, treatment should be patient centered rather than disease centered. Still, this example illustrates that most governments struggle to ensure that the money allocated for health systems is used to deliver the best possible health outcomes and high-quality care. In fact, France codified quality assurance—a medical practice supported by the government—in its creation of the National Agency for the Development of Medical Evaluation in 1990 and the Hospital Act in 1991 that made quality of care assessment mandatory. In 2004, a newer agency called the Agency for Accreditation and Evaluation of Health Care was given responsibility for these activities (Legido-Quigley et al. 2008).

Other countries have imposed on residents varying levels of **cost sharing**, the amount of which depends on income, in an attempt to reduce government expenditures while ensuring adequate care for society's poorest inhabitants. Ireland introduced a three-tiered payment system to address health equity issues. Those in the bottom tier (corresponding to the lowest-income residents) receive free health services, the middle-tier population shares some costs, and those in the highest tier overwhelmingly opt out of public insurance and buys private health insurance. Rather than providing equitable access to health services, however, this system has created increased inequality in access (Smith and Normand 2011).

These examples illustrate that an individual's income and sociodemographic status are among the most important predictors of unmet healthcare needs; that is, disparity is a multifaceted issue that extends far beyond the health system (Bryant, Leaver, and Dunn 2009). To determine the best solutions to meet these challenges, each country's

Pay for performance
Payment-related incentives often used by insurance companies or government payers to reward healthcare providers, such as physicians and hospitals, for meeting preestablished performance measures for quality and efficiency.

Clinical practice guidelines
Evidence-based and systematically developed protocols (statements) used to assist healthcare providers in making appropriate healthcare and clinical decisions regarding specific conditions or circumstances.

Evidence-based medicine
Using the best available evidence acquired through the scientific method to guide clinical decision making.

> ### ⓗ GLOBAL HEALTH IMPACT
> Pandemics: SARS, H1N1, and Avian Flu
>
> A single businessman traveling from the Guangdong province of China through Hong Kong and on to Hanoi, Vietnam, brought severe acute respiratory syndrome (SARS) to global attention. He, and the doctor who diagnosed him, died of the disease while it was spreading rapidly throughout Asia, and later to 24 other countries worldwide (*A.D.A.M. Medical Encyclopedia* 2011). The story of SARS illustrates the negative impact of globalization and migration and the ease with which a highly contagious disease can spread worldwide and cause a pandemic (Shi and Singh 2011).
>
> Threats of widespread illness from H1N1 (swine) influenza and West Nile virus evolved in similar fashion, and avian flu is the next major infectious disease to watch, according to observers (Pompe et al. 2005; CDC 2012). As of this writing, only people who work in close contact with infected birds are known to have been infected with avian flu. However, it is a highly deadly influenza virus, and if it should mutate and become easily transmitted from human to human, serious consequences will follow.
>
> In efforts to thwart pandemics, worldwide reporting systems have been developed and are improving, but many countries lack critical laboratory infrastructure and access to vaccines and antiviral medications. Any country that has not already done so should establish emergency preparedness plans that account for social distancing, travel, health system processes, and mass vaccination procedures.

Cost sharing
Refers to the obligation of patients to pay for a portion of the healthcare services they receive. It is typically used as an incentive to avoid excessive or unnecessary utilization. However, it may also deter appropriate utilization.

government must clarify its values and priorities with regard to health equity and cost sharing.

As the burden of chronic disease increases in industrialized countries, disease prevention is promoted as a way to improve public health and reduce healthcare costs. Obesity is a preventable risk factor associated with cardiovascular disease, diabetes, cancer, and premature death. The treatment, management, and health complications associated with these chronic diseases generate high healthcare expenditures (Sassi 2010). Therefore, some countries are taking a public health approach to addressing obesity by encouraging lifestyle changes. Nordic countries have placed taxes on unhealthy foods in the hope of steering consumers to healthier choices. However, the obesity epidemic is not merely a result of an individual's food choices; it also reflects broad changes that have occurred in the everyday lives of people in the modern world compared to pre-Industrial times. As such, some governments are considering new transportation and urban planning policies, among other programs, to improve health and decrease obesity rates.

UNDERLYING FACTORS

Several factors affect healthcare costs in developed countries, including the impact of aging populations and technological progress as previously discussed. Country GDP, the participation of women in the labor force, and public budgetary values are also important variables that influence cost trends (Pammolli, Riccaboni, and Magazzini 2012). For instance:

- As a country's total income rises, so do healthcare expenditures.

- As an increasing number of women enter the workforce, caregiver responsibilities shift from the private sphere to the public sphere.

- Countries tend to spend more money on those social goods most valued by society, which may or may not be related to healthcare.

UNIQUE POLICY ISSUES, BY SELECTED COUNTRY

Maintaining a healthy population should be a high priority for any nation, just as cost control should be. Taking these two constraints into consideration, countries have approached the creation and implementation of health system administration, quality, and access policies in different ways. We discuss Japan, Denmark, Canada, and South Korea to illustrate unique health policy issues addressed by developed nations.

Japan

Japan adopted universal health insurance coverage in 1961. Since that time, its model has served as a blueprint for other counties to build a successful low-cost, high-quality, and highly equitable health system. However, the Japanese system is reaching a critical crossroads. The population has been rapidly aging for the last several decades (currently, more than 20 percent of the population is 65 or older), which has enormous implications for the cost of healthcare. At the same time, the government cannot rely on increasing tax revenues to pay for the health system because population growth and, consequently, economic growth are stagnant (Shibuya et al. 2011). In response to these challenges, the Japanese government has introduced innovative ways to slow spending.

In 2000, the government instituted its Long-Term Care Insurance (LTCI) program to care for the country's aging population. The goal of LTCI is to provide institutional- and community-based long-term care services to adults over the age of 65 and to ease financial and emotional burdens for both the patient and the patient's caregivers (Tsutsui and Maramatsu 2007). To pay for LTCI, Japan diverted some general tax revenues to the program and levied a new tax on adults over the age of 40.

Compared to other industrialized countries, Japan has made few efforts to formally ensure healthcare quality. While healthcare payment is under tight control, healthcare delivery is not; providers within the system are free to deliver care as they see fit. They are reimbursed on the basis of diagnosis–procedure combination categorization, thus diluting healthcare quality data that would be available under a fee-for-service payment system; monitoring fee-for-service data is the primary way providers can be held accountable. Although its health outcomes are comparable to those of other countries, Japan has no accountability mechanism in place, such as the pay-for-performance model in the United Kingdom and the quality assurance law in France. As Japan's health system continues to undergo reform, structural measures of quality assurance might eventually be considered (Hashimoto et al. 2011).

Despite a lack of quality standards, Japan's long-standing health system has achieved successes that other developed countries are still striving toward. All of the measures described here were adopted to maintain good health outcomes and quality of life at low cost to both consumers and the government, making it a model worth consideration by other developed nations.

Denmark

The Danish parliament passed major legislation in 2007 to reorganize and consolidate the country's governmental structure; 215 local municipalities were condensed to 98, and 13 counties were reduced to 5 regions. The health system underwent a similar recentralization. Key areas in need of improvement had been identified in hospital future planning and current efficiency, primary care coordination, and public health prevention (Andersen and Jensen 2010). Denmark has one of the lowest life expectancies and highest cancer mortality rates in the European Union (Economist Intelligence Unit 2011). The population is also getting older, and as a result, the chronic disease burden is increasingly cumbersome.

Denmark's 2007 health reform legislation, called the Health Act, included several measures to address the country's pressing health policy concerns. To improve coordination of care, Danish officials put into effect a series of regulations (Andersen and Jensen 2010):

- ◆ Regional health authorities were charged with creating patient rehabilitation plans for hospital discharge.

- ◆ General practitioners were asked to participate in coordination-of-care strategies by reporting patient data in a shared database.

- ◆ The newly formed regions were required to plan hospital systems whereby all hospitals are expected to provide an array of basic, frequently needed services, accounting for about 90 percent of hospital services; one hospital per region is

> **GLOBAL HEALTH IMPACT**
> Bioterrorism
>
> A notorious example of bioterrorism is the 1995 attack in a Tokyo subway, where a domestic terrorist group released a chemical weapon called sarin. Sarin is a nerve agent that can paralyze muscles needed for breathing; in the Tokyo subway attack, 13 people were killed and 50 were severely injured. In past decades, Iraq and the former Soviet Union were found to have military bioweapons programs (Khan et al. 2000). Scientists in the United States and the Netherlands exposed the possibility of disease-related bioterrorism when they created a highly contagious strain of avian flu in late 2011 (Novossiolova, Minehata, and Dando 2012).
>
> Health policy related to bioterrorism should focus on preparedness efforts, as with natural disasters and pandemics, and the plans that are put in place must be carefully and thoroughly executed. Local jurisdictions can also take measures to reduce their vulnerability to bioterrorism by assessing the built environment, health system capacity, current infrastructures, and emergency response teams and procedures.

to provide specialized services; and a few hospitals in the country will perform a limited number of highly specialized services.

These initiatives are meant to work together to provide coordinated and high-quality care for all Danish patients, whether they have an acute condition or a chronic disease.

The implementation of Danish health reform is well under way, but it is progressing at a sluggish pace. Successful implementation seems to depend on the goals of the dominant political party in each region. Yet to be seen is how political and ideological tensions—such as those present in most countries—will affect the end result of the Danish health reform (Andersen and Jensen 2010).

Canada

Canada's health policy issues are different from those of Japan and Denmark. Its population is not aging as rapidly as Japan's, and, unlike Denmark, its provincial decentralization of the healthcare system has been stable over the past decades. However, Canada faces problems related to paying for healthcare and an increasing public health burden from preventable diseases.

Canada spends a greater percentage of its GDP, and more per capita, on healthcare than many industrialized countries do (but less than Germany, Denmark, and the United States spend). The country has taken steps over the past several decades to control healthcare spending at all levels of government. For example, Canada established the Common Drug Review in 2002 to assess the safety, clinical effectiveness, and cost-effectiveness of new drugs presented by pharmaceutical companies and provides recommendations to all participating drug plans. In this way, Canada seeks to promote the use of the most effective and least expensive pharmaceuticals.

Canada's drug plans, which are administered separately from general health services plans, attempt to use cost-sharing mechanisms to control public expenditures. For example, the province of British Columbia implemented the policy Fair PharmaCare in May 2003. It is an income-based benefits program with three main goals: (1) to keep government spending low while (2) providing access to all necessary medication in (3) a way that is equitable for people of all income levels. Analyses show that decreases in public pharmaceutical funding would work against stated policy goals and that federal money infused into the states is key to access and equity (Morgan et al. 2006).

Canada's struggle to achieve equity in medication access and affordability reflects its larger struggle with health disparities. The life expectancy at birth of an aboriginal man living on a reserve (67 years) is nine years less than that of a man in the general population (76 years). Aboriginal status and socioeconomic status are the biggest contributors to health inequities in Canada, with disadvantaged populations having increased infant mortality rates, risky health behaviors (e.g., smoking), infectious disease, and chronic disease. These disparities are primarily attributable to differences in access to resources and opportunities (Frohlich, Ross, and Richmond 2006). As with the public health agencies of other countries grappling with similar issues, research findings about Canadian health issues are slowly being translated into programs and policies designed to reduce health disparities (Health Council of Canada 2011).

South Korea

South Korea adopted universal health insurance coverage in 1989. Since that time, it has worked to improve the health system, but with minimal success. Although the country has achieved admirable gains in health outcomes (e.g., increased life expectancies), the health system is plagued with several problems:

◆ The healthcare benefits that citizens enjoy are still limited compared to those of other developed countries.

◆ The public sector has little involvement in healthcare delivery.

◆   Costs are rapidly rising.

◆   Some insurance plans are in financial distress.

These problems are caused by a diverse set of factors and will likely take significant effort over many years to resolve (Moon and Shin 2007).

From 1989 to 2000, South Koreans were covered under a multi-insurance fund that included about 370 insurers. The government instituted the National Health Insurance Corporation (NHIC) in 2000 under the Ministry of Health, Welfare, and Family Affairs. South Korea is currently working to increase health insurance benefits, which is particularly difficult because of the variety of sources from which the NHIC is funded (i.e., the public sector, out-of-pocket payments, private financing, and voluntary and charitable contributions) (Chun et al. 2009).

In the coming years, South Korea must address high utilization rates of health services and expensive medical technologies, physician shortages, and a rapidly aging population caused by low fertility rates and increasing life expectancy. To address high utilization of physician and medical technology services, South Korea piloted a diagnosis-related group financing mechanism with promising results (Moon and Shin 2007). South Korea also instituted a long-term care insurance scheme in 2006. However, more needs to be done to address the healthcare challenges the nation faces.

HEALTH POLICY ISSUES IN DEVELOPING COUNTRIES

The health policy issues of developing countries are, in many ways, fundamentally distinct from those of industrialized countries. Developing countries face a range of health problems, from communicable, highly contagious diseases to incipient, invisible problems that manifest from exposure to polluted environments. These nations must address the drivers of preventable morbidity and mortality to improve health outcomes and, relatedly, increase economic growth and development.

In this section, we discuss the policy issues shared by developing countries, including the communicable and noncommunicable diseases that cause the highest burden of disease. Because developing nations rely heavily on international governing bodies to provide assistance regarding health concerns, we also outline the types of policy actions these international agencies take to combat problems. Finally, as with the selected developed countries, we delve into the particular problems faced by China, Ukraine, Nigeria, and Colombia.

COMMON POLICY ISSUES

Distinct policy issues and risk factors related to both **communicable diseases** and **noncommunicable diseases** are common problems in developing countries. Communicable

Communicable diseases
Also called infectious diseases; refer to illnesses caused by organisms such as bacteria, viruses, fungi, and parasites. Communicable diseases may be transmitted by one infected person to another, from an animal to a human, or from some inanimate object to an individual, depending on the disease.

Noncommunicable diseases
Refer to noninfectious medical conditions or illnesses; typically of long duration and slow progression.

diseases include acute diarrheal disease, sexually transmitted diseases, HIV/AIDS, tuberculosis (TB), malaria and other tropical diseases, and other infectious diseases. Noncommunicable diseases—illnesses not traditionally seen in abundance in developing nations, such as cancer, cardiovascular disease, diabetes, chronic pulmonary disease, and mental illness—are becoming increasingly common in developing countries and come with a different set of health policy considerations.

A common theme among these diseases is the economic depression that accompanies high incidence of disease and the paradox that large economic inputs (capital, labor, and innovation) are necessary to prevent the transmission and onset of disease, which places low-income, developing countries in a particularly difficult position to solve these public health problems.

GLOBAL HEALTH IMPACT
Migration

The UN Department of Economic and Social Affairs estimates that 3.1 percent of the world's population lives outside of their country of origin. In addition, many people are internally displaced, meaning that they have been forced from their homes but remain within the country's boundaries.

People migrate for a variety of reasons, including to take advantage of economic opportunities, in reaction to political instability, and to avoid conflict. Two aspects of migrant health must be addressed. The first is the public health threat inherent in the migratory movement of people. Infectious disease concerns exist in all phases of such a journey, and the ease with which people and products can move around the world directly corresponds to the rapidity with which a disease threat may spread.

The second issue concerns the health needs of individual migrants upon reaching their destination. In many countries, the health system restricts migrants' access to healthcare or does not provide culturally appropriate care, leading to poor health outcomes (International Organization for Migration 2011). Australia, in which one-fourth of the population is foreign-born, has a well-developed system of healthcare delivery for migrants (*Bulletin of the World Health Organization* 2008). In contrast, Spain has only just begun to consider the health concerns and integration issues of migrants. Migrant health issues will grow as people continue to move around the world to find work and to escape undesirable conditions.

Communicable Diseases

Acute diarrheal disease and other diseases attributable to poor water sanitation (e.g., acute respiratory disease, some tropical diseases) account for about 10 percent of the global burden of disease. Nearly 1.7 million deaths each year are attributable to acute diarrheal disease; about 95 percent of these deaths are children under five who live in developing countries (van Minh and Hung 2011). Worldwide, about 1 billion people lack access to an improved water supply—one of the most important preventive measures that can be taken to lower mortality rates (Water Sanitation and Health 2013).

The UN has recognized this type of disease as a global public health problem. In its Millennium Development Goal (MDG) 7.C, the UN states that it aims to "halve, by 2015, the proportion of the population without sustainable access to safe drinking water and basic sanitation" toward ensuring sustainability of the environment (UN 2010). Cost–benefit analyses suggest that achieving this MDG could result in a total worldwide economic benefit of $38 billion annually (van Minh and Hung 2011). Some countries have accepted the challenge, but, as the UN has noted, "disparities in urban and rural sanitation remain daunting" (UN 2010). These challenges were illustrated by the cholera epidemic in Haiti following the devastating earthquake in 2010, which showed that poor sanitation and resulting diseases can virtually shut down entire industries (Haiti Libre 2010).

The MDG also addresses HIV/AIDS, TB (which often accompanies AIDS), malaria, and other major diseases in MDG 6 (UN 2010), as the burden of these diseases is most heavily felt in developing countries. At the same time, some global health experts argue that the attention given to HIV/AIDS prevention and treatment diverts resources from more basic public health and health system needs (Yu et al. 2008).

Noncommunicable Diseases

While much has been written about the devastating effects of communicable diseases, as well as their prevention and treatment modalities (*HIV/AIDS*: Bongaarts and Over 2010; UN Department of Public Information 2010; Potts et al. 2008; Weiss et al. 2008; Stanecki et al. 2010; Sambo and Kirigia 2011; *TB and other infectious diseases*: Kirwan 2009; Avert .org 2011; WHO 2013), noncommunicable diseases are beginning to have an equally disruptive impact on developing countries. In these nations, 80 percent of deaths related to noncommunicable diseases occur before the age of 60—the age at which people tend to reach their peak economic productivity, therefore reducing economic growth and progress in the country.

Mental Illness

Mental illnesses are a group of noncommunicable diseases responsible for about 13 percent of the global burden of disease. Mental illnesses in particular do not generally attract

GLOBAL HEALTH IMPACT
Medical Tourism

Medical tourism is an international phenomenon by which people travel to another country for medical services. Travel often occurs on a regional level, and most procedures are elective (e.g., weight loss surgery, cosmetic surgery, dental care, fertility treatment). For example, Americans travel to Mexican border towns for dental procedures that would be very expensive in the United States (*IMTJ* 2012) and seek affordable healthcare procedures, such as knee and hip replacements and cardiac surgery, outside of the country. Some countries are known to specialize in medical tourism procedures, including gender reassignment surgery offered in Thailand and cell transplants offered in China (Alleman et al. 2011; Aizura 2010; Song 2010).

Major US medical schools have partnered with foreign countries to set up tertiary/referral hospitals that provide higher-level care and procedures. These ventures can control costs for private insurers and improve the standards of care for those seeking care abroad. According to the Centers for Disease Control and Prevention, Joint Commission International has accredited nearly 300 facilities worldwide (Lee and Balaban 2011; JCI 2013). People also travel to the United States to receive healthcare at leading institutions, such as the University of Texas MD Andersen Cancer Center in Houston; Mayo Clinic in Rochester, Minnesota; and Jackson Memorial Hospital in Miami. In fact, the United States ranks second worldwide in medical tourism destinations after Thailand (Pollard 2011).

(continued)

international health policy attention. Neuropsychiatric disorders that affect people in developing countries include unipolar depressive disorder, bipolar disorder, schizophrenia, epilepsy, alcohol and drug abuse disorders, dementia, anxiety disorders, mental retardation, and some neurological disorders (Patel 2007). Those who experience mental illness often endure many years of living with a disability. In addition, the societal costs of mental disorders, such as the impact on families, social services, and the criminal justice system, are significant and essentially immeasurable.

People who are poor, are less educated, or face acute financial strain are at a greater risk for mental illness than are those who are financially secure and educated. In turn, those who suffer mental illness are likely to remain impoverished due to lost wages or the cost of medical care. Mental health disorders can be effectively treated, but policymakers in developing nations face enormous challenges in legislating and financing effective

GLOBAL HEALTH IMPACT
Medical Tourism

(continued from previous page)

Facilitators of medical tourism have established an industry focused on connecting people with medical services abroad. However, several challenges have arisen with this emerging field. Reports have surfaced of complications after surgeries that could have been avoided if proper quality standards had been followed, underscoring the need for uniform standards of care across various settings. Public health concerns also can be an issue for medical tourists, as they may become vectors, able to spread infectious agents, and/or victims of multidrug-resistant bacteria—an increasing threat as more physicians are unprincipled in their use of antimicrobial medications (Rogers, Aminzadeh, and Paterson 2011). Finally, critics have cited ethical issues regarding the use of the healthcare workforce and resources for medical tourism that takes away resources from basic local medical needs of the country. As this market continues to develop and stabilize, these and numerous other issues will need to be addressed.

interventions; in low-income countries, the average government mental health spending is US$0.25 per person per year, and half the world lives in a country where psychiatric care is highly unavailable (one or fewer professionals per 200,000 people) (WHO 2011).

To help countries identify gaps in their existing mental health system and address any deficiencies with system-level policy changes, the World Health Organization developed the WHO Assessment Instrument for Mental Health Systems (WHO-AIMS), which evaluates countries across several domains (e.g., policy/legislative framework, existing mental health services) to present a broad picture of their mental health provision capabilities. To date, more than 80 countries have used WHO-AIMS. As additional countries implement WHO-AIMS, policymakers can comprehend the state of their country's mental health services and policy as a whole.

Weak Health Infrastructure

The lack of a sound health system infrastructure affects all diseases and impedes access to essential health services. Governments in developing countries generally spend about 5 percent of their total budget on health; in contrast, the average developed country spends about 9.5 percent of its GDP on health (Nambiar et al. 2007). Low government spending leads to extremely low quality of care and creates long waiting times, constant shortages of essential drugs and supplies, and untrained staff. In addition, out-of-pocket expenses can prohibit residents of developing countries from seeking care.

Modern Environmental Hazards

In the developing world, substances such as mercury, lead, pesticides, asbestos, air toxins, and hazardous waste are commonly released into the environment by unregulated mining operations (e.g., mining for gold ore), soap product and paint manufacturers, gasoline producers, agricultural operations, emissions from automobiles, and industrial waste disposal. Such toxins are associated with a host of complicated health problems, including nerve or nerve tissue damage, birth defects, and hormone dysfunction—problems that the health systems of many developing countries are ill equipped to handle.

These and other modern environmental health hazards (MEHH) are emerging in a health environment that is already overwhelmed by poverty, malnutrition, and communicable diseases. With the understanding that governments in developing nations must take swift preventive measures, the United Nations Environment Programme has made headway with its Partnership for Clean Fuels and Vehicles (PCFV) initiative for removing lead from gasoline and sulfur from diesel fuel. Other initiatives aim to reduce or control stockpiles of harmful pesticides, introduce cleaner methods of gold mining (which is strongly associated with mercury poisoning), and initiate monitoring programs for manufacturing and other operations.

Nongovernmental organizations
Organizations that are operated independent of the government.

Most of this work has been performed by **nongovernmental organizations**, with less substantive action taken by national governments. Going forward, policymakers must take a population-level approach toward addressing MEHH "necessary to successfully alleviate the burden of avoidable ill health and premature death" (Nweke and Sanders 2009).

UNDERLYING FACTORS

These health-related challenges raise the question of how to use health policy to strengthen health systems and public health infrastructure in developing countries. Industrialized countries are seeking ways to provide aid to developing nations that will help overwhelmed ministries of health. The sector-wide approach, which focuses on centralizing public health leadership, improving health sector management, and increasing coordination, is one such method that has had some success.

In recognition of the fact that good governance is essential for overall development and an effective health system, WHO has devised a method for assessing health system governance. This framework allows researchers to assess the problems with health system leadership and governance at the policy and operational levels and to use that information to suggest improvements. Using the WHO method allows motivated governments to effectively promote and protect population health (Siddiqi et al. 2009).

Tackling noncommunicable diseases requires that health policies be designed to work together at various levels of government. For example, one policy might impose taxes to deter people from smoking cigarettes and other policies might ensure that care for chronic obstructive pulmonary disease is accessible to those who need it.

UNIQUE POLICY ISSUES, BY SELECTED COUNTRY

Many blanket statements have been made about health issues in developing countries, but it is essential to recognize the great inter- and intra-country diversity with regard to health issues and health policies. China, for example, has a huge land mass and a diverse population of urban and rural dwellers, posing health policy challenges that are unique to that country. Each country is dealing with a different set of factors that largely determine what health issues are pertinent and what policy solutions are feasible. Here we examine the unique situations of four developing countries: China, Ukraine, Nigeria, and Colombia.

China

With more than 1.3 billion residents, China has one of the largest populations in the world. The country has seen overwhelming transformations over the past several decades, which have dramatically affected population health.

Prior to 1978, the Chinese government headed up extensive public health improvements, leading to lower infant and maternal mortality rates, greater life expectancies, and improved water sanitation. The associated policy decisions emphasized disease prevention and community involvement, reflecting an approach to health rooted in basic public health principles (Gong, Walker, and Shi 2007).

A major change in China occurred in 1978, when it moved from a communism-based to a capitalism-based market economy. This shift brought many positive developments as well as a number of challenges in terms of China's health system:

- Overall spending on healthcare has rapidly increased while government funding for public health institutions has steadily fallen (Gong, Walker, and Shi 2007).

- Rates of noncommunicable diseases and health disparities are on the rise (Hu, Liu, and Willett 2011).

- The cost of healthcare has become prohibitively expensive for many, particularly those living in rural areas (Hu, Liu, and Willett 2011).

In response to these emerging issues and to create a solid health policy framework for the coming years, in 2008 the Chinese government passed the Healthy China 2020

> **GLOBAL HEALTH IMPACT**
> Technology and Innovation
>
> The advancement of information technology, and of clinical technology in particular, has greatly altered how healthcare is delivered. Examples of these innovations include health informatics, mHealth, electronic medical records, telemedicine, and virtual physician visits. Medical innovations have also brought safer surgical and imaging procedures; genetic testing and gene therapy; and therapeutic uses for vaccines to treat diseases, such as cancer and HIV/AIDS.
>
> As with any area of technological innovation, the positive aspects of clinical technology are accompanied by a number of challenges. The development of useful medical technologies often comes at a very high cost. These costs in turn may make it difficult for poorer countries to bring technological innovations to their populations. In addition, technological advances in processes can threaten the privacy of individuals and the confidentiality of their medical history because of increased access to medical records.
>
> The US Department of Health and Human Services, in its Global Health Initiatives statements, has described the need for the government to strengthen regulatory systems and to monitor the safety of the medical products, food, and feed that enter the United States through global manufacturing and supply chains (HHS 2013). Another approach to addressing the challenges brought by technology is for the health department to assess community needs and ensure that appropriate medical devices and technologies reach people in need in a cost-effective manner.

legislation to address equity and accessibility through five mandates that correspond to major health problems as identified by the Chinese Ministry of Health (Chen 2009):

◆ Health insurance must be expanded to cover 90 percent of the population.

◆ A national drug system must be established to meet basic pharmaceutical needs.

◆ Grassroots-level improvement of medical care and public health must occur.

◆ Basic public health services, including preventive health, must expand.

◆ Hospital reform must be instituted to abate the health system's increasing tendency to commercialize.

Ukraine

Over the five years following the fall of the former Soviet Union in 1991, Ukraine faced—and continues to battle—several debilitating public health issues. The population is plagued by a high rate of HIV/AIDS, which is closely associated with a TB epidemic: About 1.6 percent of the population has HIV/AIDS, with most new cases occurring among injection drug users and other high-risk populations (e.g., men who have sex with men, sex workers, prisoners), and an estimated 1.4 percent of Ukraine's population is currently living with TB, classified as an epidemic. In addition, cardiovascular disease, the biggest contributor to the country's overall mortality rate, is highly prevalent among the population, partly because of high rates of smoking and alcohol consumption.

Inconsistent health legislation and implementation, stemming from an unstable parliament, results in a difficult political environment in which to address these challenges and improve health (Lekhan, Rudiy, and Richardson 2010). For example, the Global Fund for AIDS, Tuberculosis, and Malaria initially granted $98 million to the Ukrainian government to respond to the combined AIDS/TB epidemic; however, the fund later changed its grantee to community organizations because it felt that the government was not being transparent with the use of its finances. As a result, local community organizations now provide the bulk of Ukraine's HIV/AIDS prevention and treatment services with funding provided by the Global Fund (Hurley 2010).

Poor policy development and implementation separate Ukraine's TB control from that of the rest of Europe. For example, the infection is often transmitted through the prison system, but post-incarceration treatment plans in Ukraine are not coordinated before prisoners' release. Furthermore, many ex-prisoners do not adhere to their medication plans and transmit the disease to the general public, as evidenced by higher-than-average TB infection rates in areas surrounding prisons. In addition, Ukraine does not have a centralized TB monitoring system, and most existing TB regional recording and reporting systems do not meet WHO recommendations (Atun and Olynik 2008).

Policies aimed at reducing the burden of noncommunicable disease in Ukraine have been more successful—the tobacco excise tax is one example. Estimates from 2005 suggest that 66 percent of men and 20 percent of women smoked cigarettes. Following the lead of other countries that adopted tax policy reform in response to high rates of disease, premature death, and lost productivity, Ukraine implemented excise taxes on tobacco in 2009 and 2010. Studies show that these taxes have significantly reduced tobacco consumption, illustrating that tobacco use is price sensitive (Ross, Stoklosa, and Krasovsky 2011).

In spite of this success, Ukraine still faces significant work in dealing with the burden of noncommunicable diseases, mostly to address the country's dysfunctional health system and corrupt government. Overcoming those two issues will vastly improve overall population health.

Nigeria

Nigeria's health issues are all-encompassing, ranging from communicable diseases, such as HIV/AIDS, TB, rare tropical diseases, and even poliomyelitis (polio), to noncommunicable diseases, such as cardiovascular disease and the effects of MEHH. Each of these health problems is inefficiently managed by the Nigerian government and exacerbated by a weak health system, low levels of health financing, and health professional emigration.

A few health issues set Nigeria apart from other sub-Saharan nations with otherwise similar health problems. First, it is the only African country (and one of four countries in the world) to have failed to ever eliminate polio. The failure of Nigeria to eliminate polio also led to the spread of the disease in neighboring countries. Efforts implemented by the Global Polio Eradication Initiative in 2009 did reduce the total number of cases by 50 percent—in 2011, 46 cases of polio in Nigeria were known (Global Polio Eradication Initiative 2011), and Nigeria was working toward eradication in 2012 through vaccination and monitoring efforts (Global Polio Eradication Initiative 2012).

Many nations, both developed and developing, have had to confront health issues surrounding HIV/AIDS. Nigeria, however, has encountered particular difficulty implementing key components of standard disease control protocol. For example, the country has a particularly high burden of infected pregnant women, yet just 3 percent of HIV-positive mothers receive antiretroviral treatment. Despite the fact that cost-effective interventions are available, mother-to-child transmission rates are expected to reach nearly 40 percent if no additional action is taken (Shah et al. 2011).

Despite these difficulties, the prospects for improvement are promising. The 2011 presidential election in Nigeria was deemed by some experts as the most legitimate and transparent election the country has ever held. In addition, the National Assembly passed the National Health Bill in May 2011, putting health at the top of the national agenda. The bill aims to ensure basic access to health services for all citizens, retain trained health professionals, and hold the government accountable for complete implementation of the bill's mandates (*Lancet* 2011). Because it enjoys widespread support from health professionals and the general public as well as a demonstrated commitment to health by the Nigerian president, the bill seems likely to be signed into law.

Colombia

Colombia faces challenging public health issues that are deeply rooted in an ongoing conflict and urban–rural disparities.

Insurance Scheme

The country's health disparities are evident in examinations of its universal health insurance system. Law 100 was approved in 1993, granting all citizens the right to health insurance with an essential benefits package, regardless of ability to pay. By 2009, about 80 percent of Colombians were covered under one or two health insurance schemes—the Contributory Regime (CR) or the Subsidized Regime (SR). The CR covers those who work and earn more than a set minimum level of pay, and the SR covers those who are considered poor, as determined by a means test. The SR offers a meager benefits package compared to that for the CR; for example, the SR offers only basic primary care services and catastrophic coverage, whereas the CR offers comprehensive coverage. Critics say that the managed care model used by insurers covering both CR and SR limits access to care, restricts utilization, and has changed public providers' clinical behaviors to suit a competitive market scheme, all resulting in increased health disparities (Vargas et al. 2010). Proponents argue that this universal health insurance approach improved on the previous model covering SR

GLOBAL HEALTH IMPACT
Healthcare Workforce

The structural makeup of the global healthcare workforce is undergoing significant change due to migration, globalization, and other social changes. The world's demographics are shifting, with many developed countries rapidly aging, resulting in increasing need for services for countries' aging populations (Segal and Singh 2009). WHO estimates that the world faces a shortage of 4.5 million health professionals required to deliver essential healthcare services to populations in need (Taylor et al. 2011). Developing countries in particular are experiencing "brain drain," whereby trained medical professionals leave their country of origin to pursue the better standard of living and quality of life, higher salary, increased access to advanced technology, and more stable political conditions that wealthier nations offer (Mackey and Liang 2012).

A few strategies are being employed to address deficiencies in the global healthcare workforce. In May 2010, the WHO Global Code of Practice on International Recruitment of Health Professionals was adopted by the 193 member states of the World Health Assembly (WHO 2010). This code calls for the development of measures to educate and retain health professionals and to foster sustainable health systems. Telemedicine, the provision of care at a distance using communications and information technology, is increasingly used to decrease workforce disparities, allowing exchanges of knowledge between providers across regions and even countries and lifting some of the burden placed on providers operating in remote areas of the world. Finally, some countries are increasing their use of physician extenders, such as nurse practitioners and physician assistants, to fill workforce gaps in developing nations (Roderick, Hogan, and Leeker 2007).

subscribers by increasing access and reducing catastrophic health spending (Giedion and Uribe 2009). Although the government plans to implement policies to reach 100 percent insurance coverage of the population, no concurrent strategy is in place to address the great disparities inherent in this insurance scheme.

Vector-Borne Diseases

Colombia is also working to prevent and treat vector-borne communicable diseases (diseases spread to humans by another species, often an arthropod), which are still prevalent and dangerous in about 20 percent of Colombia's land area. Vector-borne diseases include malaria, Chagas disease, and dengue fever, which are preventable through the use of proper insecticide treatment measures. However, prevention measures are not executed in a systematic, efficient way in Colombia (Castillo-Riquelme et al. 2008), and the bulk of the money allocated to vector-borne diseases is spent on treatment several years after contraction. For example, Chagas disease sufferers do not usually present with symptoms for at least a decade following exposure, and when symptoms do manifest, they often resemble other general cardiac illnesses. Significant amounts of money, at levels that far surpass prevention efforts, are needlessly spent on diagnostic testing for and treatment of cardiomyopathy (i.e., deterioration of the heart muscle) and congestive heart failure. The government then pays the majority of associated costs, as Law 100 grants universal health insurance coverage, but those with Chagas do not experience a positive outcome.

Violence

Colombia leads Latin American countries in homicides, fueled by gang activity, civil strife, and general civil disobedience exacerbated by alcohol consumption. The murder rate in 2011 was 31.4 homicides per 100,000 people, compared to the US rate of 4.8 per 100,000 in 2010 (UNODC 2012).

Law enforcement policies are in place to tackle gangs and paramilitary forces, and municipalities address the "culture of violence" through social outreach and by mitigating the effects of alcohol with restrictive policies (Ceaser 2007). For example, between 2004 and 2008, the government of Cali enacted three different policies dictating the availability of alcohol. Studies showed that when alcohol sales were stopped earlier in the night, homicide rates dropped significantly (Sánchez et al. 2011). To further reduce the homicide rate, Colombia must address underlying social factors leading to different types of violence.

Overall, Colombia's health policy issues reflect larger societal problems. Tropical diseases, health inequities, and violence must be curbed in conjunction with broader social and economic policies. The Colombian government under Alvaro Uribe, president from 2002 to 2010, began addressing these issues (especially those related to violence), and his successor, Juan Manuel Santos, has followed suit. How these measures will affect heath issues and disparate health indicators within the population remains to be seen.

KEY POINTS

➤ Although most developed nations have controlled the spread of communicable diseases, their health systems are strained by an aging population and widespread chronic disease. They must maintain an adequate, well-trained workforce and integrate new technologies while keeping costs at a manageable level.

➤ Several factors affect rising healthcare costs in developed countries, including the aging populations, rapid technological progress, the participation of women in the labor force, and public funding for healthcare.

➤ Developing countries face a range of health problems, from communicable, highly contagious diseases to incipient, invisible problems that manifest from exposure to polluted environments. These nations must address the drivers of preventable morbidity and mortality to increase economic development.

➤ The lack of a sound health system infrastructure in most developing countries affects the spread of all diseases and impedes access to essential health services. Further, low government spending leads to low quality of care and creates long waiting times, constant shortages of essential drugs and supplies, and untrained staff.

CASE STUDY QUESTIONS

On the basis of your own research of climate change and its impact on public health, answer the following questions:

1. Why are changes to the climate important for public health?
2. What potential health policies and public health strategies could mitigate the effects of climate change?

FOR DISCUSSION

1. What are the primary health policy issues in industrialized countries? In developing countries?
2. What are the specific health challenges in Japan?
3. What has Denmark's health reform accomplished?
4. What is Canada's health policy agenda?
5. What are the challenges facing South Korea?

6. What goals is China's Healthy China 2020 attempting to accomplish?
7. What are the public health challenges faced by Ukraine?
8. What are the health issues of Nigeria?
9. What factors do Colombia's health policies focus on?

REFERENCES

A.D.A.M. Medical Encyclopedia. 2011. "Severe Acute Respiratory Syndrome (SARS)." Updated February 19. www.ncbi.nlm.nih.gov/pubmedhealth/PMH0004460/.

Aizura, A. Z. 2010. "Feminine Transformations: Gender Reassignment Surgery in Thailand." *Medical Anthropology* 29 (4): 424–43.

Alleman, B. W., T. Lugar, H. S. Reisinger, R. Martin, M. D. Horowitz, and P. Cram. 2011. "Medical Tourism Services Available to Residents of the United States." *Journal of General Internal Medicine* 26 (5): 492–97.

Andersen, P. T., and J. Jensen. 2010. "Healthcare Reform in Denmark." *Scandinavian Journal of Public Health* 38 (3): 246–52.

Atun, R., and I. Olynik. 2008. "Resistance to Implementing Policy Change: The Cast of Ukraine." *Bulletin of the World Health Organization* 86: 147–54.

Avert.org. 2011. "Fact Sheet: Tuberculosis." Accessed December 21. www.avert.org/tuberculosis.htm.

Bongaarts, J., and M. Over. 2010. "HIV/AIDS Policy in Transition." *Science* 328 (5984): 1359–60.

Bryant, T., C. Leaver, and J. Dunn. 2009. "Unmet Healthcare Need, Gender, and Health Inequalities in Canada." *Health Policy* 91 (1): 24–32.

Bulletin of the World Health Organization. 2008. "Overcoming Migrants' Barriers to Health." Published in August. www.who.int/bulletin/volumes/86/8/08-020808/en/index.html.

Castillo-Riquelme, M., F. Guhl, B. Turriago, N. Pinto, F. Rosas, M. F. Martinez, J. Fox-Rushby, C. Davies, and D. Campbell-Lendrum. 2008. "The Costs of Preventing and Treating Chagas Disease in Colombia." *PLoS Neglected Tropical Diseases* 2 (11): e336.

Ceaser, M. 2007. "Colombia Continues to Struggle with Violence." *Lancet* 370 (9599): 1601–2.

Centers for Disease Control and Prevention (CDC). 2012. "Information on Avian Influenza." Updated June 22. www.cdc.gov/flu/avianflu/.

Chen, Z. 2009. "Launch of the Health-Care Reform Plan in China." *Lancet* 373 (9672): 1322–24.

Chun, C. B., S. Y. Kim, J. Y. Lee, and S. Y. Lee. 2009. "Republic of Korea: Health System Review." *Health Systems in Transition* 11 (7): 1–184.

Clement, F. M., A. Harris, J. J. Li, K. Yong, K. M. Lee, and B. J. Manns. 2009. "Using Effectiveness and Cost-Effectiveness to Make Drug Coverage Decisions: A Comparison of Britain, Australia, and Canada." *Journal of the American Medical Association* 302 (13): 1437–43.

Cumming, J., and N. Mays. 2011. "New Zealand's Primary Health Care Strategy: Early Effects of the New Financing and Payment System for General Practice and Future Challenges." *Health Economics, Policy and Law* 6 (1): 1–21.

Dalal, S., J. J. Beunza, J. Volmink, C. Adebamowo, F. Bajunirwe, M. Njelekela, D. Mozaffarian, W. Fawzi, W. Willett, H.-O. Adami, and M. D. Holmes. 2011. "Non-communicable Diseases in Sub-Saharan Africa: What We Know Now." *International Journal of Epidemiology* 40 (4): 885–901.

Economist Intelligence Unit. 2011. "Denmark: Healthcare and Pharmaceuticals Report." Published January 27. [Log-in required.] http://viewswire.eiu.com/index.asp?layout=ib3Article&article_id=1027773887&pubtypeid=1152462500&country_id=1330000133&category_id=775133077.

Frohlich, K. L., N. Ross, and C. Richmond. 2006. "Health Disparities in Canada Today: Some Evidence and a Theoretical Framework." *Health Policy* 79 (2–3): 132–43.

Giedion, U., and M. V. Uribe. 2009. "Colombia's Universal Health Insurance System." *Health Affairs* 28 (3): 853–63.

Global Polio Eradication Initiative. 2012. "Nigeria." Published in October. www.polioeradication .org/Infectedcountries/Nigeria.aspx.

———. 2011. "Deliberations of the 22nd Meeting of the Expert Review Committee on Polio Eradication and Routine Immunization in Nigeria (ERC)." Presented October 13–14 in Abuja, Nigeria. www.polioeradication.org/Portals/o/Document/Resources/Advisory Certification/TAG/22ERCMeeting_Report_2011101314.pdf.

Gong, S., A. Walker, and G. Shi. 2007. "From Chinese Model to U.S. Symptoms: The Paradox of China's Health System." *International Journal of Health Services* 37 (4): 651–72.

Haiti Libre. 2010. "Agriculture: Cholera Threatens Food Security in Haiti." Published December 29. www.haitilibre.com/en/news-2001-haiti-agriculture-cholera-threatens-food-security-in-haiti.html.

Hashimoto, H., N. Ikegami, K. Shibuya, N. Izumida, H. Noguchi, H. Yasunaga, H. Miyata, J. M. Acuin, and M. R. Reich. 2011. "Cost Containment and Quality of Care in Japan: Is There a Trade-off?" *Lancet* 378 (9797): 1174–82.

Health Council of Canada. 2011. "Understanding and Improving Aboriginal Maternal and Child Health in Canada: Conversations About Promising Practices Across Canada." Published in August. http://publications.gc.ca/collections/collection_2011/ccs-hcc/H174-23-2011-eng.pdf.

Hu, F. B., Y. Liu, and W. C. Willett. 2011. "Preventing Chronic Diseases by Promoting Healthy Diet and Lifestyle: Public Policy Implications for China." *Obesity Reviews* 12 (7): 552–59.

Hurley, R. 2010. How Ukraine Is Tackling Europe's Worst HIV Epidemic." *BMJ* 341: c3538.

International Medical Travel Journal (*IMTJ*). 2012. "GLOBAL: Which countries do people select as a medical tourism destination?" *International Medical Travel Journal: News.* Published January 13. www.imtj.com/news/?entryid82=332786.

International Organization for Migration. 2011. "Migration Initiatives 2012." Published in December. www.iom.int/jahia/webdav/site/myjahiasite/shared/shared/mainsite/published_docs/books/Migration-Initiatives-Appeal.pdf.

Joint Commission International (JCI). 2013. "JCI Accredited Organizations." Accessed March 21. www.jointcommissioninternational.org/JCI-Accredited-Organizations/.

Khan, A. S., A. M. Levitt, M. J. Sage, and the CDC Strategic Planning Workgroup. 2000. "Biological and Chemical Terrorism: Strategic Plan for Preparedness and Response." Published April 21. www.cdc.gov/mmwr/preview/mmwrhtml/rr4904a1.htm.

Kirwan, D. 2009. "Global Health: Current Issues, Future Trends, and Foreign Policy." *Clinical Medicine* 9 (3): 247–53.

Koplan, J. P., T. C. Bond, M. H. Merson, K. S. Reddy, M. H. Rodriguez, N. K. Sewankambo, J. N. Wasserheit, and the Consortium of Universities for Global Health Executive Board. 2009. "Towards a Common Definition of Global Health." *Lancet* 373 (9679): 1993–95.

Lancet. 2011. "Hope for Health in Nigeria" [editorial]. *Lancet* 377 (9781): 1891.

Lee, C. V., and V. Balaban. 2011. "Medical Tourism." Published July 1. wwwnc.cdc.gov/travel/yellowbook/2012/chapter-2-the-pre-travel-consultation/medical-tourism.htm.

Legido-Quigley, H., M. McKee, E. Nolte, and I. A. Glinos. 2008. *Assuring the Quality of Health Care in the European Union: A Case for Action.* Geneva, Switzerland: World Health Organization.

Lekhan, V., V. Rudiy, and E. Richardson. 2010. "Ukraine: Health System Review." *Health Systems in Transition* 12 (8): 1–183.

Mackey, T. K., and B. A. Liang. 2012. "Rebalancing Brain Drain: Exploring Resource Reallocation to Address Health Worker Migration and Promote Global Health." *Health Policy* 107 (1): 66–73.

McMichael, A. J., and E. Lindgren. 2011. "Climate Change: Present and Future Risks to Health, and Necessary Responses." *Journal of Internal Medicine* 270 (5): 401–13.

McMichael, A. J., D. H. Campbell-Lendrum, C. F. Corvalán, K. L. Ebi, A. Githeko, J. D. Scheraga, and A. Woodward (eds.). 2003. *Climate Change and Human Health—Risks and Responses*. World Health Organization. Accessed February 25, 2013. www.who.int/globalchange/publications/cchhbook/en/.

Moon, S., and J. Shin. 2007. "Performance of Universal Health Insurance: Lessons from South Korea." *World Health and Population* 9 (2): 95–113.

Morgan, S., R. G. Evans, G. E. Hanley, P. A. Caetano, and C. Black. 2006. "Income-Based Coverage in British Columbia: Lessons for BC and the Rest of Canada." *Health Policy* 2 (2): 116–27.

Nambiar, B., S. Lewycka, C. Mwansambo, and A. Costello. 2007. "Planning Healthcare in Developing Countries." *Anaesthesia* 62 (Suppl. 1): 5–10.

Navarro, A. M., K. P. Voetsch, L. C. Liburd, H. W. Giles, and J. L. Collins. 2007. "Charting the Future of Community Health Promotion: Recommendations from the National Expert Panel on Community Health Promotion." Published in July. www.cdc.gov/pcd/issues/2007/jul/07_0013.htm.

Novossiolova, T., M. Minehata, and M. Dando. 2012. "The Creation of a Contagious H5N1 Influenza Virus: Implications for the Education of Life Scientists." *Journal of Terrorism Research* 3 (1).

Nweke, O. C., and W. H. Sanders. 2009. "Modern Environmental Health Hazards: A Public Health Issue of Increasing Significance in Africa." *Environmental Health Perspectives* 117 (6): 863–70.

Organisation for Economic Co-operation and Development (OECD). 2011. "Spending Continues to Outpace Economic Growth in Most OECD Countries." Published June 30. www.oecd.org/document/38/0,3746,en_21571361_44315115_48289894_1_1_1_1,00.html#.

Pammolli, F., M. Riccaboni, and L. Magazzini. 2012. "The Sustainability of European Health-care Systems: Beyond Income and Aging." *European Journal of Health Economics* 13 (5): 623–34.

Patel, V. 2007. "Mental Health in Low and Middle Income Countries." *British Medical Bulletin* 81–82: 81–96.

Pollard, K. 2011. "Medical Tourism: Past, Present, and Future." Presentation at the International Health Tourism Conference, Istanbul, October. www.imtj.com/resources/?entryid115=316569.

Pompe, S., J. Simon, P. M. Wiedemann, and C. Tannert. 2005. "Future Trends and Challenges in Pathogenomics." *European Molecular Biology Organization* 6 (7): 600–606.

Potts, M., D. T. Halperin, D. Kirby, A. Swidler, E. Marseille, J. D. Klausner, N. Hearst, R. G. Wamai, J. G. Kahn, and J. Walsh. 2008. "Reassessing HIV Prevention." *Science* 320 (5877): 749–50.

Roderick, S. H., K. Hogan, and E. Leeker. 2007. "The Globalization of the Physician Assistant Profession." *Journal of Physician Assistant Education* 18 (3): 76–85.

Rogers, B. A., Z. Aminzadeh, and D. L. Paterson. 2011. "Country-Country Transfer of Patients and the Risk of Multi-drug Resistant Bacterial Infection." *Clinical Infectious Diseases* 53 (1): 49–56.

Ross, H., M. Stoklosa, and K. Krasovsky. 2011. "Economic and Public Health Impact of 2007–2010 Tobacco Tax Increases in Ukraine." *Tobacco Control* 21 (4): 429–35.

Sambo, L. G., and J. M. Kirigia. 2011. "Africa's Health: Could the Private Sector Accelerate the Progress Towards Health MDGs?" *International Archives of Medicine* 4: 39.

Sánchez, A. I., A. Villaveces, R. T. Krafty, T. Park, H. B. Weiss, A. Fabio, J. C. Puyana, and M. I. Gutierrez. 2011. "Policies for Alcohol Restriction and Their Association with Interpersonal Violence: A Time-Series Analysis of Homicides in Cali, Colombia." *International Journal of Epidemiology* 40 (4): 1037–46.

Sassi, F. 2010. *Obesity and the Economics of Prevention: Fit Not Fat.* Paris: Organisation for Economic Co-operation and Development.

Segal, L., and D. A. Singh. 2009. "Issues Facing the Future of Healthcare: The Importance of Demand Modeling." *Australia and New Zealand Health Policy* 6: 12.

Shah, M., B. Johns, A. Abimiku, and D. G. Walker. 2011. "Cost-Effectiveness of New WHO Recommendations for Prevention of Mother-to-Child Transmission of HIV in a Resource-Limited Setting." *AIDS* 25 (8): 1093–102.

Shi, L., and D. A. Singh. 2011. *Delivering Health Care in America: A Systems Approach,* 5th ed. Sudbury, MA: Jones and Bartlett.

Shibuya, K., H. Hashimoto, N. Ikegami, A. Nishi, T. Tanimoto, H. Miyata, K. Takemi, and M. R. Reich. 2011. "Future of Japan's System of Good Health at Low Cost with Equity: Beyond Universal Coverage." *Lancet* 378 (9798): 1265–73.

Siddiqi, S., T. I. Masud, S. Nishtar, D. H. Peters, B. Sabri, K. M. Bile, and M. A. Jama. 2009. "Framework for Assessing Governance of the Health System in Developing Countries: Gateway to Good Governance." *Health Policy* 90 (1): 13–15.

Singh, S., U. Mushtaq, C. Holm-Hansen, D. Milan, A. Cheung, and N. Watts. 2011. "The Importance of Climate Change to Health." *Lancet* 378 (9785): 29–30.

Smith, S., and C. Normand. 2011. "Equity in Healthcare: The Irish Perspective." *Health Economics, Policy and Law* 6 (2): 205–17.

Song, P. 2010. "Biotech Pilgrims and the Transnational Quest for Stem Cell Cures." *Medical Anthropology* 29 (4): 384–402.

Stanecki, K., J. Daher, J. Stover, M. Beusenberg, Y. Souteyrand, and J. M. García Calleja. 2010. "Antiretroviral Therapy Needs: The Effect of Changing Global Guidelines." *Sexually Transmitted Infections* 86 (Suppl. 2): ii62–ii66.

Starfield, B., and D. Mangin. 2010. "An International Perspective on the Basis for Payment for Performance." *Quality in Primary Care* 18 (6): 399–404.

Taylor, A. L., L. Hwenda, B.-I. Larsen, and N. Daulaire. 2011. "Stemming the Brain Drain—A WHO Global Code of Practice on International Recruitment of Health Personnel." *New England Journal of Medicine* 365 (25): 2348–51.

Tediosi, F., S. Gabriele, and F. Longo. 2009. "Governing Decentralization in Healthcare Under Tough Budget Constraint: What Can We Learn from the Italian Experience?" *Health Policy* 90 (2): 303–12.

Tsutsui, T., and N. Maramatsu. 2007. "Japan's Universal Longer Term Care System Reform of 2005: Containing Costs and Realizing a Vision." *Journal of the American Geriatrics Society* 55 (9): 1458–63.

UN Department of Public Information. 2010. "Goal Six: Combat HIV/AIDS, Malaria and Other Diseases: Fact Sheet." Published in September. www.un.org/millenniumgoals/pdf/MDG_FS_6_EN.pdf.

United Nations Office on Drugs and Crime (UNODC). 2012. "UNODC Homicide Statistics." Accessed March 8, 2013. www.unodc.org/unodc/en/data-and-analysis/homicide.html.

US Department of Health and Human Services (HHS). 2013. "Global Programs & Initiatives." www.globalhealth.gov/global-programs-and-initiatives/index.html.

Van Minh, H., and N.-V. Hung. 2011. "Economic Aspects of Sanitation in Developing Countries." *Environmental Health Insights* 5: 63–70.

Vargas, I., M. L. Vázquez, A. S. Mogollón-Pérez, and J.-P. Unger. 2010. "Barriers of Access to Care in a Managed Competition Model: Lessons from Colombia." *BMC Health Services Research* 10: 297.

Wagner, K. H., and H. Brath. 2012. "A Global View on the Development of Non-communicable Diseases." *Preventive Medicine* 54 (Suppl.): S38–S41.

Water Sanitation and Health, World Health Organization. 2013. "Facts and Figures on Water Quality and Health." Copyright 2013. www.who.int/water_sanitation_health/facts_figures/en/index.html.

Weiss, H. A., D. Halperin, R. C. Bailey, R. J. Hayes, G. Schmid, and C. A. Hankins. 2008. "Male Circumcision for HIV Prevention: From Evidence to Action?" *AIDS* 22 (5): 567–74.

World Health Organization (WHO). 2013. "Dracunculiasis: The Global Eradication Campaign." Copyright 2013. www.who.int/dracunculiasis/eradication/en/.

———. 2011. *Mental Health Atlas 2011.* Accessed March 8, 2013. http://whqlibdoc.who .int/publications/2011/9799241564359_eng.pdf.

———. 2010. "WHO Global Code of Practice on the International Recruitment of Health Personnel." Accessed March 9, 2013. www.who.int/hrh/migration/code/WHO_global_code_of_practice_EN.pdf.

———. 2005. "Rethinking 'Diseases of Affluence': The Economic Impact of Chronic Diseases." Accessed March 8, 2013. www.who.int/chp/chronic_disease_report/media/Factsheet4.pdf.

Yu, D., Y. Souteyrand, M. A. Banda, J. Kaufman, and J. H. Perriëns. 2008. "Investment in HIV/AIDS Programs: Does It Help Strengthen Health Systems in Developing Countries?" *Global Health* 4: 8.

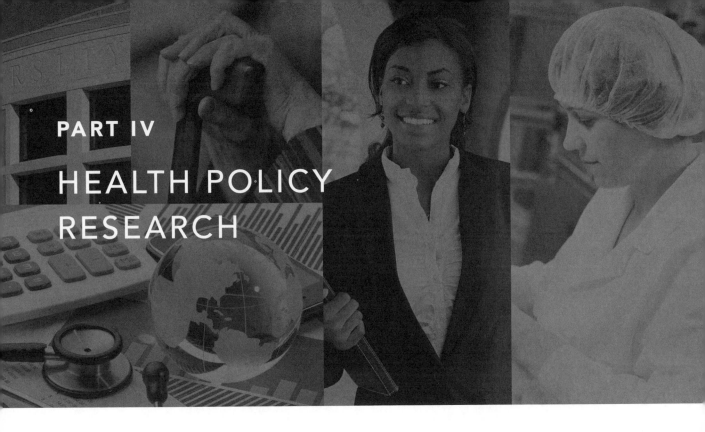

PART IV

HEALTH POLICY RESEARCH

Part IV of this book consists of three chapters that describe how policy issues can be studied and analyzed. Specifically, Chapter 8, "Overview of Health Policy Research," provides an introduction to the field of health policy research, including definitions and general characteristics. Chapter 9, "Health Policy Research Methods," illustrates some commonly used methods—both quantitative and qualitative—for conducting health policy research. Chapter 10, "An Example of Health Policy Research," concludes the book with an example of an application of health policy research. The introductory and illustrative materials presented in this part may stimulate students to delve further into health policy at an advanced level.

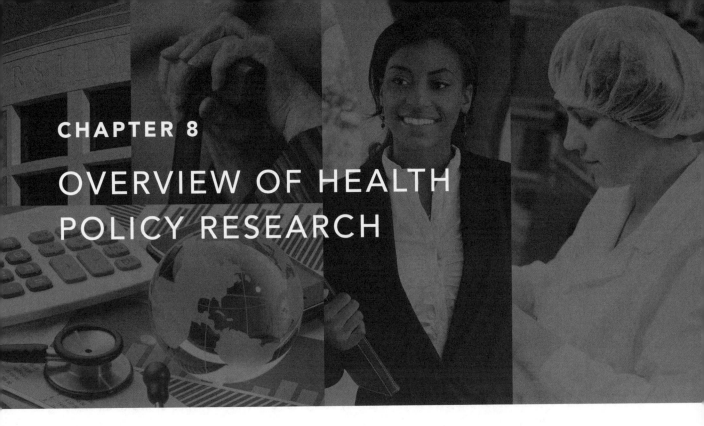

CHAPTER 8

OVERVIEW OF HEALTH POLICY RESEARCH

Honesty is the best policy.

— Benjamin Franklin

LEARNING OBJECTIVES

Studying this chapter will help you to

➤ define and understand the characteristics of health policy research,

➤ describe the research process as applied to health policy,

➤ discuss how to communicate findings from health policy research, and

➤ appreciate the challenges in implementing findings from research to health policy.

CASE STUDY

THE RAND HEALTH INSURANCE EXPERIMENT

The RAND Health Insurance Experiment (HIE) (www.rand.org/health/projects/hie.html) was one of the largest and most comprehensive health policy studies carried out in the United States. The HIE was a randomized experiment conducted between 1971 and 1982. A total of 2,750 families, including more than 7,700 individuals under age 65, were chosen from six sites across the country to participate. The study answered two questions regarding the financing of healthcare:

1. If medical care is free, how much more will patients use?

2. Are patient health outcomes impacted by the cost of medical care?

The study subjects were randomly assigned to one of five types of health insurance plans:

- Free care

- 25 percent coinsurance

- 50 percent coinsurance

- 95 percent coinsurance

- An HMO that provided care free of charge

The key findings of the study, as noted by Brook et al. (2006), were the following:

- Patients having to contribute toward the cost of medical care used fewer services than did those who received services free of charge.

- Coinsurance equally reduced patient utilization of highly effective and less effective medical care.

- The quality of medical care was not significantly affected by coinsurance.

- Overall, coinsurance was not shown to negatively affect patients' health; however, medical care provided free of charge brought about improvements in hypertension, dental and vision health, and other serious conditions. This difference was found to be the greatest among patients with poor health and low income.

The study's findings provided input for policymaking related to restructuring private insurance and strengthening managed care.

Now that we have a basic understanding of the policymaking process and major health issues in the United States and elsewhere, we continue with an overview of the field of health policy research (HPR), which contributes significantly to policy development and improvement. In this chapter, HPR is defined and its unique characteristics highlighted. The process of HPR is then summarized, followed by a discussion on how to communicate findings from HPR. The chapter concludes by underscoring the challenges in implementing HPR.

DEFINING HEALTH POLICY RESEARCH

Health policy research is the process of scientific investigation that applies various health-related and social science methodologies to formulate and evaluate health policies (WHO 2005). The goal of HPR is to improve the health of populations through needs assessment, policy and program development, implementation, and evaluation.

Harrison (2001) identifies the following aspects of the policy process that researchers actively investigate:

◆ How issues come to be seen and defined as problems

◆ How some issues reach policy agendas and others do not

◆ How policies and decisions are made, and why proposed options are rejected

◆ The normative and explanatory theories espoused by researchers

◆ The impact that implementation attempts have on the policy itself

◆ Why policies survive or are abandoned

◆ The factors that contribute to successful interventions

Although this book does not make the distinction (i.e., the two terms are used interchangeably), *health policy research* is technically different than *health policy analysis*: Although both disciplines address a particular health problem, policy research tends to be conducted in a rigorous and systematic fashion, whereas **policy analysis** is time sensitive and relies on existing and current information.

In the second edition of the classic text *A Practical Guide to Policy Analysis*, Bardach (2005, 13) elaborates on the multiple roles and tasks of policy analysts:

Policy analysts help in planning, budgeting, program evaluation, program design, program management, public relations, and other functions. They work alone, in teams, and in loose networks that cut across organizations. They work in the public, nonprofit, and for-profit spheres. Although their work is ideally distinguished by transparency of method and inter-

Policy analysis
A systematic approach by which to assess problems and guide decision making.

pretation, the analysts themselves may explicitly bring to their jobs the values and passions of advocacy groups as well as "neutral" civil servants. The professional networks in which they work may contain—in most cases, do contain—professionals drawn from law, engineering, accounting, and so on and in those settings the policy-analytic point of view has to struggle for the right to counter—or better yet, synthesize—the viewpoints of the other professionals. Although policy-analytic work products typically involve written reports, they may also include briefings, slide presentations, magazine articles, and television interviews. The recipients of these products may be broad and diffuse audiences as well as narrowly construed paying clients or employers.

As Bardach describes, the work of policy analysts informs the decision making of, and guides program implementation for, policymakers and professionals in other fields. Policy analysts often follow a five-step framework to assess problems (Stokey and Zeckhauser 1978): (1) establishing the context and goals for a particular issue, (2) identifying alternative approaches to addressing the issue, (3) evaluating alternatives and predicting the consequences, (4) valuing the outcomes, and (5) making a choice.

Health policy analysis is performed by a wide array of researchers and research organizations, including academics, government officials, think tanks, and consulting firms, each yielding different types of policy analysis products. For example, academic researchers tend to produce scholarly articles or policy analysis books for publication; government officials, policy memos or briefs to inform policymakers; and think tanks and consulting firms, reports tailored to the needs of particular clients. For example, the not-for-profit think tank RAND Corporation released a report on the diffusion of health information technology (HIT) (Taylor et al. 2005). In this study, RAND performed classic policy analysis by summarizing the current state of HIT adoption by the US healthcare system, identifying factors predicting its adoption, determining policy alternatives to improve HIT diffusion, discussing the alternatives, and making policy recommendations regarding HIT.

CHARACTERISTICS OF HEALTH POLICY RESEARCH

Health policy research can be characterized by five main attributes: its nature as an applied field, its ethics framework, the multidisciplinary input it enjoys, its basis in science, and its focus on population.

Applied Field

Health policy research is an applied field in which objectives are largely determined by priorities within health systems and concerns of society. To illustrate this point, researcher Anderson (1985, 237) wrote: "Research in the field of health services has generally stemmed not from curiosity, but from a need to have facts on which to base organization, administration, and legislation and this search for facts has been frankly for public policy purposes, to provide a factual basis for a given policy."

Health policy research aims to address problems related to specific populations, such as pregnant women, the elderly, or migrants, and to enhance health interventions at local, national, and international levels. Findings from HPR are used by clinicians, healthcare administrators, and formulators of healthcare policy, and researchers must often frame findings in a way that will be useful for various stakeholders.

The objectives of researchers and policymakers are not always complementary. This view is echoed in the work of Lavis and colleagues (2002), who used organizing frameworks from three disciplines—organizational behavior and management research, knowledge utilization, and political science research—to study the role of health policy research in public policy formulation in Canada. They found that interactions between researchers and policymakers can affect the amount of influence research has on policymaking.

For example, small-scale, content-driven policies (e.g., HIV prenatal testing, needs-based funding formulas) appeared to be particularly amenable to recommendations from research findings, but larger-scale policy decisions (e.g., broad healthcare financing schemes) seemed less affected because of various conflicting and influential political factors.

The practical application and problem-solving orientation of health policy research must remain balanced with theory-driven standards. Theory and systematic methodologies provide the framework within which healthcare problems are modeled. Health policy researchers should ensure that their techniques and the findings they uncover are generalizable beyond specific populations or settings to properly assess the quality of research and corresponding findings.

Policy-Relevant Applied HPR

Exhibit 8.1 shows the policymaking process as developed by Longest (2010). Health policy research and analysis may occur at several points throughout the policy process. For example, HPR often comes into play as the life of a policy begins—at the policy formulation stage, during which problems and possible solutions are evaluated against the current political and social climate. Researchers may investigate successful (or failed) policies to inform policymakers or offer suggestions for the direction of future efforts. As mentioned in earlier chapters, a window of opportunity must exist for a policy to be fully developed, which is determined by the current landscape of social, economic, political, ethical, and legal factors. Regardless of the amount and quality of evidence gathered by researchers, this window of opportunity must be present for successful acceptance and implementation.

Once a policy is implemented and appropriate regulatory rules are in place for it to function, policy researchers may conduct evaluations to assess whether the policy and asso-

Exhibit 8.1

A Model of the Public Policymaking Process in the United States

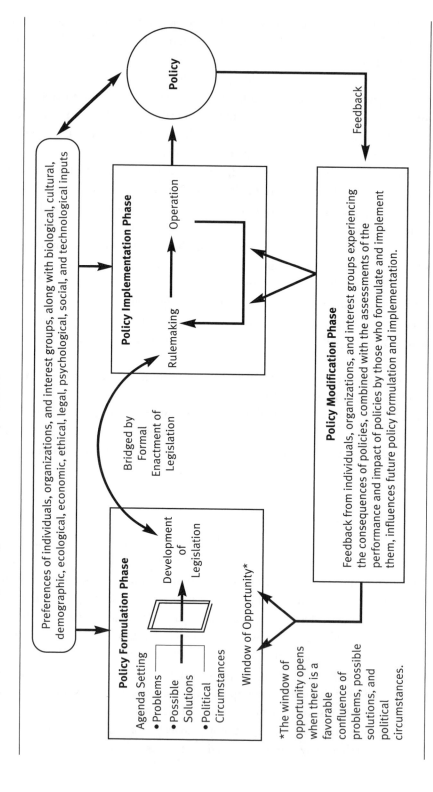

SOURCE: Longest (2010). Reprinted with permission from Health Administration Press, Chicago. © 2010 Health Administration Press. www.ache.org/hap.cfm.

ciated programs are meeting objectives and the needs of target populations. Policy researchers may also compare the current policy's performance against existing or past efforts.

On the basis of findings from policy researchers or of feedback from individuals, organizations, or interest groups, a policy may enter the policy modification stage, during which it is further evaluated and assessed for impact. Thus, the policy process is a feedback cycle that is constantly informed by policy research.

Framework of Ethics

Ethical standards dictate the proper conduct of research, including accommodation of the interests of research subjects. Health policy analysts must consider all relevant ethical issues when developing research plans to ensure the safety and rights of study participants. The organization that sponsors the research typically has an **institutional review board (IRB)** in place, whose responsibility is to review the study design before the research begins to ensure that researchers have thoroughly considered all ethical implications of their work and to consider potential legal implications should ethical negligence occur.

Institutional review board (IRB)
A committee that examines the ethical implications of research to protect study subjects from physical or psychological harm.

For example, study designs should not place participants at risk for potential physical or psychological harm. Researchers must seek voluntary participation and disclose any associated risks. Ethical standards for research are particularly important to follow when dealing with "captive audiences," such as students or prisoners.

Throughout the duration of the study, the privacy of subjects should be protected through anonymity (i.e., participants remain anonymous throughout the study, even to the researchers) or confidentiality (i.e., identifying information is not made available to anyone who is not directly involved in the study).

Multidisciplinary Approach

HPR incorporates a wide variety of social and biomedical sciences in its approach to finding the best solutions to complex health-related problems—particularly disciplines used in problem solving and public decision making (Bice 1980). In fact, many health policy researchers are trained in social science disciplines, including sociology, economics, law, psychology, and political science, and often incorporate the theories and methods from these areas when addressing health policy concerns.

For example, knowledge from the biological sciences is often applied in the beginning stages of policy analysis, during which an existing health issue or program must be analyzed. The biological sciences include the study of biological determinants, risk factors, and consequences of health processes—as well as methods and techniques to characterize such phenomena—to contribute to the understanding of human populations (IOM 1979). Examples of research that involves the biological sciences include the study of the prevalence or incidence of a given condition and the genetic makeup of a certain population.

Health policy researchers also benefit from knowledge of demography, or population studies. Facts about population size, composition, and growth rates are needed for the early stages of program planning. Mapping technologies can be particularly helpful for health policy researchers. For example, using data on hospital patients and estimates of population size, local health researchers can compute hospital discharge rates for their local geographic or service areas. Such information might be used to guide funding decisions and allocation of resources to areas of need.

Economics is another area of expertise that is critical to health policy research, particularly with regard to cost–benefit and cost-effectiveness analyses of healthcare interventions. Findings from health economics–related research enables decision makers to best allocate limited resources.

Finally, the behavioral sciences are crucial to HPR, drawing from epidemiological studies that identify behavioral determinants of illness, such as diet and smoking habits, and examining the social and psychological components of these determinants.

Although many biomedical and social science disciplines are incorporated into HPR, true multidisciplinary research is not common. Researchers from the various fields do not often collaborate when conducting health-related research that could affect policy. For example, economic theory and methodologies have been used in research on prospective payment systems to assess the systems' impact on hospital cost containment, but knowledge that is often closely related, such as research from the behavioral sciences about patient characteristics or research from population studies on the community, is not usually considered. Such fragmentation of knowledge and disciplines restricts the impact that research toward problem solving and decision making can have on policy solutions.

Scientific Basis

Theories from the social sciences and methodologies used in empirical research can provide guidance for HPR and include problem conceptualization, data collection, analysis, and interpretation. Incorporating scientific methodologies can also help health policy researchers maintain objectivity about their work.

Although such methods could be useful to health policy researchers, the application of scientific principles is often constrained due in part to the complex nature of health-related problems. HPR often examines specific settings and populations; thus, findings from a particular study are not always generalizable. For example, the policy decisions that apply to healthcare delivery in rural areas are usually drastically different than those that emerge in urban areas in terms of access issues and financing (Humphreys et al. 2009).

The types of data available often impose limitations on HPR, which must rely on information from existing population surveys, records, and documents as well as direct observation. Seeking information beyond these sources is usually outside the scope of the study design because it can be an expensive and time-consuming activity. For example, health policy researchers studying the effect of technological advances on healthcare spending among cancer patients may be limited to the data contained in the annual series of national healthcare expenditure estimates produced by the Centers for Medicare & Medicaid Services (i.e., annual healthcare expenditures by type of service and source of funding [CMS 2012]) or reports from the National Health Care Survey (i.e., national estimates of the prevalence of illness and the use of various health services [NCHS 2011]), which could be outdated or not fully applicable to the researchers' populations of interest.

The gold standard for scientific research is the randomized controlled trial, in which research subjects are randomly assigned to an experimental group or a control group. This experimental design is often incompatible with HPR because researchers must consider determinants of health and environmental factors beyond those captured under strict experimental conditions. Furthermore, ethical standards of HPR do not allow experimental research on humans, and the effects of bias introduced into study results, due to the inability to control outside influences, can skew findings. To address these concerns, health policy researchers typically use quasi-experimental designs, cohort studies, longitudinal analyses, survey analyses, and multidisciplinary approaches (discussed later in this book).

Population Focus

Health policy research differs from other health-related research in that it focuses on healthcare solutions for the population rather than for the individual. In contrast, clinical research primarily focuses on the efficacy of the preventive, diagnostic, and therapeutic services applied to individual patients (IOM 1979). In addition, biomedical research is largely concerned with the conditions, processes, and mechanisms of health and illness at the biological level within the human body (Frenk 1993).

Epidemiological research investigates questions at the population level, focusing on frequency distribution and determinants of health and disease among populations. In other words, epidemiological research begins with a specific condition and studies its various determinants.

Bioepidemiology, clinical epidemiology, decision analysis, and technology assessment are some examples of disciplines that are similar to HPR in that they also deal with connections and interfaces among the major types of health-related research.

THE PROCESS OF HEALTH POLICY RESEARCH

HPR or analysis can be undertaken in a number of ways. The most widely used approach is a rationalist model (see Exhibit 8.2), similar to the five-step framework outlined earlier in this chapter, in which problem definition leads to the identification and evaluation of alternatives followed by policy implementation. (See Chapter 9 for a more detailed discussion of this approach.)

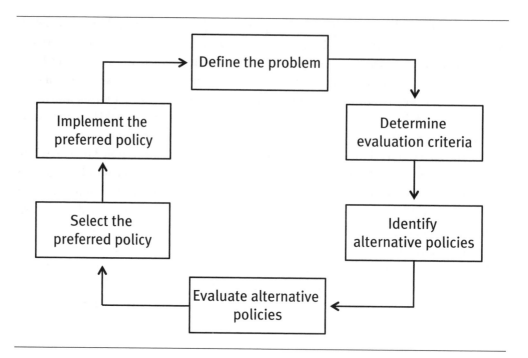

A more formal approach to conducting HPR is presented in Exhibit 8.3, which displays the steps involved in systematically conducting health policy research. This approach is similar to that followed when conducting health science–related research. Exhibit 8.4 breaks down these steps into their critical elements. Although the sequencing is not fixed, the stages are interdependent, and some stages must be conducted before others are initiated.

For example, an adequate hypothesis cannot be formulated without a proper understanding of the underlying subject matter. Similarly, the early steps of the research process must be executed properly to achieve a successful study. Writing an untestable hypothesis and securing an inadequate sample are two examples of execution errors that prevent successful completion of a study.

CONCEPTUALIZATION

The conceptualization stage of the research process requires the researcher to understand the general purpose of the research, determine the specific research topic, identify theories and literature relevant to the topic, specify the meaning of the concepts and variables to be studied, and formulate general hypotheses or research questions. Research hypotheses differ from research questions in that hypotheses suggest relationships between the variables.

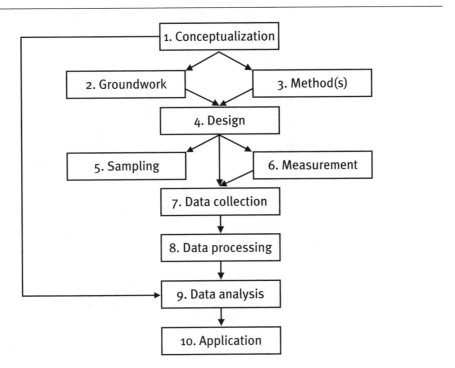

EXHIBIT 8.3
Steps in
Conducting Health
Policy Research

Theoretical research generally involves the testing of hypotheses developed from theories that are intellectually interesting to the researcher, whereas research questions typically arise from current social problems. Applied policy research focused on current social problems generally specifies its purpose through research questions. Hypotheses may be formulated if current knowledge (from theories and evidence) indicates an anticipated direction of the relationships among the variables of interest.

The conceptualization phase completes the development of a *conceptual framework*, which is a preliminary model of the problem under study that depicts relationships among critical variables of interest and between variables and concepts of interest. This phase, which is founded in literature and existing theory, helps researchers synthesize and guide the course of research and its subsequent analysis.

Conducting a literature review is a critical step within the conceptualization component. Literature reviews inform researchers about the current state of the study on the topic as well as the existing limitations in the body of research. Findings from literature reviews can be used to direct research efforts to areas yet to be explored or to those with conflicting results.

In addition to helping researchers narrow and refine a topic, literature reviews facilitate the identification of theories and provide guidance in the formulation of hypotheses

EXHIBIT 8.4
Key Elements
of the Research
Process Steps

Conceptualization
– Research aims and objective
– Problem statement and significance
– Literature and theory
– Conceptual framework
– Research hypotheses and/or questions

Groundwork
– Data
– Funding
– Proposal
– Infrastructure

Methods
– Research review
– Secondary analysis
– Qualitative research
– Experiment/quasi-experiment
– Survey
– Evaluation
– Longitudinal study

Design
– Choices of methods
– Validity threats
– Designs and pitfalls

Sampling
– Random/probability (simple, systematic, stratified, cluster)
– Nonrandom/nonprobability (convenience, quota, purposive, snowball)
– Sample size

Measurement
– Levels (nominal, ordinal, interval)
– Validity (construct, content, concurrent, predictive)
– Reliability (test-retest, split-half, interrater
– New measures and validation

Data collection
– Available versus empirical
– Published versus unpublished
– Instrument versus observation
– Impact on research projects
– Impact on respondents
– Impact on interviewers
– Impact on instrument
– Choices among methods
– Improving response rate

(continued)

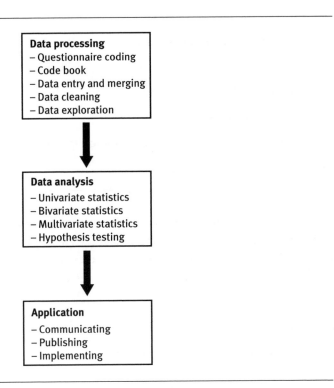

Exhibit 8.4
Key Elements
of the Research
Process Steps
(continued)

to be tested. As a result, researchers do not need to confine themselves to the generally accepted practices of their discipline when searching for relevant theories. They can use alternative approaches and theories to stimulate their research and generate more thorough findings than they might otherwise.

Another benefit of literature reviews is that they help identify relevant study and control variables to be included in the analysis. Exhibit 8.5 illustrates this process. The initial topic of interest is represented by the variable Y, and researchers are interested in finding out the causes of Y. The variable X is identified as a potential cause on the basis of the researchers' experience or the observed evidence; however, these researchers have limited experience with Y and thus are unable to consider all potential causes of Y. A literature review helps identify not only the potential causes (i.e., variable Xs) but also other potential factors (variable Zs). Furthermore, a literature review may suggest different dimensions of the topic (variable Ys). In short, a literature review enables researchers to operationalize abstract concepts—a prerequisite for empirical research.

Literature reviews also suggest pertinent research design, procedures, and analyses by indicating how other researchers have addressed a given topic. Researchers may use a previous investigator's method, revise the research design, or even replicate an earlier study. (See the Learning Point box for a summary description of the systematic research literature review process.)

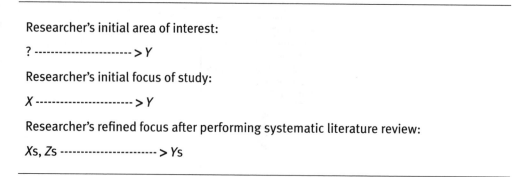

Researcher's initial area of interest:

? ----------------------- > Y

Researcher's initial focus of study:

X ----------------------- > Y

Researcher's refined focus after performing systematic literature review:

Xs, Zs ----------------------- > Ys

Policy-oriented reviews summarize current knowledge of a topic to draw out the policy implications of study findings. Such reviews require knowledge of the major policy issues and debates and common research expertise. (See the For Your Consideration box for the steps involved in synthesizing policy research findings.)

GROUNDWORK

In the groundwork stage, the researcher

- identifies relevant data sources,

- explores potential funding,

- develops a research plan or proposal by which to obtain funding, and

- makes organizational and administrative preparations to carry out the research.

Choosing a data source for policy research can be a difficult endeavor; policy-related evidence is not as clearly available as is evidence from experimental research in the life sciences. For example, a researcher planning to investigate the effects of tobacco control policies might need to examine economic data on tobacco taxes as well as health outcome information from local healthcare systems.

Those engaged in policy research often use a range of data types, including quantitative, qualitative, experimental, and descriptive data. Although it is difficult to fully assess the quality of data sources that might be used for policy research, investigators should weigh the positive and negative factors associated with using each relevant data source.

LEARNING POINT
Conducting a Systematic Literature Review

1. Identify the Topic

The choice of a topic for review is influenced by the interests of the policy community. A topic is probably not suitable for independent review unless sufficient research activity already surrounds it.

2. Prepare a Coding Sheet

Once the topic is identified and refined, a coding sheet should be constructed to collect relevant information from articles to be reviewed. A coding sheet enables the researcher to collect all needed information during the first reading. The preparation of a coding sheet is even useful for reviewing a small number of studies because the information collected will assist the investigator in analyzing and reporting those studies.

The information to be collected in the coding sheet should be determined on the basis of the preliminary review and the strategy to be adopted in analyzing and synthesizing studies. Generally, any information that may be analyzed and used in the review should be collected at the time of the review, because it is better to collect too much information than to have to re-read.

The general categories of information related to empirical research in which an investigator is likely to be interested include a study's background, design, measurement, and outcome characteristics.

In the background category, the source indicates the media or information channel from which a study is retrieved.

In the design category, the general categorization as presented may not be sufficient to generate information. Researchers may then include additional design characteristics (e.g., whether restrictions were placed on the types of individuals sampled in the original study, when and where the study was conducted, whether time series or longitudinal designs were used).

In the measurement category, investigators may document the use of particular scales, available instruments, and specific features of the analytic models (e.g., number of variables used, types of measures implemented for the same construct, tests of interaction terms and nonlinearity).

(continued)

> ### ✳ LEARNING POINT
> Conducting a Systematic Literature Review
>
> *(continued from previous page)*
>
> In the outcome category, if more quantitative analysis is envisioned, precise statistical information related to study results may be recorded. Examples include means, standard deviations, sample sizes for each comparison group (to be used for effect size calculation), association between variables (e.g., correlation coefficient), values of inferential test statistics (e.g., c^2, t ratio, F ratio), and the strength of an F ratio (e.g., regression, R^2).
>
> It bears reemphasizing that the construction of a coding sheet is the result of, rather than a prelude to, preliminary review. The development of a coding sheet forces researchers to think ahead about the review and analysis strategy and to be precise in their approach to gathering the information.
>
> #### 3. Search Research Publications
> Four major sources of literature are available for reviewers to retrieve: (a) books; (b) journals, including professional journals, published newsletters, magazines, and newspapers; (c) theses, including doctoral, master's, and bachelor's degree theses; and (d) unpublished work, including monographs, technical reports, grant proposals, conference papers, personal manuscripts, and other unpublished materials.
>
> #### 4. Synthesize Research Publications
> The relationship between synthesizing and coding studies is a close one. Before studies can be synthesized, they need to be properly coded. The proper coding of studies relies on knowledge about how the studies will eventually be analyzed and synthesized. Thus, although analysis and synthesis are performed much later in the literature review process, the strategy needs to be delineated before the coding sheet is designed.
>
> Synthesizing research entails categorizing a series of related studies, analyzing and interpreting their findings, and summarizing those findings into unified statements about the topic being reviewed.

RESEARCH METHODS

After completing the groundwork stage, the researcher must choose the appropriate research methods with which to conduct the study. Many methods are available for researchers undertaking policy analyses, such as research review (e.g., meta-analysis), secondary analysis (e.g., research analysis of administrative records), qualitative research (e.g., case study), experimental methods, survey methods (e.g., longitudinal study), and evaluation research. Each method has strengths and weaknesses, and the best strategy often is a combination of methods. There are three categories of research methods: exploratory, descriptive, and explanatory. The appropriate application of the various research methods varies according to these categories. Researchers should carefully consider the field of supporting evidence, research questions, and funding and administrative resources prior to choosing one or more methods.

Exploratory research methods are used to learn more about a little-known topic or to test new research methods. Examples of exploratory research include qualitative efforts, such as case studies or focus groups. Although it is among the least expensive research methods (due, in part, to the frequent use of small sample sizes), exploratory research is also considered the least rigorous, and findings may not be generalizable to other contexts or research questions.

Descriptive research methods are used to investigate study characteristics among subjects; one example is the administration and analysis of survey data. Although descriptive research methods are considered more rigorous than exploratory methods, they can be expensive to conduct because they often require large sample sizes.

The final type of research method, *explanatory research*, includes experimental studies—considered the gold standard among research study methods—as well as case control studies and longitudinal research. These methods are among the most rigorous in design, and thus, findings have the greatest level of generalizability compared with other research methods. Still, it can be expensive, requiring large sample sizes and complex statistical analysis.

> **? FOR YOUR CONSIDERATION**
> Steps in Synthesizing Policy Research Studies
>
> 1. Compile an inventory of public policies that might address the health problem under study.
> 2. Determine the policy that will be the focus of your synthesis.
> 3. Detail the sequence of effects that you expect will link the policy to the problem.
> 4. Synthesize data on the impact of this policy in areas of previous implementation (e.g., effectiveness, unintended effects, effects related to equity) and on related issues (e.g., cost, feasibility, acceptability).
> 5. Consider the data drawn from the literature review in terms of the present context under study.
>
> *SOURCE:* Adapted from NCCHPP (2010).

RESEARCH DESIGN

Once the research problem has been identified, the researcher develops an overall framework for investigation. Research design addresses the planning of scientific inquiry by

- anticipating subsequent stages of the research project, including choosing the research method;

- identifying the unit of analysis and the variables to be measured;

- establishing procedures for data collection; and

- devising an analysis strategy.

Potential implementation strategies must also be considered because much of the value of HPR lies in using research to bring effective and targeted programs and resources to populations in need (Atkins and Kupersmith 2011). Problems that arise in the future would necessitate changes to the research plan.

SAMPLING

In the sampling stage, the researcher must clearly define the population of interest in the study. It is not feasible to study every individual in the population; thus, a sample must be taken to draw conclusions about that population.

Random selection
Methods by which subjects from a sampling frame are randomly selected to create a representative sample.

Four types of sampling methods—often referred to as probability sample designs because each subject in a sampling frame has a known probability of being selected for the sample—incorporate varying degrees of **random selection**:

- *Simple random sampling* is the most basic method, in which every subject in the sampling frame has an equal probability of being selected.

- *Systematic sampling* is a bit more complicated. Every kth subject from the sampling frame is selected (e.g., every fifth subject is selected from the sampling frame). The interval between selected subjects (k) is chosen by the researcher.

- *Cluster sampling* involves the distribution of subjects in the sampling frame into heterogeneous clusters, which are then randomly selected to comprise a sample of clusters. Cluster sampling can be a cost-effective way to conduct research over a broad geographic area.

- *Stratified sampling* is similar to cluster sampling in that subjects from the sampling frame are divided into groups; however, these groups (known as strata) are homogeneous. Once strata are chosen, simple random sampling is used for each stratum to select a final sample. Stratified sampling is chosen to ensure that the sample is representative of the population about which a researcher hopes to draw inferences in terms of characteristics of interest.

See Exhibit 8.6 for an evaluation of probability sampling designs.

	Simple random sampling	Systematic sampling	Cluster sampling	Stratified sampling
Precise	Highest	Moderate	Lowest	Highest
Able to capture groups of interest	No	No	Yes	Yes
Cost-efficient	No	No	Yes	Yes
Requires knowledge of population in advance	No	No	Yes	Yes
Allows for disproportionate sampling	No	No	Yes	Yes
Involves complex data analysis	No	No	Yes	Yes

EXHIBIT 8.6
Trade-offs of Commonly Used Random Sampling Methods

A number of nonprobability sampling methods are also available, such as convenience sampling, quota sampling, purposive sampling, and snowball sampling. The probability of subject selection in a sample is unknown when these methods are used. Although nonprobability sampling methods can be less expensive to employ than probability sampling methods, nonprobability methods cannot be used to make inferences about a population and are subject to research bias.

MEASUREMENT

The measurement, or operationalization, stage involves devising measures that link concepts of interest to empirically observable events or variables. The **measurement's validity** and **reliability** should also be ascertained. Because survey research is frequently used, health policy researchers should be knowledgeable of the general guidelines and specific techniques for writing survey questionnaire instruments.

DATA COLLECTION

Data for HPR can come from a variety of sources, typically categorized as *primary sources* and *existing sources* (see Exhibit 8.7). The research method chosen often influences the method used for data collection. Two commonly used primary data collection tools are interviews and administration of questionnaires. Primary data are collected by researchers for the purpose of their specific study, so primary data tend to be more valid than existing data. Researchers can design the questions they use to gather primary data specifically ac-

Measurement reliability
The extent to which results are similar if the measurement tool is reapplied in a consistent way.

Measurement validity
The extent to which the measurement tool accurately measures the intended concepts.

cording to the study objectives, while existing data from another study may not contain all of the information desired for analysis. However, existing, or secondary, data are widely used in HPR because they tend to be more generalizable and are more efficient in terms of saving time and cost than are primary data.

DATA PROCESSING AND ANALYSIS

Generally, data in their raw format are difficult to analyze and interpret. Before data can be interpreted, the researcher must transform or process the data into a format that can be analyzed. For example, the data may need to be converted into numerical values or "cleaned" to identify data entry errors. In addition, the researcher may need to identify missing data and account for them. The researcher then employs statistical procedures to manipulate the processed data and draw conclusions about the study population.

APPLICATION

The final stage of research deals with the interpretation and use of research. Applying research findings to scientific theory and policy formulation can be the most satisfying step in the research process (see detailed discussion in the next sections). Researchers should also provide recommendations for further research on the subject and outline limitations that may be avoidable in future studies.

EXHIBIT 8.7
Health Policy
Research Data
Sources

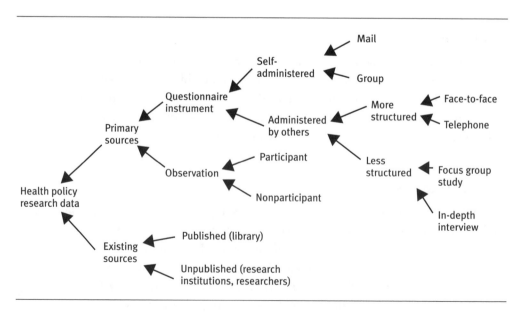

COMMUNICATING HEALTH POLICY RESEARCH

The way in which evidence is disseminated depends on the intended audience. Potential audiences may be divided into three groups: the research community, stakeholders, and the public. The research community includes scientists or others who share similar research interests. Stakeholders are those who provide funding or have a key role in implementing research findings. The public is the population at large affected by the findings of the research who are neither researchers nor stakeholders. Investigators should adapt their communications to specific audiences in order to maximize comprehension and acceptance.

RESEARCH COMMUNITY

When the intended audience is part of the research community, certain assumptions can be made about prior knowledge. Research findings may be summarized, rather than explained in great detail, and technical terms may be used. Researchers must also be as transparent as possible, clearly explaining methods and the reasons behind them. Transparency is even more important regarding studies that employ modeling because the findings that a researcher chooses to include or omit in a study can have an enormous impact on the results (Søgaard and Lindholt 2011).

The most common way of communicating results to the scientific community is by publishing an article on the research in a peer-reviewed scientific journal. Prior to submitting a paper for publication, researchers should be aware of the manuscript preparation guidelines of the journal in question. Because it often takes months for an article to publish from the time of submission and publication, researchers often seek out other ways to publicize research findings.

Professional conferences are another common way to present findings. Professional associations generally hold periodic conferences that offer members the opportunity to present their research. Conferences are an excellent outlet because it is often much easier to get a paper selected for a conference than to have an article accepted by a journal for publication and because results can be presented sooner than in a journal. Conferences also enable the researcher to receive comments, suggestions, and criticism that may be useful for later submission of a research article to a journal.

Working papers and monographs are a third way in which results can be presented to the research community. The implication of calling a document a working paper is that the article is in progress. It is typically circulated among those with the same research interests, with an implicit request for comments and suggestions. Because professional reputations are not at stake when distributing a working paper, tentative analyses and interpretations can be included. Similar to working papers, which are preludes to journal articles, monographs are drafted in preparation for writing books. Monographs are usually written for large, complex projects and may also be circulated among peers for suggestions.

STAKEHOLDERS

When stakeholders are the intended audience, investigators cannot assume any prior knowledge of the research subject and terminology. Stakeholders include funders or sponsors, people affected by the research results, and primary users of the research results. It is important to consider how to best translate research findings for these different stakeholders (Milstein, Wetterhall, and CDC Evaluation Working Group 1999).

A research proposal is often the first point of contact a researcher has with the sponsor or funders. A research proposal is written by the investigator to convince a potential sponsor of his or her qualifications for performing research and to answer questions that are important to a sponsor or funder.

Perhaps the most common means of communicating with stakeholders is through technical reports required by funders and sponsors. Reports often serve the additional purpose of informing policymakers, administrators, and other groups interested in study results. The report should directly address the questions posed by sponsors or funders and be consistent with the intended use and audience of the research. If applicable, it also may summarize the ways in which the research has advanced scientific knowledge.

Stakeholders such as sponsors and policymakers may also be invited to symposiums where the research and its implications for decision makers are discussed. Symposiums provide a forum where the research and its importance to the stakeholders can be fleshed out.

PUBLIC

When the intended audience is the general public, investigators can rely on the mass media to publicize significant research findings. In this instance, presentations to the press should avoid technical language and clearly explain any key terms or concepts. No assumptions should be made about the audience's existing knowledge of the research topic.

Fact sheets and issue briefs are other ways to synthesize and communicate research findings to the public. Many government and private research agencies regularly disseminate summaries of major studies or analyses through fact sheets and issue briefs. For example, the Henry J. Kaiser Family Foundation has produced periodic issue briefs and fact sheets on such topics as Medicaid, the Children's Health Insurance Program (CHIP), Medicare, the uninsured, prescription drugs, HIV/AIDS, minority health, and women's health (www.kff.org).

Researchers must expend more effort to educate the public on HPR. With improved dissemination of research results, the public may take more notice of healthcare findings and implement policy research into their healthcare decision making.

In some cases, the use of community-based participatory research, where members of the community are involved in the actual research study, can lead to the dissemination of research to the public. For example, a study of the cardiovascular risks among Mexican

Americans living along the Mexico–United States border not only collected data on the cardiovascular risks of the population but also informed them of the study results through the community-based researchers (Balcazar et al. 2009).

For researchers conducting studies in the field of health services, the ultimate challenge is to see their findings through to implementation in policy decisions. Because of the applied nature of health services research, a major goal is to apply disciplinary knowledge to solve current and emerging health-related problems. The synthesis and dissemination of health services research have played, and continue to play, an important role in health policy formulation (Ginzberg 1991). Historically, health services research has influenced early health policy formulation, implementation, and clinical practice with respect to HIV/AIDS-related illness and primary care (AHRQ 1990; National Center for Health Services Research and Health Care Technology Assessment 1985).

IMPLEMENTING HEALTH POLICY RESEARCH

The impact of HPR on health policy has grown since that time. For example, research identifying large gaps in access to healthcare has compelled the formulation of policies aimed at healthcare reform to reduce these gaps. The Robert Wood Johnson Foundation's Covering Kids and Families (CKF) initiative represents an elegant integration of HPR and practice (Morgan, Ellis, and Gifford 2005). The CKF initiative aimed to improve states' reenrollment processes for children and families covered by Medicaid and CHIP. An evaluation of the initiative found that it had a positive impact on reenrollment in 45 states and allowed states that have succeeded in improving their reenrollment processes to advise struggling states (Morgan, Ellis, and Gifford 2005).

Research is often dismissed or improperly reflected in policy efforts, leaving investigators frustrated. The remainder of this section identifies several barriers to the implementation of research in policy and some ways to overcome these barriers.

RELEVANCE

Sometimes a scientifically significant study may not have immediate or obvious policy significance. Further investigation may be necessary to make these studies more relevant from both a clinical and a health policy perspective. Studies that translate scientific discoveries into practical (e.g., clinical) applications are termed *translational research*.

TYPE OF STUDY

Adoption of research findings by policymakers and practitioners is also influenced by the type of study conducted. Research with a clinical focus is typically adopted more quickly than that focused on organization because of the importance that evidence plays in clinical practice. Research related to organization is often slowly adopted because organizational practices require more time to change. An emphasis on quality improvement within an organization will often speed up an organization's propensity to change.

Research focused on a national health problem or need takes much longer to influence policy. Often, national policies are formulated through political processes in which stakeholders strongly advocate for their own interests. In this context, research is merely one form of advocacy that competes with other influencers for the attention of policymakers.

PRIORITIES

A potential conflict exists between policy priorities and research priorities. Decision makers, who choose a course of action in response to a given health problem, are generally concerned with the most pressing and current issues. Researchers, who are generally at liberty to choose their research focus, often study problems that do not align with the concerns of decision makers, limiting the reach of useful HPR.

Increasing the frequency of meetings between investigators and decision makers would facilitate the communication process and, in turn, enhance the applicability of research. One way to achieve this increase is by ensuring the presence of decision makers in the governing or consultative bodies of research institutions. Their access to the institutions may more easily bring their needs to the attention of researchers as possible projects.

Community-based participatory research, mentioned earlier, in which academics partner with community leaders who have direct knowledge of community health issues, is becoming increasingly important (O'Brien and Whitaker 2011). The practicality of this type of research is enhanced by including not only decision makers but also stakeholders and community leaders as contributors to the study.

TIMETABLE

Another potential area of conflict between decision makers and investigators is their respective expectations regarding the research timetable. Decision makers facing a pressing problem expect research results immediately. Researchers, on the other hand, are concerned with the validity of the study design and findings and often require more time to complete the research than decision makers are willing to give.

This discrepancy can be reduced by involving decision makers in the research planning phase so that more realistic expectations are set. This gap can also be shortened by producing a series of progress reports outlining intermediate results from the study. During data collection, the participation of respondents and their characteristics can be summarized and reported. Also, immediately after data collection, descriptive summaries can be shared with decision makers before in-depth analyses are conducted.

COMMUNICATION

To enhance the comprehension of decision makers about study findings, research results must be expressed accurately without using technical terms. Investigators are trained to communicate results with specific scientific terms, in part to adhere to scientific journal guidelines, but decision makers often have trouble understanding study design descriptions or statistics used in data analysis. Researchers should help decision makers reach a clear understanding of results by providing them with nontechnical reports.

SCOPE

Differences between policy scope and research scope are another barrier to the implementation of research findings. Because of the inherent complexity of social problems, decision makers require research to provide broad, integrated results that account for all dimensions of the problem. To deliver such results, investigators must overcome their tendency to focus on a well-defined subject and provide broad results instead.

Researchers must be knowledgeable about the context of the problems under investigation so that an integrated project that takes into account all important policy issues can be designed. Effective research will include an analysis that reflects the multiple interests in both the political system and the healthcare system.

VALUES

Researchers and decision makers often place different values on research. Investigators may desire publication in a prestigious scientific journal, whereas decision makers are focused on the applicability of the research to problem solving. Decision makers should, at a minimum, value the contribution that scientific inquiry has made toward improved decision making and understand the criteria for judging quality research. In turn, the scientific community must accept that excellence in research is defined not only as scientific knowledge but also as application for health policies and problem solving.

Because of the role that funding agencies play in the research process, they can often serve as intermediaries between policymakers and researchers. Funding agencies take into account the importance of political needs while balancing a desire to gain advances in science. In short, funding agencies often shape the direction of policy and science by accommodating the values of both the policymakers and the researchers (Braun 1998).

LEADERSHIP

While investigators may provide valid and practical research, leadership is required to transfer HPR into politically acceptable policy. The development and implementation of policy depend on the initiatives taken by decision makers across all levels of society. For example, leaders must promote local ownership of the clinical effectiveness agenda among clinicians and managers, make better use of the skills and expertise available in higher education organizations, increase understanding of the mechanisms that encourage the adoption of new interventions, and facilitate organizational receptivity of new research (Harvey et al. 2011).

RAPPORT

Researchers and decision makers operate interdependently. Decision makers rely on investigators to assist them in making sound and legitimate decisions on the basis of scientific evidence. Researchers need decision makers to help identify research problems, obtain funding, gain access to research sites and subjects, and implement findings. By cooperating, decision makers and researchers increase the potential impact of health services research on policymaking.

SKILLS

Although researchers may possess some background in related disciplines, such as medicine, public health, and political science, they must be competent in several specific skill areas. These skill areas are relevant to each stage of HPR and include knowledge about the subject matter under study, methodology, statistics, computer applications (i.e., software), writing, and public relations. If investigators lack any of these skills, proper steps must be taken to ensure that a member of the research team is able to compensate for the lack of expertise. Many of these skills can be acquired in the classroom, but proficiency in research can be achieved only through experience in the field of HPR.

Subject Matter

The most important research skill is subject knowledge. In-depth knowledge of the subject matter, research data, instruments, funding sources, and survey design is critical to the conceptualization, groundwork, and measurement steps in HPR. For example, conceptualization requires an investigator to clearly understand the topic and purpose of the research, relevant theories and literature, and the process of formulating hypotheses and research questions.

Methodology

The second critical research skill is a command of general research methods. Without a clear understanding of the general approaches to research, the investigator will be unable to select the appropriate research method, study design, sampling model, and type of data collection.

Statistics

The third important research skill is statistical knowledge. This skill is particularly critical in the data analysis, design, sampling, and measurement phases of research. Knowledge of the choice and appropriate application of statistical procedures enable the investigator to conduct research independently.

Computer Application Software

The fourth research skill—knowledge of computer applications—is especially critical for analyses of large data sets. This skill is particularly useful in the data processing and analysis stages of HPR.

Writing

The ability to write is another critical research skill. Whether drafting proposals for funding or reports for publication, investigators must properly convey their research goals. In many cases, they can follow established formats (e.g., research proposals, journal articles). However, the ability to write concise and clear sentences is extremely valuable in producing reports.

Public Relations

Finally, public relations skills are particularly useful in the groundwork, data collection, and application stages of research, as well as for project management. Excellent people skills are essential to acquiring potential funds for a study, obtaining access to research sites and subjects, and successful collaboration with decision makers for policy formulation.

KEY POINTS

➤ HPR can be characterized by five main attributes: its nature as an applied field, its ethics framework, the multidisciplinary input it enjoys, its basis in science, and its focus on population.

➤ Formal approaches to HPR typically include ten steps: conceptualization, groundwork, method(s), design, sampling, measurement, data collection, data processing, data analysis, and application.

➤ HPR findings should be communicated to the research community, stakeholders, and the public.

➤ Barriers constrain the implementation of research in policy. However, researchers and decision makers should operate interdependently.

CASE STUDY QUESTIONS

On the basis of your research of the Rand HIE, answer the following questions:

1. How does the RAND study illustrate the characteristics of health policy research?
2. What specific contributions did the RAND study make to health policies regarding health insurance?

FOR DISCUSSION

1. Define HPR, and describe the difference between HPR and health policy analysis.
2. Discuss the differences and trade-offs between the sampling methods commonly used in HPR.
3. Identify the difference between the reliability and validity of measurements.
4. Discuss the skills needed to become a health policy researcher and why these skills are important.

REFERENCES

Agency for Healthcare Research and Quality (AHRQ). 1990. *Health Services Research on HIV/AIDS-Related Illness*. Rockville, MD: AHRQ.

Anderson, O. W. 1985. *Health Services in the United States*. Chicago: Health Administration Press.

Atkins, D., and J. Kupersmith. 2011. *Implementation Research: A Critical Component of Realizing the Benefits of Comparative Effectiveness Research*. Washington, DC: Office of Research and Development, US Department of Veterans Affairs.

Balcazar, H., L. Rosenthal, H. De Heer, M. Aguirre, L. Flores, E. Vasquez, M. Duarte, and L. Schulz. 2009. "Use of Community-Based Participatory Research to Disseminate Baseline Results from a Cardiovascular Disease Randomized Community Trial for Mexican Americans Living in a U.S.-Mexico Border Community." *Education for Health (Abingdon, England)* 22 (3): 279.

Bardach, E. 2005. *A Practical Guide in Policy Analysis: The Eightfold Path to More Effective Problem Solving*, 2nd ed. Washington, DC: CQ Press.

Bice, T. W. 1980. "Social Science and Health Services Research: Contributions to Public Policy." *Milbank Memorial Fund Quarterly: Health and Society* 58 (2): 173–200.

Braun, D. 1998. "The Role of Funding Agencies in the Cognitive Development of Science." *Research Policy* 27 (8): 807–21.

Brook, R., E. Keele, K. Lohr, J. P. Newhouse, J. E. Ware, W. H. Rogers, A. R. Davies, C. D. Sherbourne, G. A. Goldberg, P. Camp, C. Kamberg, A. Leibowitz, J. Keesey, and D. Reboussin. 2006. "The Health Insurance Experiment: A Classic RAND Study Speaks to the Current Health Care Reform Debate." [Research brief.] Accessed January 20, 2012. www.rand.org/pubs/research_briefs/RB9174.html.

Centers for Medicare & Medicaid Services (CMS). 2012. "National Health Expenditure Data." Accessed March 30, 2013. www.cms.gov/Research-Statistics-Data-and-Systems/Statistics-Trends-and-Reports/NationalHealthExpendData/index.html.

Frenk, J. 1993. "The New Public Health." *Annual Review of Public Health* 14: 469–90.

Ginzberg, E. 1991. *Health Services Research: Key to Health Policy*. Cambridge, MA: Harvard University Press.

Harrison, S. 2001. "Policy Analysis." In *Studying the Organization and Delivery of Health Services,* edited by P. Allen, N. Black, A. Clarke, N. Fulop, and S. Anderson. New York: Routledge.

Harvey, G., L. Fitzgerald, S. Fielden, A. McBride, H. Waterman, D. Bamford, R. Kislov, and R. Boaden. 2011. "The NIHR Collaboration for Leadership in Applied Health Research and Care (CLAHRC) for Greater Manchester: Combining Empirical, Theoretical and Experiential Evidence to Design and Evaluate a Large-Scale Implementation Strategy." *Implementation Science* 23 (6): 96.

Humphreys, J. S., P. Kuipers, J. Wakerman, R. Wells, J. A. Jones, and L. D. Kinsman. 2009. "How Far Can Systematic Reviews Inform Policy Development for 'Wicked' Rural Health Service Problems?" *Australian Health Review* 33 (4): 592–600.

Institute of Medicine (IOM). 1979. *Health Services Research*. Washington, DC: National Academies Press.

Lavis, J. N., S. E. Ross, J. E. Hurley, J. M. Hohenadel, G. L. Stoddart, C. A. Woodward, and J. Abelson. 2002. "Examining the Role of Health Services Research in Public Policymaking." *Milbank Quarterly* 80 (1): 125–54.

Longest, B. 2010. *Health Policymaking in the United States*, 5th ed. Chicago: Health Administration Press.

Milstein, R. L., S. F. Wetterhall, and the CDC Evaluation Working Group. 1999. *Framework for Program Evaluation in Public Health*. Published September 17. www.cdc.gov/mmwr/preview/mmwrhtml/rr4811a1.htm.

Morgan, G., E. Ellis, and K. Gifford. 2005. *Areas of CKF Influence on Medicaid and SCHIP Programs*. Washington, DC: Mathematica Policy Research.

National Center for Health Services Research and Health Care Technology Assessment. 1985. *Health Services Research on Primary Care*. Rockville, MD: National Center for Health Services Research.

National Center for Health Statistics (NCHS). 2011. *Health, United States*. Hyattsville, MD: Public Health Service.

National Collaborating Centre for Health Public Policy (NCCHPP). 2010. "Methods for Synthesizing Knowledge for Public Policies." Quebec, Canada: NCCHPP.

O'Brien, M. J., and R. C. Whitaker. 2011. "The Role of Community-Based Participatory Research to Inform Local Health Policy: A Case Study." *Journal of General Internal Medicine* 26 (12): 1498–501.

Søgaard, R., and J. Lindholt. 2011. "Evidence for the Credibility of Health Economic Models for Health Policy Decision-Making: A Systematic Literature Review of Screening for Abdominal Aortic Aneurysms." *Journal of Health Services Research and Policy* 17 (1): 44–52.

Stokey, E., and R. Zeckhauser. 1978. *A Primer for Policy Analysis*. New York: W. W. Norton.

Taylor, R., A. Bower, F. Girosi, J. Bigelow, K. Fonkych, and R. Hillestad. 2005. "Promoting Health Information Technology: Is There a Case for More-Aggressive Government Action?" *Health Affairs (Millwood)* 24 (5): 1234–45.

World Health Organization (WHO). 2005. "Sustainable Development and Healthy Environments Highlights 2004." Retrieved April 11, 2013. http://whqlibdoc.who.int/hq/2005/WHO_SDE_05.1.pdf.

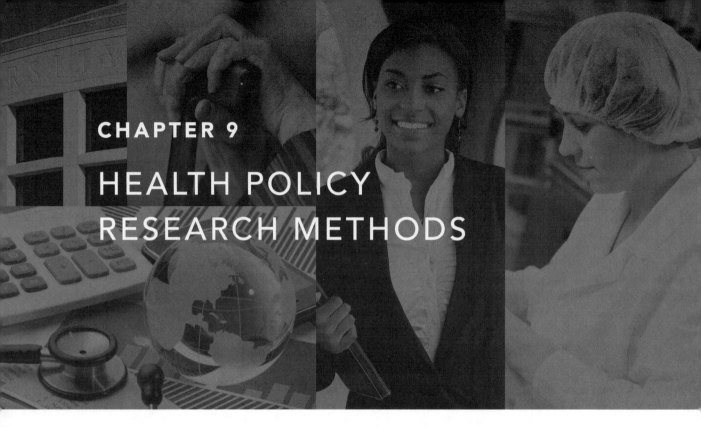

CHAPTER 9
HEALTH POLICY RESEARCH METHODS

Facts, and facts alone, are the foundation of science. . . . When one devotes oneself to experimental research it is in order to augment the sum of known facts, or to discover their mutual relations.

— François Magendie

LEARNING OBJECTIVES

Studying this chapter will help you to

➤ appreciate commonly used methods for health policy research,

➤ discuss experimental research,

➤ understand survey research,

➤ describe the process of conducting evaluation research,

➤ differentiate between cost–benefit analyses and cost-effectiveness analyses, and

➤ appreciate qualitative research methods.

CASE STUDY

HEALTH CENTERS AND THE FIGHT AGAINST HEALTH DISPARITIES IN THE UNITED STATES

The United States has experienced a long history of inequality among its citizens. From civil rights violations and suffrage restrictions, which only began to be resolved in the past 60 years, to the widening income gap between the poor and rich into the early twenty-first century, inequality continues to pervade many aspects of modern life, including education, employment, housing, and other means for fulfilling life necessities. Those most deeply affected are groups delineated by race or ethnicity, socioeconomic status, immigration status, culture and language, and sexual orientation (Shi and Stevens 2010). Perhaps the most persistent manifestation of inequality has been an ongoing and, in some cases, growing disparity in health and well-being across these social divisions. Today it is not unusual to see major health differences between whites and African Americans, the wealthy and poor, or the insured and uninsured. Although the United States spends by far the highest per capita amount on healthcare in the world (Anderson et al. 2006), it ranks in the middle of the pack in international comparisons of quality of care and health status (Hussey et al. 2004; Reinhardt, Hussey, and Anderson 2002; Macinko, Starfield, and Shi 2003).

Recognizing the inefficiencies and injustices created by health disparities, the US Department of Health and Human Services (HHS 2000), through its decennial *Healthy People* publication, seeks to eliminate these disparities. Similarly, the Institute of Medicine publishes reports aiming to increase awareness of these issues, including *Crossing the Quality Chasm* (2001) and *Unequal Treatment* (2003). Research on the various domains of primary care (i.e., accessibility, continuity, comprehensiveness, and coordination) shows that high-quality primary care can attenuate, if not eliminate, the adverse impact of income and racial or ethnic inequality on health (Gaston et al. 2001; Shi, Stevens, and Politzer 2007; Starfield and Shi 2007). In response to these findings, the federal government launched the health center (HC) model as a primary care approach to improving equity.

The HC model features community, migrant, homeless, and public housing health centers, which are also collectively known as federally qualified health centers. They are not-for-profit, community-directed healthcare providers that offer primary and preventive care to predominantly low-income, medically underserved urban and rural communities. HCs are governed by boards whose membership is composed of at least 51 percent (a majority) HC patients, and these centers have served as a crucial component of the nation's safety net system for more than four decades (BPHC 2011; Lefkowitz 2007; Sardell 1988).

In addition to clinical care, HCs provide enabling services, such as transportation, translation, and health education, to facilitate access to care for vulnerable populations. Approximately 1,400 HCs deliver care in every state and territory to more than 20 million people nationwide who are disproportionately low income (greater than 70 percent), uninsured (about 40 percent) or publicly insured (35 percent Medicaid and 8 percent Medicare), and racial and ethnic minorities (64 percent) (BPHC 2011).

Several studies have demonstrated that HCs improve access and deliver high-quality, cost-effective care (Shi, Stevens, and Politzer 2007; Shi and Stevens 2010; Shin, Markus, and Rosenbaum 2006; O'Malley et al. 2005; Proser 2005; Hadley and Cunningham 2004; Politzer et al. 2003; Frick and Regan 2001; Hadley, Cunningham, and Hargraves 2006; Landon et al. 2007). In addition, a number of studies have found that patient outcomes and quality of care in HCs are comparable to or better than those in the private sector (Falik et al. 2006; Hicks et al. 2006; Shin et al. 2008; Ulmer et al. 2000). However, limited research has been conducted to examine whether HCs are able to overcome health disparities, that is, to narrow the differences in healthcare access, quality, and outcomes across racial, ethnic, and socioeconomic population groups.

F ollowing an overview of health policy research from the previous chapter, this chapter illustrates methods commonly used in health policy research. Examples of both quantitative and qualitative methods are provided.

QUANTITATIVE METHODS

Quantitative methods in health policy research include experimental or quasi-experimental research, survey research, evaluation research, and cost–benefit and cost-effectiveness analysis.

EXPERIMENTAL RESEARCH

The purpose of experimental research is to study causal relationships between independent and dependent variables—testing hypotheses under predefined intervention settings to either establish a direct link between two factors or measure the magnitude of the association between them (Broota 1989; Campbell and Stanley 1966; Cochran 1957; Kirk 1994). The Learning Point box provides a definition and characteristics of causal relationships.

Essential Elements of Experimental Research

The ultimate goal of experimental research is to enable inferences to be drawn between the independent and dependent variables in different intervention conditions. In both the natural and social sciences, four elements must be present for research to qualify as experimental: (1) experimental and control groups, (2) randomization, (3) pre- and posttesting, and (4) application of the intervention.

Experimental and Control Groups

Test groups are defined by the service or intervention received; in other words, the experimental group includes those individuals who receive the intervention, and the control group includes those who do not receive the intervention (or who receive an alternative form of intervention).

The main purposes of a control group are to assess the true impact of the service or intervention being studied and to account for possible effects on the outcome that may come from participation in the experimental intervention. In social science experiments, control groups are also used to account for events occurring outside of the experimental setting. In this case, both experimental and control groups are subject to the effects of outside events, but the control group helps ensure that potential biases are accounted for and the true effects of the experiment determined. Although ideally subjects within the control group should be as similar as possible to those in the experimental group on key characteristics (except receipt of the experimental intervention), in reality the degree of similarity varies between groups. Control groups are either *true control groups* (i.e., made equivalent by random assignment, generally ensuring a nonbiased distribution of the various characteristics) or *comparison groups* (i.e., nonequivalent in terms of assignment) (Fitz-Gibbon and Morris 1987).

Randomization

Randomization refers to allocating a set of subjects to either an experimental or a control group by means of some random procedure. Under the best randomization method, each subject has an equal chance of being assigned to either group.

In a pure experimental design, random sampling is used to select a representative number of study subjects from a target population to ensure that study results are generalizable to the population. Randomization procedures are then used to allocate each member of the sample to an experimental or control group, ensuring internal validity of the study.

⊛ LEARNING POINT
Causal Relationship

An association between variables must have three characteristics to be considered a causal relationship:

1. Statistical association—two variables must have a statistically significant relationship, or correlation, for causality to be present.
2. Sequence of influence—a clear temporal sequence must exist between the two variables to determine a cause–effect relationship. The causal factor must occur first, before the effect.
3. Nonspuriousness—a change in one variable results in a change in another regardless of the actions of other variables. Nonspuriousness can occur when an association or a correlation between variables cannot be explained by a variable other than the two involved in the relationship.

Randomization also eliminates potential bias from self-selection, taking into account that people who volunteer for a study are likely to be different than those choosing not to volunteer. Randomization is the most effective way to eliminate alternative explanations of an intervention effect, because it helps account for a variety of characteristics (including those not explicitly captured in the study itself) that may influence study results.

Pre- and Posttesting

Experimental and control groups are typically tested or observed before (pretest) and after (posttest) the intervention at identical points in time (Fitz-Gibbon and Morris 1987). Pretest and posttest results are then compared to assess the impact of the intervention. In the simplest experimental design, a single pretest measurement is taken prior to the subjects' exposure to an intervention and a single posttest measurement is taken following the intervention.

Researchers may make additional observations while the intervention is taking place to measure the impact of the intervention over time. Similarly, a series of measurements or tests may be conducted after a program concludes to measure the long-term impact—called a *time series test* if measurements are taken at equal intervals before and after the program. Often, a time series test can eliminate the need for a control group because results from pretests may project the outcome without the intervention.

Application of the Intervention

The main **independent variables** in an experiment typically take the form of the experimental stimulus, or intervention, that is either present or absent. It is essential that both independent and **dependent variables** be operationally defined for the purpose of the experiment. Examples of common interventions include taking a therapeutic drug, undergoing a treatment procedure, becoming eligible for a service, or responding to a questionnaire.

Types of Experiments

We discuss four types of experiments in which interventions may be applied: (1) laboratory (or controlled) experiments, (2) field experiments, (3) natural experiments, and (4) simulations.

Laboratory Experiments

Laboratory experiments are conducted in artificial settings in which researchers have complete control over the random allocation of subjects to treatment and control groups and

Independent variable
The variable representing the treatment, characteristic, exposure, or other intervention that is being examined to determine its effect on the dependent variable.

Dependent variable
The variable that is examined to determine whether its observed value changes when the independent variable is present or when exposed to the independent variable.

over the degree of intervention applied. This is the ideal type of scientific experiment; however, laboratory experiments are rarely used in policy research because the ability to randomly assign subjects is limited and manipulation of interventions caused by social-, economic-, or health-related factors causes practical and ethical difficulties.

Field Experiments

Health policy studies often employ field experiments, which are conducted outside of laboratories in natural, real-life settings. For example, researchers may study the triage system in emergency departments of urban hospitals, unobtrusively making experimental observations of the normal activities of subjects. Field experiments have high external validity, generally yield generalizable results, and are particularly suitable for applied research focused on problem solving because they enable the researcher to gain insight into how complex problems unfold in the real word.

A major weakness of field experiments is the low level of control the researcher has over experimental conditions (as compared to having complete control over laboratory experiments). Furthermore, because random assignment to study groups may not be possible due to ethical considerations or subject preferences, systematic differences may result between control and experimental groups in terms of participant characteristics and levels of exposure to independent variables and other environmental factors. See the Research from the Field box for an example of a field experiment.

Natural Experiments

Natural experiments are defined by complete lack of control over experimental conditions (as compared to field experiments, which retain some level of research artificiality [i.e., experiments occur purely for research purposes] and in which researchers have control over the random allocation of subjects to treatment and control groups). In studies such as those assessing the effects of lack of access to care on health status, researchers must often rely on truly naturally occurring events in which different levels of exposure exist.

Simulations

Simulation, or modeling, is a special type of experiment that does not rely on subjects or a true intervention (Stokey and Zeckhauser 1978). Simulations are dynamic models that operate over a specified period to demonstrate the structure of the system being studied and the effects on system components when one or more of those components are altered. It is a powerful method that enables researchers to artificially observe what a world exhibiting the study factors of interest might look like as it moves into the future, giving users the opportunity to intervene and attempt to make improvements to system performance (Dooley 2002).

RESEARCH FROM THE FIELD
Experimental Research: Field Experiment

HealthPlus, a not-for-profit organization that provides HMO coverage for Michigan residents and employers, initiated a program in 2008 that gave members online access to performance and quality reports on their plan physicians. To examine how effectively the reports helped members select high-quality physicians, researchers from RAND Corporation conducted a randomized controlled field experiment of new enrollees (Martino et al. 2012).

In 2009 and 2010, the researchers randomly assigned new HealthPlus enrollees to either the experimental group or the control group. The researchers randomized participants who had yet to select a primary care physician by batches on a weekly basis, using an adapted coin-flip technique. Participants in the control group were not encouraged to view the online reports, while participants in the experimental group were encouraged to do so. The encouragement—the intervention in this experiment—comprised a letter from the plan's chief medical officer outlining the importance of the reports and a follow-up phone call.

Randomization of participants to an experimental or a control group, application of an intervention, and observation in a real-world setting are key features of field experiments. Because they examine the real-world impact of an intervention, field experiments are critical to health policy research.

The major advantages of simulations are their high economic feasibility (compared to other types of experiments), ability to magnify visibility of a certain phenomenon, ability to control and manipulate conditions, and availability as a safe alternative to experimentation that may be dangerous or potentially unethical (Fone et al. 2003). The major downside to simulations is their artificiality. The possibility always exists that a simulation is inaccurate or incomplete and that conclusions garnered from a working model are not applicable to the phenomena of interest. Simulation is thus more useful when a significant amount of empirical knowledge is already available because a model is only as good as the assumptions used in its construction.

As this discussion demonstrates, trade-offs are inherent in each experimental technique, and in certain situations, a combination of modeling and real-life experiments is necessary. For example, simulation can illuminate the effects of a program's intervention because it allows greater control over certain factors, but field experiments can reveal the degree to which the actual environment may alter the intervention. Policymakers can benefit from using both modeling and studies conducted in the environment when examining certain topics of interest (Chen et al. 2009).

Perhaps the most well-known health policy experiment is the RAND Health Insurance Experiment (HIE). See the discussion of RAND in Chapter 3, in the "Private Health Foundations" section, and the case study presented in Chapter 8 on the HIE for more detailed information about the organization and this experiment.

QUASI-EXPERIMENTAL RESEARCH

Although randomization is crucial for valid experimental results, in many situations (as in health policy research), it is not always feasible to use for practical and ethical reasons. For example, people may object to being randomly assigned to interventions that will significantly affect their lives. In addition, withholding certain interventions from a control group may be deemed unethical. To avoid these issues, researchers may employ quasi-experimental research methods. Quasi-experimental research is similar to controlled laboratory experiments in that researchers are concerned with the effect of a treatment or intervention but do not randomly assign participants to treatment groups. Because quasi-experimental studies lack the element of random assignment essential to true experimentation (Rossi, Lipsey, and Freeman 2004), researchers must use other methods to ensure some level of comparability between study groups, such as propensity score matching (Fitz-Gibbon and Morris 1987).

Matching is a strategy commonly used for nonrandom assignment of subjects to study groups. Under this approach, researchers attempt to create a control group that is as similar as possible to the experimental group by controlling for one or more major characteristics of the two groups. For example, if demographic characteristics are important, researchers select control group subjects on the basis of how their demographic characteristics compare to the experimental group. As a result, the average demographic characteristics of the experimental group (i.e., age, gender, racial composition) are comparable to those of the control group. Characteristics should only be matched if they are expected to affect the outcome of the intervention (if not taken into account in the study design). Matching ensures some level of similarity between characteristics of the experimental and control groups (other than the intervention) and helps yield more valid findings than would be obtainable by assessing the effect of treatment on unmatched groups.

Stratified random sampling is a similar strategy that combines elements of matching and randomization and may be employed in studies where the sample size is small and the population is **heterogeneous**. Beginning with a pool of subjects, researchers first create **strata** of subjects who are similar in characteristics that need to be matched. Next, subjects are chosen from each stratum and randomly assigned to experimental and control groups.

Matching
The process of ensuring equal representation among experimental and control groups by matching participants or proportions of participants on the basis of selected characteristics.

Stratified random sampling
A random selection of individual subjects from sampling frame subgroups, where each subgroup is made up of individuals who share a characteristic of interest.

Heterogeneous
Consisting of different types; a term used to describe a sample or a population composed of subjects that have dissimilar characteristics.

Strata
Levels into which a population or a sample is divided on the basis of selected characteristics.

Survey Research

The administration of surveys is the most common method of data collection (Converse 1987; Houser and Bokovoy 2006; Miller and Brewer 2003) and is used extensively both inside and outside the scientific community for various purposes (Bailer and Lanphier 1978; Dillman 2000; Fowler 2002; Miller and Salkind 2002; Singleton and Straits 2005). Its application is also widespread among health policy researchers. Those conducting qualitative research (e.g., case studies; see the discussion later in this chapter) may integrate a survey component into the data collection process. Researchers conducting experimental research commonly use surveys to collect additional information on the impact of an intervention. Similarly, survey findings are often used in evaluation research to fully assess a program's impact.

Survey research is defined as (1) the use of a systematic method to collect data directly from respondents that is of interest to researchers and (2) the subsequent analysis of those data using quantitative methods. It aims to measure the distribution of certain characteristics or results among a study sample to provide a detailed description of the population.

Survey administration is popular with researchers because it enables a wide range of topics to be covered. It may be used to discover factual information, such as age and income, or to ascertain beliefs, opinions, or values. When properly constructed, surveys can help researchers explore factors associated with a phenomenon of interest and later test a particular hypothesis.

Typically, survey research consists of the following characteristics (Fowler 2002; Miller and Salkind 2002; Singleton and Straits 2005):

- ◆ Large and randomly chosen samples

- ◆ Systematic instruments

- ◆ Quantitative analysis

A large sample of respondents that is randomly chosen from the population of interest produces survey findings that are more representative and generalizable than are results from small, nonrandom groups. Survey research uses a systematic questionnaire or interview guide to ask questions of respondents. Questions are carefully considered and written beforehand, and they are asked in the same order for all respondents. Interviewers are trained to present questions with exactly the same wording and in the same manner. Standardization of surveys and their administration is of upmost importance because it enhances data reliability by minimizing measurement error.

Cross-sectional survey
A descriptive research method used to examine characteristics of a population within a short time frame.

Survey Types

Surveys may be cross-sectional (capturing one point in time) or longitudinal (providing a series of observations over a period of time). The **cross-sectional survey** is by far the most commonly used survey design. In a cross-sectional survey, data from a cross-section of respondents that represent a target population are acquired within a short period.

The cross-sectional survey method has two major limitations. First, data collected using these surveys do not reveal causal relationships because the data are acquired within a short and limited period. Second, the risk of bias is inherent in study results because the quality of cross-sectional survey data depends on the accuracy with which individuals recall information.

One example of a cross-sectional survey is the 2009 Community Health Center User Survey, conducted by the Bureau of Primary Health Care (BPHC) of the Health Resources and Services Administration. The Community Health Center User Survey collected information on demographics and health status, healthcare utilization, and quality of services received among patients who visit community health centers (HCs). All HCs that received BPHC funding and provided primary care at the time the Community Health Center User Survey was administered were included in the survey's **sampling frame**. The content and sampling strategy of the survey produced a nationally representative snapshot of HCs' characteristics and those of the patients they serve.

Longitudinal surveys follow a single sample, or another similar sample with repeated (at least two) surveys, over a specified period. Data may be collected at predetermined intervals (e.g., at three, six, and nine months over a one-year period) or continuously (e.g., monthly over two years). Longitudinal surveys often are initiated when cross-sectional surveys or other sources of data reveal new trends. They enable researchers to investigate questions about causes and consequences associated with the data of interest and form stronger inferences about causal direction, potentially providing a basis that can substantiate theory.

The use of longitudinal surveys is limited by two factors. First, they are relatively expensive to conduct (due to the need for repeated follow-up), and continual implementation requires long-term funding and a secure organizational base from which the researchers can operate. Second, they are prone to **attrition**—subjects often drop out of the study at some point during the study period. The difficulty with following individuals over time is that the researcher is often left with a smaller subgroup at the completion of the study than at its onset. This subgroup may not be representative of the full population, threatening the validity of study conclusions. Because of the expense associated with conducting longitudinal surveys, many are designed to be multipurpose, asking a variety of questions related to other topics in addition to a core set of questions addressing the topic of interest.

The two major types of longitudinal surveys are trend studies and panel studies. A **trend study** includes a series of cross-sectional surveys used to collect data on the same items within randomly selected samples of a single population. Trend studies can also take on the appearance of cohort studies when the impact of an intervention or a program on a certain group is to be studied. A *cohort* is a group of individuals who experience the same significant event within a specified period or who share some major characteristic. See the Research from the Field box for an example of a longitudinal trend survey.

Sampling frame
The population from which a sample is selected.

Longitudinal survey
A survey administered to the same sample or similar samples at repeated intervals over a predetermined length of time.

Attrition
Loss of participants during a study that measures outcomes over time.

Trend study
A series of cross-sectional studies examining how a characteristic or set of characteristics changes over time through repeated sampling from the overall population.

Most national health surveys sponsored by the federal government are longitudinal trend surveys. One example is the National Health Interview Survey (NHIS), conducted by the National Center for Health Statistics, which is an annual survey of the US noninstitutionalized population that includes detailed questions on health conditions, doctor visits, hospital stays, and personal characteristics. Analyses of NHIS data have informed policy decisions on health insurance mandates and programs to increase access to care for vulnerable populations,

A **panel study** follows a representative sample of the group of interest over time by administering a series of surveys. Whereas trend studies focus on variables and their changes over time, panel studies focus on individuals and how they change over time. For example, the Medical Expenditure Panel Survey (MEPS), conducted by the Agency for Healthcare Research and Quality and the National Center for Health Statistics, is a well-known longitudinal panel survey used to collect information on the financing and utilization of medical services in the United States. The MEPS consists of three major components:

◆   The Household Component Survey—collects medical expenditure data at the personal and household levels

Panel study

A study in which data are collected repeatedly over time from the same sample selected from the overall population to examine how individuals change over time.

RESEARCH FROM THE FIELD
Survey Research: Longitudinal Trend Survey

Beginning in 2006, a longitudinal trend survey of clinician attitudes toward the implementation, use, and impact of electronic health record systems (EHRs) was administered to a network of health centers participating in Atrius Health, a multicenter group practice (El-Kareh et al. 2009). The objective of the longitudinal study was to examine whether clinician attitudes toward the use of EHR would change over the course of time.

Clinicians, nurse practitioners, and physician assistants practicing at selected health centers that were implementing EHR systems were included in this study. Cross-sectional surveys measuring perceptions of the EHR system were administered to all participants 1 month following EHR implementation and then again at 3, 6, and 12 months following implementation. All participants experienced the same intervention (EHR implementation) and were repeatedly surveyed on the same measures to determine changes over the course of one year.

◆   The Medical Provider Component Survey—surveys medical providers and pharmacies identified by household respondents

◆   The Insurance Component Survey—collects data on health insurance plans obtained through private- and public-sector employers

EVALUATION RESEARCH

Evaluation research is most often used for two purposes: (1) program monitoring and improvement or (2) policy application and expansion (Herman, Morris, and Fitz-Gibbon 1987; Stecher and Davis 1987). When researchers apply evaluation research to program monitoring and improvement, they are usually interested in assessing the effectiveness of the program in terms of its implementation, components, participants, cost-effectiveness, and areas for improvement. In contrast to program monitoring and improvement, which assess a program in one particular setting, evaluation research performed for policy application and expansion is intended to assess how well a policy can be applied to other settings (Bissell, Lee, and Freeman 2011). Investigators who engage in evaluation research are typically interested in studying organizational cultures, target populations, resources, financing, or effects on communities.

Evaluation research is most useful when resource constraints exist and the need arises to prioritize problem areas and select those programs that can most effectively and efficiently address health or social problems.

It is also a key methodology by which to fulfill funding requirements. For example, evaluation of health programs and policies is often required to receive funding (CDC 1999), as the Government Performance and Results Act of 1993 mandates that federal agencies set performance goals and measure results. Private sources of funding routinely require performance evaluations as well.

Evaluation research is a form of systematic, applied research conducted to assess programs and policies or their components (Rossi, Lipsey, and Freeman 2004). When used in health policy research, evaluation is performed on a particular product (e.g., therapeutic drug), service (e.g., family planning), or health or social problem (e.g., lack of access to healthcare) to study policy or program components, operation, overall impact, or generalizability to other settings and populations.

A hallmark of evaluation research is the objectivity with which it is performed. Typically, an outside investigator who has no involvement in the implementation of the program or policy is charged with conducting an evaluation through the following activities:

1.   Determining the scope of evaluation

2.   Becoming acquainted with the program

3. Choosing the methodology for evaluation

4. Collecting the data

5. Analyzing the data

6. Reporting findings

Often working with the program or policy sponsor and its staff, an investigator delineates the general purpose of the evaluation, specific components to be assessed, goals and objectives of the evaluation, study design, and evaluation budget. In addition, an investigator may outline the respective roles of researchers and staff in conducting the evaluation and delegate the responsibility for distributing evaluation results to an appropriate research team member (Nelson et al. 2011).

When choosing a study design for evaluation research, both quantitative and qualitative methods may be used, depending on the goals of the evaluation. Quantitative approaches (e.g., administering surveys, recording information from administrative records) are used to measure, summarize, and analyze outcomes or effects and to generalize program or policy results to a population. Qualitative approaches (e.g., conducting focus groups) can offer another dimension through which to properly understand a program or policy, uncover nuances that may not be captured by quantitative data methods, or identify unanticipated outcomes (Alkin et al. 1974; Brownson et al. 2003; Campbell and Stanley 1966; Cook and Campbell 1976; Fitz-Gibbon and Morris 1987; Rossi, Lipsey, and Freeman 2004).

Whether using one or both of these approaches, the following measures are typically examined:

◆ Participant characteristics

◆ Characteristics of the program structure or context that might affect the intervention (e.g., staff characteristics, organizational setting, environmental impact)

◆ Characteristics of program implementation or processes (e.g., types of intervention, activities, staffing, resources)

◆ Characteristics of program outcomes, both long term and short term (e.g., measures of program goals and objectives, including health status, condition, knowledge, satisfaction, behavior changes, and unanticipated outcomes—positive and negative)

◆ Costs and benefits associated with the program and outcomes

Types of Evaluation Research

The main types of evaluation research are needs assessments, process evaluations, and outcome evaluations (Brownson et al. 2003; Herman, Morris, and Fitz-Gibbon 1987; Neutens and Rubinson 1997; Patton 2002; Rossi, Lipsey, and Freeman 2004; Stokey and Zeckhauser 1978).

Needs Assessment

The purposes of a needs assessment are to identify areas of weakness or deficiency (i.e., needs) in a program that can be remedied and to anticipate future conditions to which a program might need to adjust (Herman, Morris, and Fitz-Gibbon 1987).

Needs assessments can be performed at the organization or community level (Brownson et al. 2003; Farley 1993; Green and Kreuter 1991; Herman, Morris, and Fitz-Gibbon 1987). Data are typically obtained from a variety of sources and used to identify problems, prioritize these problems, and determine which outcomes should be pursued.

In an organizational needs assessment, investigators focus on the key components of a program to identify any problems, such as the absence or inadequacy of necessary services, a lack of efficiency, or the delivery of ineffective or superfluous services. Investigators must also carefully consider the effects of proposed solutions on compatibility with program objectives, staff, clients, and finances. Ultimately, it is the job of the investigator, working with evaluation sponsors and program staff, to account for the consequences of alternative solutions and select one that offers the greatest net benefit.

A community needs assessment is more expansive than an organizational needs assessment in terms of the scope of issues that must be considered. Investigators must examine the social, medical, and health characteristics of the population and understand its relationship with the community's health system. When conducting a community needs assessment of vulnerable populations, common problems that are revealed include gaps between services and needs, a lack of knowledge of programs on the part of providers and patients, a lack of coordination between health entities and providers, poor patient education, and maldistribution of necessary services.

Community needs assessments can be especially useful for policymakers. One example is an assessment conducted in Louisiana in 2004. Researchers investigated tobacco use among ninth-grade students in south central Louisiana by surveying more than 4,800 students about their tobacco habits (Johnson et al. 2004). The study team confirmed self-reported survey results by collecting saliva samples from a subset of students. According to the study, more than half of all the students who participated reported smoking a cigarette at some point in time; additionally, researchers were able to identify which racial and ethnic groups were most likely to smoke and what types of social relationships and attitudes were associated with smoking. The results from this needs assessment provided

RESEARCH FROM THE FIELD
Evaluation Research: Community Needs Assessment

Following the World Trade Center attacks on September 11, 2001, a community needs assessment was done to assess the health status and use of mental health services by New York City residents (Boscarino, Adams, and Figley 2004). To collect data, the researchers conducted a telephone survey of 2,368 adults selected through the use of random-digit dialing. Participants were asked a series of questions measuring service utilization, medication usage, mental health status, and general health status. Researchers also asked participants a series of questions regarding their demographic background and social support networks. By examining participants' demographic, social, and health characteristics, the researchers were able to identify gaps in service use among resident subpopulations.

state lawmakers with data to guide tobacco-control efforts, focusing on policies and funding of programs targeted to smoking prevention and cessation among youth. See the Research from the Field box for an example of a community needs assessment.

Process Evaluation

The purpose of a process evaluation is to monitor and improve ongoing programs or policies. A process evaluation usually considers those components that are essential to the implementation and success of a program. For example, it may be used to assess operations by studying the staffing structure, budget, critical activities and services, and administration of a program. It may also be used to ensure that resources are being allocated in the proper and most efficient way or that a program is compliant with legal and regulatory requirements.

Rossi, Lipsey, and Freeman (2004) note that process evaluation can

♦ help investigators ascertain the efficiency with which program administrators conduct their day-to-day activities and identify ways to enhance efficiency;

♦ help investigators identify unexpected problems with program implementation;

♦ provide evidence to funders, sponsors, and other stakeholders that a program is being implemented according to predetermined goals and objectives;

♦ help researchers monitor costs and resource expenditures associated with a program—information that can be crucial for conducting cost–benefit analyses; and

♦ serve as a prerequisite for planning and conducting an outcome evaluation of a program or policy.

Outcome Evaluation

The purpose of an outcome evaluation, also called an *impact assessment*, is to examine the impact of a service, program, or policy and its effectiveness in attaining intended results

(Herman, Morris, and Fitz-Gibbon 1987). Program results are compared with either the status quo or an alternative program with similar goals. To complete an outcome evaluation, a researcher must address many aspects of a program by understanding how its goals and objectives are measured, how its essential components are related to achieving those goals, and how its level of success in accomplishing its intended results can be measured. With this information, the program can be compared with an alternative. After changes are identified that may lead to increased attainment of goals and objectives, a final decision can be made on whether to continue, expand, or modify a program.

Common outcome measures seen in the public health literature include health status, health-related behaviors, performance (e.g., smoking cessation), and effectiveness (e.g., participants' satisfaction on completion of a program). Outcome measures in the field of health services generally refer to the health status of patients (Greenfield and Nelson 1992) and include the traditional outcome measures of mortality and morbidity as well as assessments of physical function, mental well-being, and other aspects of health-related quality of life (Bergner 1985; Greenfield and Nelson 1992; Steinwachs 1989; Ware 1986).

A variety of structured instruments are available for assessing many dimensions of health status, such as measures for general health, pain, social health, and quality of life. These instruments are listed in the Research from the Field box.

Outcomes research conducted at the patient level, called **medical outcomes research** or *effectiveness research*, has become increasingly important in recent years because of the growing number of therapeutic options available to patients, the concomitant increase in healthcare costs, and the resulting need for healthcare reform to control these costs (Parkerson, Broadhead, and Tse 1995). This research typically focuses on the most prevalent or costly medical conditions for which alternative clinical strategies or pathways are available that may be more cost-effective. At the patient level, outcomes research involves linking positive and negative outcomes to the type of care (e.g., drug therapies, surgical procedures, diagnostic care, preventive care, rehabilitative care) received by a variety of patients with a particular condition to identify what treatment works best for which patients (Guadagnoli and McNeil 1994).

Both the public and private sectors are interested in outcomes research focused on measuring health-related outcomes and their predictors. In both sectors, payers are charged with controlling expenditures and helping to

> *Medical outcomes research*
> Research that examines the comparative effectiveness of available treatments for a patient with specified characteristics.

RESEARCH FROM THE FIELD
Health Status Dimensions Assessment Instruments

The following are examples of assessment instruments used to determine a variety of health status dimensions. See the reference citations that accompany each assessment for more information.

- Nottingham Health Profile: Hunt and McEven (1985, 1980)
- Sickness Impact Profile: Bergner et al. (1981, 1976)
- Medical Outcomes Study: 36-Item Short Form Survey: Riesenberg and Glass (1989); Tarlov et al. (1989)
- McGill Pain Questionnaire: Melzack (1983)
- Social Health Battery: Williams, Ware, and Donald (1981)
- Four Single Items of Well-Being: Andrews and Grandall (1976)
- Quality of Life Index: Spitzer, Dobson, and Hall (1981)

improve the quality of care (Bailit, Federico, and McGivney 1995). These aims can be achieved in part by allocating resources to treatments that have been established as effective (Kitzhaber 1993), making outcomes research invaluable to public policymakers and private payers.

Results from outcome evaluations can also enable sponsors to decide whether to continue, expand, or reduce the scope of programs or policies by providing information on the financial implications of different clinical strategies.

Such studies are key drivers in the continued support and funding of the nation's HC network (see the case study at the beginning of this chapter). Community health centers receive a significant portion of their operating budget from the federal government, and outcome evaluations have shown these HCs to provide high-quality, cost-efficient primary and preventive healthcare (e.g., Falik et al. 2006; O'Malley et al. 2005; Shin, Markus, and Rosenbaum 2006). In addition, outcome evaluations have shown that expansion of the HC network is a promising strategy for reducing racial and ethnic disparities in health and healthcare (Shi, Tsai, and Collins 2009; Shi et al. 2004).

Strengths and Weaknesses of Evaluation Research

The major strength of evaluation research is its potential for making an impact on policy. Findings from evaluation research can lead to improved design and implementation of health programs and interventions in the field of public health. Evaluation research offers practical and tangible evidence for policymakers and other decision makers to act on.

It can, however, suffer from selection bias and differential attrition rates (i.e., subjects drop out of each study group at varying rates) due to an inability to randomly assign subjects to study groups. In addition, results from evaluation studies often have limited generalizability; that is, the success of a particular program or policy may not be guaranteed in other environments or settings. Finally, time constraints, financial constraints, and an unfavorable political climate are limitations that can affect the scope and depth of program evaluation.

Key Health Services Evaluation Studies

Examples of important evaluation research related to health services abound in the literature. One of the most notable is the Women's Health Initiative, which evaluated the health risks and benefits of hormone replacement therapy (HRT) for postmenopausal women (Writing Group for the Women's Health Initiative 2002). For decades, HRT was routinely prescribed to this population to help prevent coronary heart disease despite the lack of evidence of HRT's long-term effects. Beginning in 1993, the Women's Health Initiative conducted a rigorous randomized controlled trial with an enrollment of more than 16,000 women to assess the associations between HRT and coronary heart disease, breast cancer, stroke, pulmonary embolism, endometrial cancer, colorectal cancer, and hip fracture. After approximately five years of follow-up study, the trial was abruptly halted in response to the finding that women using HRT experienced unacceptably high rates of invasive breast cancer.

COST–BENEFIT ANALYSIS AND COST-EFFECTIVENESS ANALYSIS

Cost–benefit analysis (CBA) and cost-effectiveness analysis (CEA) are methods by which to analyze or judge the efficiency and net impact of programs. These analyses are particularly useful during evaluation of policy or programs and when considering alternative programs. Following are definitions of CBA and CEA (Guttentag and Struening 1975; Rossi, Lipsey, and Freeman 2004; Stokey and Zeckhauser 1978), and Exhibit 9.1 compares the methods on the basis of key characteristics.

CBA is a type of **efficiency analysis** in which a program's benefits are compared with its costs (direct and indirect) in monetary terms. Benefits and costs may be projected into the future to reflect the lifetime of a program, or the future benefits and costs may be discounted to reflect present values.

CEA is a type of efficiency analysis in which a program's benefits are compared with its costs, but only the costs of the program are monetized. Program benefits in CEA are expressed in outcome units, such as the quality-adjusted life year, which integrates a measure of quality or desirability of a health state for the duration of survival (Haddix, Teutsch, and Corso 2003). CEA is often used to compare the efficiency of programs that share similar goals and outcome measures.

Because both CBA and CEA provide insight on efficiency levels, these analyses are crucial for decisions related to the planning, implementation, continuation, and expansion of health programs. Resource constraints force program directors to measure programs' effectiveness to determine whether or not they should be continued. See the Research from the Field box for an example of cost-effectiveness research.

Efficiency analysis
Analysis of the overall direct and indirect costs and benefits of an intervention; can be used to compare interventions or programs with similar goals.

RESEARCH FROM THE FIELD
Cost-Effectiveness Research

The Health Disparities Collaborative (HDC) is a program that was initiated by the Health Resources and Services Administration (HRSA) Bureau of Primary Health Care (BPHC) to improve the quality of care for chronically ill patients receiving primary care services at HRSA health centers. Various HDCs have been established to focus on specific chronic conditions. To examine the efficiency of the Diabetes HDC, researchers conducted a cost-effectiveness study of the program, using data collected between 1998 and 2002 on a randomly chosen sample of 80 patients with diabetes from a selection of health centers (Huang et al. 2007). The data included information on patient demographics and receipt of services as well as clinical information. Using these data and a simulation model, the researchers determined the resulting quality-adjusted life years (QALYs) and calculated the costs associated with the patients' treatments. The QALYs and costs then were compared to determine the cost-effectiveness of care received through the Diabetes HDC.

Exhibit 9.1

Comparisons
Between Cost–
Benefit Analysis
(CBA) and Cost-
Effectiveness
Analysis (CEA)

(1) Steps	(2) Considerations	(3) CBA	(4) CEA
Specify the accounting perspectives to influence what items are chosen and how items are valued	Decide whether to consider costs and benefits from the perspective of program participants, the program sponsor/funder, or society as a whole	√	
Identify costs and benefits	Include all relevant cost and benefit components to ensure valid results	√	√
Measure costs and benefits (in terms of a common monetary unit) and specify measurement method	Consider opportunity costs (to reflect alternative ways that resources can be used) and externalities (unintended spillover consequences)	√	√
Value costs and benefits; compare total program costs to total program benefits	May employ discounting, a technique used to reduce costs and benefits that are spread out over time to their present or future values	√	√
Assess effectiveness of the program and compare results to similar programs	Measure program benefits in terms of whether the program reached its substantive goals		√

SOURCES: Adapted from Blaney (1988); VA (1989); Drummond et al. (2005); Patrick (1993); Pearce (1981); Rossi, Lipsey, and Freeman (2004); Rowland (1995); Stokey and Zeckhauser (1978); Veney and Kaluzny (2005).

QUALITATIVE METHODS

Qualitative research can serve as a critical complement or alternative to quantitative research. It is particularly useful as an exploratory study method when little is known about a program or its outcomes. In contrast to quantitative research, in which numbers represent the bulk of an analysis, qualitative research attempts to embody observations and analyses captured in statements and concepts obtained from open-ended responses and quotes from participants.

The goal of qualitative research is to gain individual accounts of actions, knowledge, thoughts, and feelings. Researchers attempt to understand the perspective of a program insider by capturing the participant's view of reality. By examining the program from this perspective, qualitative researchers hope to gain insight into a complicated event or problem.

TYPES OF QUALITATIVE RESEARCH

Many types of qualitative methods are used in research; in fact, a number of terms are commonly applied to the methodological approaches examined here (Patton 2002). For example, qualitative research is often referred to as *field research* because the study often takes place in a natural social setting to allow researchers direct and close contact with subjects and situations under study.

The three most widely used qualitative approaches are participant observation, the in-depth interview, and the case study (Babbie 2006; Patton 2002; Rubin 1983; Singleton and Straits 2005; Yin 2003).

Participant Observation

Direct participation and close observation are critical methodologies by which to understand a program, enabling researchers to go beyond the selective perceptions of others and experience a program firsthand. Qualitative observation differs from other forms of scientific observation because it takes place in a natural setting (rather than a controlled setting or laboratory) and requires the researchers to be physically present for direct observation (rather than participating in an indirect capacity, such as through the use of surveys).

Often referred to as *observational research*, participant observation allows researchers to become part of the group or setting of interest. Participation can either be open, with investigators making known their role as researchers, or disguised, with only group leaders or the heads of organizations being made aware that the observation is taking place. The selection of open versus disguised participation depends on whether knowledge that an observer is present will significantly affect normal behavior.

As participants, researchers pay close attention to the physical, social, and human environment; formal and informal interactions; and unplanned activities surrounding the topic under study. By directly observing operations within the research setting, researchers gain a better understanding of the context and process of the environment.

In-Depth Interview

An in-depth interview can take one of three forms: the informal conversational interview, the general interview guide approach, and the standardized open-ended interview (Patton 2002).

Informal conversational interview
An interview conducted in observational studies that does not follow a prescribed set of questions.

An **informal conversational interview** is the most unstructured of the three types. Often occurring during the course of fieldwork, informal conversational interviews do not include specific predetermined questions or presentation of general topics. The interaction is organic, allowing researchers to spontaneously generate questions depending on the flow of conversation.

The **general interview guide approach** is more structured than an informal conversational interview but allows the researcher some flexibility in conducting an in-depth interview. Under this methodology, a researcher follows an outline listing the issues to be explored during the interview; however, the interviewer's approach to raising the issues is unstructured and the questions asked are open-ended and vary in length. The outline ensures that no major issues are omitted. The general interview guide approach often yields new findings that may determine subsequent interview questions.

General interview guide approach
An approach to conducting interviews that provides an outline of subjects the interviewer is required to cover but allows the interviewer flexibility with regard to the type and order of questions asked.

The **standardized open-ended interview** is the most structured of the three in-depth interview types. The interview is based on a questionnaire that contains a set of carefully worded and sequenced questions. Each respondent is asked the same set of questions in the same sequence. Although the standardized open-ended interview affords the researcher less flexibility and spontaneity, it minimizes variation in the questions asked.

In-depth interviews may be conducted with an individual or a group of individuals. The latter is often referred to as a focus group study, or merely focus group (Morgan 1997). A focus group typically consists of 6 to 12 people who are brought together to engage in a guided discussion of a topic. Participants are selected on the basis of their experience with the topic rather than through the use of probability sampling methods, as in experimental and quasi-experimental research. Conducting a focus group can be an efficient way to gather information that would be difficult to capture through a survey or an individual interview because a focus group establishes a context for the perspectives of group members and allows researchers to assess whether these perspectives are consistent among the target population. Focus groups are often used to assess outreach efforts of programs and policies, such as health insurance coverage programs aimed at vulnerable populations.

Standardized open-ended interview
A structured interview that is conducted by reciting predetermined open-ended questions verbatim in a specified order.

The use of in-depth interviews offers several advantages, including flexibility in how and where an interview is conducted, high face validity in terms of interview responses, and low associated costs (Patton 2002). However, in-depth interviews have several limitations. Researchers often confront time limits that may affect the number of questions asked or issues explored. The less structured formats of the informal conversational interview, general interview approach, and focus group study allow the researcher less control than more structured methods provide. Furthermore, data from in-depth interviews can be a challenge to analyze because the process of conducting and transcribing the interview demands considerable time and requires that the investigator remain objective to capture the participant's statements accurately. See the Research from the Field box for an example of an in-depth interview.

RESEARCH FROM THE FIELD
Qualitative Research: In-Depth Interviews

To assess the capabilities of community health centers (CHCs) to respond to emergency and disaster situations, researchers conducted a series of focus groups between 2006 and 2007 with CHC staff in New York City (Ablah et al. 2008). Focus groups are a qualitative research method used to conduct open-ended, in-depth interviews.

The researchers did not randomly choose participants; administrators and medical directors who were members of the Community Health Care Association of New York State Emergency Preparedness Advisory Committee were recruited and assigned to one of three focus groups of 6 to 12 participants each. A predeveloped script of questions was used to direct the participants' conversation toward discussion of New York CHCs' competency in responding to emergency situations and the use of/further need for emergency preparedness training. The use of this method enabled the researchers to gain an in-depth understanding of the capacity of multiple CHCs and collect information that could be used to develop future programming and training.

Case Study

A case study may be defined as an empirical inquiry that uses multiple sources of evidence to investigate a real-life social entity or phenomenon (Yin 2003). A case study typically takes place in a single social setting, such as an organization, a community, or an association. Case studies can be especially valuable when the researcher is trying to make distinctions between different environments, as they can provide rich detail so that in-depth, comprehensive understanding of programs may be achieved.

The case study method is flexible and diverse; the type and quantity of data collected and analyzed can vary greatly. Researchers typically use several methods of data collection, including the analysis of administrative records, in-depth interviews, structured surveys, and participant observation. Multiple data sources enable researchers to construct a more complete account of the issues under study than does a single source. These characteristics make case studies useful in both qualitative and quantitative research.

The ways that researchers can define *cases* are equally as diverse as the potential data sources that may be used in case study. Types of cases may include a person, an event, a program, a critical incident, or a community.

During a case study of an individual, interviews are typically conducted over an extended period to obtain detailed accounts of a personal history. Individual case studies are commonly used to study ethnic or cultural groups with distinctive experiences. In addition to the individual's account, interviews of family and friends and observations of relevant social settings or events can provide an enhanced picture of an individual's history.

In contrast, case studies that focus on a particular social entity or group seek to describe certain aspects of community life. For example, a community case study can provide a detailed account of a community's organization and needs for assessing a community-based healthcare network.

A case study may also be conducted for organizations or institutions, such as health services organizations, schools, or regulatory agencies. For example, a case study of a health maintenance organization may reveal its impact on cost containment and quality of care. Similarly, a political interest group case study can help measure the group's influence on health policies of interest.

QUALITATIVE STUDY DESIGN

Similar to quantitative methods, qualitative research should begin with a review of the relevant literature and background information so that researchers may become familiar with the population, the setting, and issues of relevance in a field study. Investigators must also ensure that they can gain the desired level of access to study participants and a research setting that will fulfill the research inquiry. In qualitative research, investigators often work closely with program administrators and other staff; such entities are crucial to facilitating access to study participants (Grady and Wallston 1988).

As previously stated, the primary difference between quantitative and qualitative research is that in the latter, investigators do not attempt to manipulate the research setting. Qualitative study—and thus qualitative study design—depends on the changing nature of the setting, and in many cases, the design is not finalized until the major issue of study and potential opportunities and obstacles are identified.

The next several paragraphs describe a number of design considerations unique to qualitative study, including the unit of analysis, preliminary sampling procedures, the researcher's role in the study, ethical implications, data collection, and analysis strategy.

Unit of Analysis

In qualitative research, the unit of analysis selected depends on the research goals for the study. Units of analysis may include individuals; groups; incidents or longer-term actions, such as events and activities; or the research setting itself. The unit of analysis in turn determines the researcher's strategies for data collection, analysis, and reporting.

Sampling

The sites and subjects from which the qualitative research investigator can select a sample are typically determined on the basis of their availability and accessibility. Researchers must rely on alternatives to probability sampling in order to choose a sample that is as representative as possible to the population. One such method is **purposive**, or **quota**, **sampling**, which is used to ensure that a small sample of individuals or entities is similar to the target population of interest in terms of important characteristics. For example, if qualitative research is conducted to investigate statewide hospital conditions, limitations on funding and other resources may only allow for a few sites to be included. A purposive sampling technique may help researchers choose hospitals that share certain characteristics with the average hospitals in the state, such as an urban or rural location, socioeconomic status of the patients in the community, or size. Thus, the use of this method ensures that the results of this qualitative research will be generalizable.

Other commonly used qualitative sampling methods are time sampling, typical case sampling, extreme (deviant) case sampling, intensity sampling, and stratified purposeful sampling (Patton 2002). Time sampling is based on sampling periods (e.g., months of the year) or units of time (e.g., hours of the day) and is used when activities are believed to vary significantly from one period to the next. Typical case sampling gives the researcher the ability to compile a profile of one or more typical cases to determine the major characteristics of the study. In contrast, extreme case sampling focuses on cases that are vastly different from typical cases, providing examples of unusual or extreme situations. Intensity sampling uses the most information-rich cases to provide researchers with detailed accounts of events or situations of interest. Finally, stratified purposeful sampling combines typical and extreme case sampling to produce samples that fall along an entire spectrum of characteristics.

Purposive (quota) sampling
A nonprobability sampling technique whereby the investigator selects among accessible sites or participants to establish proportions of characteristics in the sample that are similar to the proportions found in the population.

Role of Researchers

The role of investigators and the degree to which they reveal themselves during the study must be clearly defined during the preliminary stages of a study. The researcher's role may range from solely observation (i.e., the investigator simply watches events) to full participation (i.e., the investigator interacts as a member of the group).

Ethical Implications

Ethical considerations are extremely important when designing and implementing qualitative research. Potential risks, such as bodily harm, side effects, legal liabilities, and ostracism by colleagues, must all be taken into account. (See the discussion in Chapter 8 on the ethical framework of health policy research.)

Data Collection

In general, qualitative researchers use multiple sources of evidence to address a broad range of issues related to a topic and to validate study findings. As previously described, the most common methods of data collection are observations, interviews, and case studies.

To properly collect data, researchers must be adept interviewers. Even during informal conversational interviews, certain protocols must be followed. Prior to the interview, the interviewer must have a general understanding of the topic and issues under study as well as the type of information desired. During the interview, the investigator must maintain neutrality by avoiding leading questions or mentioning personal opinions. Finally, the interviewer must listen to the complete, detailed answers while also understanding that the interview setting may influence those answers.

Technology is becoming increasingly useful in the data collection process, which has important implications for qualitative research. First, a larger amount of data for future analysis can be collected by technological means than can be gained manually, allowing for a more comprehensive qualitative study (Peacock et al. 2011). Technology can also facilitate the participation of program staff and support future evaluation efforts.

Analysis Strategy

Through descriptions, field notes, and coding schemes, researchers must not only produce detailed descriptions of subjects' perspectives through anecdotes, examples, and quotes but must further organize these descriptions into a comprehensible framework suitable for analysis. Descriptions may be organized by the various periods and processes they cover, the level of importance to the study, the extent to which they focus on critical events, or how they fall within the major unit of analysis.

Researchers are also responsible for explaining and interpreting the actions, activities, and beliefs described by participants and assigning significance to the results, themes, and concepts identified as possible components of grounded theories.

The frequent review and editing of field notes is one way to facilitate later analysis. The coding can begin with a small segment of data (e.g., with interview or observational notes) for which the researcher identifies each unique response, theme, or concept. Coding strategies act as a foundation for analyzing the next segment of data and can later be refined when a better understanding of the data is reached. When new categories no longer present themselves during data collection, the researcher can develop instructions for coding. After this step, all of the data should be recoded using the same instructions and framework.

While an exhaustive overview of the approaches used to analyze qualitative data is beyond the scope of this book, two central methods—constant comparative analysis and narrative analysis—are described below.

Constant Comparative Analysis

Glaser and Strauss (1967) first developed constant comparative analysis in their seminal text, *The Discovery of Grounded Theory*. The constant comparative process involves comparing one piece of data (e.g., a single interview or statement) to others in order to develop an understanding of the relationships between different pieces of data (Thorne 2000). This method enables the researcher to identify similarities and differences across data sets and potentially develop theories about the relationships and patterns that emerge from the data. The use of constant comparative analysis produces an enhanced understanding of a human phenomenon within a specific context, enabling the researcher to develop theories about basic social processes and factors that may account for variation in people's experiences of these processes (Thorne 2000).

One example of this type of analysis is a study conducted at the Washington Diabetes Care Center in Seattle by researchers who used constant comparative methods to explore issues of trust and collaboration in the healthcare setting (Ciechanowski and Katon 2006). First, 27 diabetic patients completed a self-report measure of "attachment style," which captured the level of trust patients felt toward the healthcare system. The set of patient responses was used to capture a wide range of attachment styles among the group, allowing for comparisons within the group. Researchers then interviewed the patients, asking questions about their experiences within the healthcare setting and their interactions with providers. By comparing the interview results of patients with varying levels of attachment style, the investigators were able to develop theories about how patients with different levels of trust in the healthcare system could be better served.

Narrative Analysis

Narrative analysis involves generating, interpreting, and representing people's stories (Thorne 2000). As Chase (2005, 657) explains, narrative analysis as a method of qualitative research is distinguished by its ability to "highlight the uniqueness of each human action and event rather than their common properties." In contrast to constant comparative analysis, which aims to identify similarities across groups, narrative analysis aims to identify patterns and themes within each narrative. Thus, rather than create generalizations, the goal of narrative research is to emphasize the particularity of each narrative and to place each into a broader frame (Chase 2005).

In health policy research, narrative analysis can help improve understanding in areas such as patients' personal experiences with disease. For instance, noting the small amount of literature that addresses living with lupus (a chronic autoimmune disease), one researcher conducted a narrative analysis using interview data from lupus patients (Mendelson 2006). Seven women with lupus participated in three interviews, conducted one month apart, and maintained a daily symptom journal. Accounts were also gathered from 23 additional women. Using narrative analysis, the researcher identified patterns and themes within each narrative and noted many overlapping themes across the narratives, such as feelings of uncertainty, a shifting sense of identity, and experiences of financial stress related to living with lupus. Such research is important in shaping programs and funding therapies both in and beyond the healthcare setting.

Ensuring Rigor in Qualitative Research

Devers (1999) and Bowling (1997) cite several criteria for ensuring the rigor and quality of qualitative research. First, the research question, theoretical framework, methods of the research process, and context of the research should be clearly defined. The research study design should reflect the researcher's understanding of the implications of choosing a particular sample. Similarly, researchers must choose an appropriate sample size that will ensure that useful information is collected, while avoiding the saturation point, at which similar ideas are repeated by study participants. In fact, qualitative researchers have increasingly called for a more rigorous definition of what saturation entails, as this concept has been invoked to justify small samples with inadequate data for explanation (Charmaz 2006).

Data collection methods, data types and sources, and analysis methods must also be described and justified. Ideally, an independent investigator should be able to replicate the data collection and analysis to produce similar results. The validity and reliability of qualitative research can also be improved through triangulation methods, in which several quantitative and qualitative methods may be used to study the same topic. Other strategies for enhancing the rigor of qualitative research include searching for evidence that may disprove results, carrying out data archiving, and conducting a peer review. Finally, researchers must carefully consider the information they or their colleagues present in a final report and how that information will be interpreted by sponsors and other stakeholders. For example, presenting adequate amounts of raw data (e.g., transcripts of interviews) in the final report supports the researcher's claim that interpretations of the data are based on evidence rather than subjective impressions.

Key Points

➤ Quantitative methods in health policy research include experimental or quasi-experimental research, survey research, evaluation research, and cost–benefit and cost-effectiveness analysis.

➤ The main difference between experimental and quasi-experimental research is that in the latter, there is no random assignment of participants to treatment groups; thus, researchers must use other methods to ensure that study groups are comparable.

➤ Survey research is a popular approach to studying health policy. It provides a systematic way to capture data from a large sample.

➤ Evaluation in health policy research allows researchers to objectively assess policy or program components, operations, or impacts associated with a particular product, service, or problem.

➤ Qualitative research is performed to capture and categorize observations and thoughts into cohesive themes and concepts; the most widely used types are participant observation, the in-depth interview, and the case study.

CASE STUDY ASSIGNMENT

Using one quantitative and one qualitative health policy research method described in this chapter, design a study to examine whether health centers are able to reduce or eliminate health disparities (i.e., differences in access, quality, and health outcomes) across racial or ethnic and socioeconomic subpopulations.

FOR DISCUSSION

1. What methods are commonly used in health policy research?
2. What are the conditions for causal relationship?
3. What are the essential elements for experimental research?
4. Describe different types of experimental research and situations where they are most appropriately used.
5. What is survey research?
6. What is the difference between a cross-sectional survey and a longitudinal survey?
7. What is a panel study?
8. What is evaluation research?
9. Differentiate needs assessments, process evaluations, and outcome evaluations.
10. Differentiate cost–benefit analysis and cost-effectiveness analysis.
11. What methods are commonly used in qualitative research?
12. Describe the case study method.
13. Describe the process of designing a qualitative study.
14. What steps can be taken to enhance rigor in conducting qualitative research?

REFERENCES

Ablah, E., A. M. Tinius, L. Horn, C. Williams, and K. M. Gebbie. 2008. "Community Health Centers and Emergency Preparedness: An Assessment of Competencies and Training Needs." *Journal of Community Health* 33 (4): 241–47.

Alkin, M. C., J. Kosecoff, C. T. Fitz-Gibbon, and R. Seligman. 1974. *Evaluation and Decision-Making: The Title VII Experience*. CSE Monograph Series in Evaluation No. 4. Los Angeles: Center for the Study of Evaluation.

Anderson, G. F., B. K. Frogner, R. A. Johns, and U. E. Reinhardt. 2006. "Health Care Spending and Use of Information Technology in OECD Countries." *Health Affairs* 25 (1): 819–31.

Andrews, F., and R. Grandall. 1976. "The Validity of Measures of Self-Reported Well-Being." *Social Indications Research* 3: 1–19.

Babbie, E. 2006. "Field Research." In *The Practice of Social Research*, 11th ed., chap. 11. Belmont, CA: Thomson/Wadsworth.

Bailer, B., and C. Lanphier. 1978. *Development of Survey Research Methods to Assess Survey Practices*. Washington, DC: American Statistical Association.

Bailit, H., J. Federico, and W. McGivney. 1995. "Use of Outcomes Studies by a Managed Care Organization: Valuing Measured Treatment Effects." *Medical Care* 33 (4, Suppl.): AS216–AS225.

Bergner, M. 1985. "Measurement of Health Status." *Medical Care* 23: 696–704.

Bergner, M., R. Bobbitt, W. B. Carter, and B. S. Gilson. 1981. "The Sickness Impact Profile: A Development and Final Revision of a Health Status Measure." *Medical Care* 19 (8): 787–805.

Bergner, M., R. Bobbitt, S. Kressel, W. E. Pollard, B. S. Gilson, and J. R. Morris. 1976. "The Sickness Impact Profile: Conceptual Formulation and Methodology for the Development of a Health Status Measure." *International Journal of Health Services* 6: 393–415.

Bissell, K., K. Lee, and R. Freeman. 2011. "Analysing Policy Transfer: Perspectives for Operational Research." *International Journal of Tuberculosis and Lung Disease* 15 (9): 1140–48.

Blaney, D. R. 1988. *Cost-Effective Nursing Practice: Guidelines for Nurse Managers*. Philadelphia: Lippincott.

Boscarino, J. A., R. E. Adams, and C. R. Figley. 2004. "Mental Health Service Use 1-Year After the World Trade Center Disaster: Implications for Mental Health Care." *General Hospital Psychiatry* 26 (5): 346–58.

Bowling, A. 1997. *Research Methods in Health: Investigating Health and Health Services.* Buckingham, UK: Open University Press.

Broota, K. D. 1989. *Experimental Design in Behavioral Research.* New York: Wiley.

Brownson, R. C., E. A. Baker, T. L. Leet, and K. N. Gillespie. 2003. *Evidence-Based Public Health.* Oxford, UK: Oxford University Press.

Bureau of Primary Health Care (BPHC), Health Resources and Services Administration. 2011. "Health Center Data." Accessed March 27, 2013. http://bphc.hrsa.gov/healthcenterdata-statistics/index.html.

Campbell, D. T., and J. C. Stanley. 1966. *Experimental and Quasi-experimental Designs for Research.* Chicago: Rand McNally.

Centers for Disease Control and Prevention (CDC). 1999. "Framework for Program Evaluation in Public Health." *Morbidity and Mortality Weekly Report* 48 (RR-11).

Charmaz, K. 2006. *Constructing Grounded Theory: A Practical Guide Through Qualitative Analysis.* London: Sage.

Chase, S. E. 2005. "Narrative Inquiry: Multiple Lenses, Approaches, Voices." In *The Sage Handbook of Qualitative Research*, 3rd ed., chap. 25, edited by N. K. Denzin and Y. S. Lincoln. Thousand Oaks, CA: Sage.

Chen, J., A. Flabouris, R. Bellomo, K. Hillman, S. Finfer; MERIT Investigators for the Simpson Centre, and ANZICS Clinical Trial Group. 2009. "Baseline Hospital Performance and the Impact of Medical Emergency Teams: Modelling vs. Conventional Subgroup Analysis." *Trials* 10: 117.

Ciechanowski, P., and W. J. Katon. 2006. "The Interpersonal Experience of Health Care Through the Eyes of Patients with Diabetes." *Social Science and Medicine* 63 (12): 3067–79.

Cochran, W. G. 1957. *Experimental Designs*. New York: Wiley.

Converse, J. 1987. *Survey Research in the United States*. Berkeley: University of California Press.

Cook, T. D., and D. T. Campbell. 1976. "The Design and Conduct of Quasi-experimental and True Experiments in Field Settings." In *Handbook of Industrial and Organizational Psychology*, edited by M. Dunnette. Chicago: Rand McNally.

Devers, K. J. 1999. "How Will We Know 'Good' Qualitative Research When We See It? Beginning the Dialogue in Health Services Research." *Health Services Research* 34 (5, Pt. 2): 1153–87.

Dillman, D. A. 2000. *Mail and Internet Surveys: The Tailored Design Method*, 2nd ed. New York: Wiley.

Dooley, K. 2002. "Simulation Research Methods." In *The Blackwell Companion to Organizations*, edited by J. Baum, 829–48. Oxford, UK: Blackwell.

Drummond, M. F., M. J. Sculpher, G. W. Torrance, B. J. O'Brien, and G. L. Stoddard. 2005. *Methods for the Economic Evaluation of Health Care Programmes*, 3rd ed. New York: Oxford University Press.

El-Kareh, R., K. G. Tejal, E. G. Poon, L. P. Newmark, J. Ungar, S. Lipsitz, and T. D. Sequist. 2009. "Trends in Primary Care Clinician Perceptions of a New Electronic Health Record." *Journal of General Internal Medicine* 24 (4): 464–68.

Falik, M., J. Needleman, R. Herbert, B. Wells, R. M. Politzer, and M. B. Benedict. 2006. "Comparative Effectiveness of Health Centers as Regular Source of Care: Application of Sentinel ACSC Events as Performance Measures." *Journal of Ambulatory Care Management* 29 (1): 24–35.

Farley, S. 1993. "The Community as Partner in Primary Health Care." *Nursing and Health Care* 14: 244–49.

Fitz-Gibbon, C. T., and L. L. Morris. 1987. *How to Design a Program Evaluation*. Newbury Park, CA: Sage.

Fone, D., S. Hollinghurst, M. Temple, A. Round, N. Lester, A. Weightman, K. Roberts, E. Coyle, G. Bevan, and S. Palmer. 2003. "Systematic Review of the Use and Value of Computer Simulation Modeling in Population Health and Health Care Delivery." *Journal of Public Health Medicine* 25 (4): 325–35.

Fowler, F. J. 2002. *Survey Research Methods*, 3rd ed. Thousand Oaks, CA: Sage.

Frick, K. D., and J. Regan. 2001. "Whether and Where Community Health Centers Users Obtain Screening Services." *Journal of Healthcare for the Poor and Underserved* 12 (4): 429–45.

Gaston, M. H., R. G. Hughes, R. M. Politzer, J. Regan, L. Shi, and J. Yoon. 2001. "Inequality in America: The Contribution of Health Centers in Reducing and Eliminating Disparities in Access to Care." *Medical Care Research and Review* 58 (2): 234–48.

Glaser, B. G., and A. L. Strauss. 1967. *The Discovery of Grounded Theory*. Hawthorne, NY: Aldine.

Grady, K. E., and B. S. Wallston. 1988. *Research in Health Care Settings*. Newbury Park, CA: Sage.

Green, L., and M. Kreuter. 1991. *Health Promotion Planning: An Educational and Environmental Approach*. Mountain View, CA: Mayfield.

Greenfield, S., and E. C. Nelson. 1992. "Recent Developments and Future Issues in the Use of Health Status Assessment Measures in Clinical Settings." *Medical Care* 30 (Suppl.): MS23–MS41.

Guadagnoli, E., and B. J. McNeil. 1994. "Outcomes Research: Hope for the Future or the Latest Rage?" *Inquiry* 31 (1): 14–24.

Guttentag, M., and L. Struening (eds.). 1975. *Handbook of Evaluation Research*, Vol. 2. Beverly Hills, CA: Sage.

Haddix, A. C., S. M. Teutsch, and P. S. Corso. 2003. *Prevention Effectiveness: A Guide to Decision Analysis and Economic Evaluation*. Oxford, UK: Oxford University Press.

Hadley, J., and P. Cunningham. 2004. "Availability of Safety Net Providers and Access to Care of Uninsured Persons." *Health Services Research* 39 (5): 1527–46.

Hadley, J., P. Cunningham, and J. L. Hargraves. 2006. "Would Safety-Net Expansions Offset Reduced Access Resulting from Lost Insurance Coverage? Race/Ethnicity Differences." *Health Affairs* 25 (6): 1679–87.

Herman, J. L., L. L. Morris, and C. T. Fitz-Gibbon. 1987. *Evaluator's Handbook*. Newbury Park, CA: Sage.

Hicks, L. S., A. J. O'Malley, T. A. Lieu, T. Keegan, N. L. Cook, B. J. McNeil, B. E. Landon, and E. Guadagnoli. 2006. "The Quality of Chronic Disease Care in U.S. Community Health Centers." *Health Affairs* 25 (6): 1713–23.

Houser, J., and J. L. Bokovoy. 2006. *Clinical Research in Practice: A Guide for the Bedside Scientist*. Sudbury, MA: Jones and Bartlett.

Huang, E. S., Q. Zhang, S. E. S. Brown, M. L. Drum, D. O. Meltzer, and M. H. Chin. 2007. "The Cost-Effectiveness of Improving Diabetes Care in U.S. Federally Qualified Community Health Centers." *Health Services Research* 42 (6): 2174–93.

Hunt, S., and J. McEven. 1985. "Measuring Health Status: A New Tool for Clinicians and Epidemiologists." *Journal of Royal College General Practitioners* 35: 185–88.

———. 1980. "The Development of a Subjective Health Indicator." *Social Health and Illness* 2 (3): 231–46.

Hussey, P. S., G. F. Anderson, R. Osborn, C. Feek, V. McLaughlin, J. Millar, and A. Epstein. 2004. "How Does the Quality of Care Compare in Five Countries?" *Health Affairs* 23 (3): 89–99.

Institute of Medicine (IOM). 2003. *Unequal Treatment: Confronting Racial and Ethnic Disparities in Healthcare*. Washington, DC: National Academies Press.

———. 2001. *Crossing the Quality Chasm: A New Health System for the 21st Century*. Washington, DC: National Academies Press.

Johnson, C. C., L. Myers, L. S. Webber, and N. W. Boris. 2004. "Profiles of the Adolescent Smoker: Models of Tobacco Use Among 9th Grade High School Students: Acadiana Coalition of Teens Against Tobacco (ACTT)." *Preventive Medicine* 39 (3): 551–58.

Kirk, R. E. 1994. *Experimental Design: Procedures for the Behavioral Sciences*, 3rd ed. Belmont, CA: Wadsworth.

Kitzhaber, J. A. 1993. "Prioritizing Health Services in an Era of Limits: The Oregon Experience." *BMJ* 307 (6900): 373–77.

Landon, B. E., L. S. Hicks, A. J. O'Malley, T. A. Leiu, T. Keegan, B. J. McNeil, and E. Guadagnoli. 2007. "Improving the Management of Chronic Disease at Community Health Centers." *New England Journal of Medicine* 356 (9): 921–34.

Lefkowitz, B. 2007. *Community Health Centers: A Movement and the People Who Made It Happen*. New Brunswick, NJ: Rutgers University Press.

Macinko, J., B. Starfield, and L. Shi. 2003. "The Contribution of Primary Care Systems to Health Outcomes Within Organization for Economic Cooperation and Development (OECD) Countries, 1970–98." *Health Services Research* 38 (3): 831–65.

Martino, S. C., D. E. Kanouse, M. N. Elliott, S. S. Teleki, and R. D. Hays. 2012. "A Field Experiment on the Impact of Physician-Level Performance Data on Consumers' Choice of Physician." *Medical Care* 50 (Suppl.): S65–S73.

Melzack, R. (ed.). 1983. *Pain Measurement and Assessment*. New York: Raven Press.

Mendelson, C. 2006. "Managing a Medically and Socially Complex Life: Women Living with Lupus." *Qualitative Health Research* 16 (7): 982–97.

Miller, D. C., and N. J. Salkind. 2002. *Handbook of Research Design and Social Measurement*, 6th ed. Thousand Oaks, CA: Sage.

Miller, R. L., and J. D. Brewer. 2003. *The A–Z of Social Research: A Dictionary of Key Social Science Research Concepts*. Thousand Oaks, CA: Sage.

Morgan, D. L. 1997. *Focus Groups as Qualitative Research*. Newbury Park, CA: Sage.

Nelson, A., R. Lewy, T. Dovydaitis, F. Ricardo, and C. Kugel. 2011. "Promotores as Researchers: Expanding the Promotor Role in Community-Based Research." *Health Promotion Practice* 12 (5): 681–88.

Neutens, J. J., and L. Rubinson. 1997. *Research Techniques for the Health Sciences*. Needham Heights, MA: Allyn & Bacon.

O'Malley, A. S., C. B. Forrest, R. M. Politzer, J. T. Wulu, and L. Shi. 2005. "Health Center Trends, 1994–2001: What Do They Portend for the Federal Growth Initiative?" *Health Affairs* 24 (2): 465–72.

Parkerson, G. R., Jr., W. E. Broadhead, and C. K. Tse. 1995. "Health Status and Severity of Illness as Predictors of Outcomes in Primary Care." *Medical Care* 33 (1): 53–66.

Patrick, D. 1993. *Health Status and Health Policy: Quality of Life in Health Care Evaluation and Resource Allocation*. New York: Oxford University Press.

Patton, M. Q. 2002. *Qualitative Evaluation and Research Methods*, 3rd ed. Thousand Oaks, CA: Sage.

Peacock, N., L. M. Issel, S. J. Townsell, T. Chapple-McGruder, and A. Handler. 2011. "An Innovative Method to Involve Community Health Workers as Partners in Evaluation Research." *American Journal of Public Health* 101 (12): 2275–80.

Pearce, D. W. 1981. *The Social Appraisal of Projects: A Text in Cost-Benefit Analysis*. London: Macmillan.

Politzer, R. M., A. H. Schempf, B. Starfield, and L. Shi. 2003. "The Future Role of Health Centers in Improving National Health." *Journal of Public Health Policy* 24 (3/4): 296–306.

Proser, M. 2005. "Deserving the Spotlight: Health Centers Provide High-Quality and Cost-Effective Care." *Journal of Ambulatory Care Management* 28 (4): 321–30.

Reinhardt, U. E., P. S. Hussey, and G. F. Anderson. 2002. "Cross-National Comparisons of Health Systems Using OECD Data." *Health Affairs* 21 (3): 169–81.

Riesenberg, D., and R. M. Glass. 1989. "The Medical Outcomes Study." *Journal of the American Medical Association* 262 (7): 943.

Rossi, P. H., M. W. Lipsey, and H. E. Freeman. 2004. *Evaluation: A Systematic Approach*, 7th ed. Thousand Oaks, CA: Sage.

Rowland, N. 1995. *Evaluating the Cost-Effectiveness of Counseling in Health Care*. New York: Routledge.

Rubin, H. J. 1983. *Applied Social Research*. Columbus, OH: Charles E. Merrill.

Sardell A. 1988. *The U.S. Experiment in Social Medicine: The Community Health Center Program, 1965–1986*. Pittsburgh: University of Pittsburgh Press.

Shi, L., and G. D. Stevens. 2010. *Vulnerable Populations in the United States*, 2nd ed. San Francisco: Jossey-Bass.

Shi, L., G. D. Stevens, J. T. Wulu Jr., R. M. Politzer, and J. Xu. 2004. "America's Health Centers: Reducing Racial and Ethnic Disparities in Perinatal Care and Birth Outcomes." *Health Services Research* 39 (6): 1881–901.

Shi, L., G. D. Stevens, and R. Politzer. 2007. "Access to Care for U.S. Health Center Patients and Patients Nationally—How Do the Most Vulnerable Populations Fare?" *Medical Care* 45 (3): 206–13.

Shi, L., J. Tsai, and P. Collins. 2009. "Racial/Ethnic and Socioeconomic Disparities in Access to Care and Quality of Care for U.S. Health Center Patients Compared to Non-Health Center Patients." *Journal of Ambulatory Care Management* 32 (4): 342–50.

Shin, P., A. Markus, and S. Rosenbaum. 2006. *Measuring Health Centers Against Standard Indicators of High Quality Performance: Early Results from a Multi-site Demonstration Project.* [Interim report.] Minnetonka, MN: United Health Foundation.

Shin, P., A. Markus, S. Rosenbaum, and J. Sharac. 2008. "Adoption of Health Center Performance Measures and National Benchmarks." *Journal of Ambulatory Care Management* 31 (1): 69–75.

Singleton, R. A., and B. C. Straits. 2005. *Approaches to Social Research*, 4th ed. New York: Oxford University Press.

Spitzer, W. O., A. J. Dobson, and J. Hall. 1981. "Measuring Quality of Life of Cancer Patients: A Concise QL-Index for Use by Physicians." *Journal of Chronic Disease* 34: 585–97.

Starfield, B., and L. Shi. 2007. "The Impact of Primary Care and What States Can Do." *North Carolina Medical Journal* 68 (3): 204–7.

Stecher, B. M., and W. A. Davis. 1987. *How to Focus an Evaluation*. Newbury Park, CA: Sage.

Steinwachs, D. M. 1989. "Application of Health Status Assessment Measures in Policy Research." *Medical Care* 27 (Suppl.): S12–S26.

Stokey, E., and R. Zeckhauser. 1978. *A Primer for Policy Analysis*. New York: W. W. Norton.

Tarlov, B. R., J. E. Ware, S. Greenfield, E. C. Nelson, and E. Perrin. 1989. "The Medical Outcomes Study." *Journal of the American Medical Association* 262 (7): 925–30.

Thorne, S. 2000. "Data Analysis in Qualitative Research." *Evidence-Based Nursing* 3: 68–70.

Ulmer, C., D. Lewis-Idema, A. M. Von Worley, J. Rodgers, L. Berger, E. Darling, and B. Lefkowitz. 2000. "Assessing Primary Care Content: Four Conditions Common in Community Health Center Practice." *Journal of Ambulatory Care Management* 23 (1): 23–28.

US Department of Health and Human Services (HHS). 2000. *Healthy People 2010: Understanding and Improving Health*, 2nd ed. Washington, DC: US Government Printing Office.

US Department of Veterans Affairs (VA). 1989. *Cost-Benefit Analysis Handbook*. Washington, DC: Office of Planning and Management Analysis.

Veney, J. E., and A. D. Kaluzny. 2005. *Evaluation and Decision Making for Health Services*, 3rd ed. Frederick, MD: Beard Books.

Ware, J. E. 1986. "The Assessment of Health Status." In *Applications of Social Science to Clinical Medicine and Health Policy*, edited by L. H. Aiken and D. Mechanic. New Brunswick, NJ: Rutgers University Press.

Williams, A., J. Ware, and C. Donald. 1981. "A Model of Mental Health, Life Events and Social Supports Applicable to General Populations." *Journal of Health and Social Behavior* 22: 324–36.

Writing Group for the Women's Health Initiative. 2002. "Risks and Benefits of Estrogen Plus Progestin in Healthy Postmenopausal Women: Principal Results from the Women's Health Initiative Randomized Controlled Trial." *Journal of the American Medical Association* 288 (3): 321–33.

Yin, R. K. 2003. *Case Study Research: Design and Methods*. Thousand Oaks, CA: Sage.

Additional Resources

Bailey, K. D. 1994. "Observation." In *Methods of Social Research*, 4th ed., chap. 10. New York: Free Press.

Barker, J. B., T. Bayne, Z. R. Higgs, S. A. Jenkin, D. Murphy, and G. Synoground. 1994. "Community Analysis: A Collaborative Community Practice Project." *Public Health Nursing* 11, 113–18.

Cox, B. G., and B. S. Cohen. 1985. *Methodological Issues for Health Care Surveys*. New York: Marcel Dekker.

Denzin, N. K., and Y. S. Lincoln (eds.). 2005. *The Sage Handbook of Qualitative Research*, 3rd ed. Thousand Oaks, CA: Sage.

Dignan, M., and P. Carr. 1987. *Program Planning for Health Education and Health Promotion*. Philadelphia: Lea and Febiger.

Dixon, J. S., and H. A. Bird. 1981. "Reproducibility Along a 10cm Vertical Visual Analogue Scale." *Annals of Rheumatic Diseases* 40: 87–89.

Kark, S. L. 1981. *The Practice of Community-Oriented Primary Health Care*. New York: Appleton-Century-Crofts.

Scott, J., and E. C. Huskisson. 1979. "Vertical or Horizontal Visual Analogue Scales." *Annals of Rheumatic Diseases* 38 (6): 560.

Shi, L., and G. D. Stevens. 2007. "The Role of Community Health Centers in Delivering Primary Care to the Underserved: Experiences of the Uninsured and Medicaid Insured." *Journal of Ambulatory Care Management* 30 (2): 159–70.

Sterk, C. E., and K. W. Elifson. 2004. "Qualitative Methods in Community-Based Research." In *Community-Based Health Research: Issues and Methods*, chap. 7, edited by D. S. Blumenthal and R. J. DiClemente. New York: Springer.

Young, K. R. 1994. "An Evaluative Study of a Community Health Service Development." *Journal of Advanced Nursing* 19: 58–65.

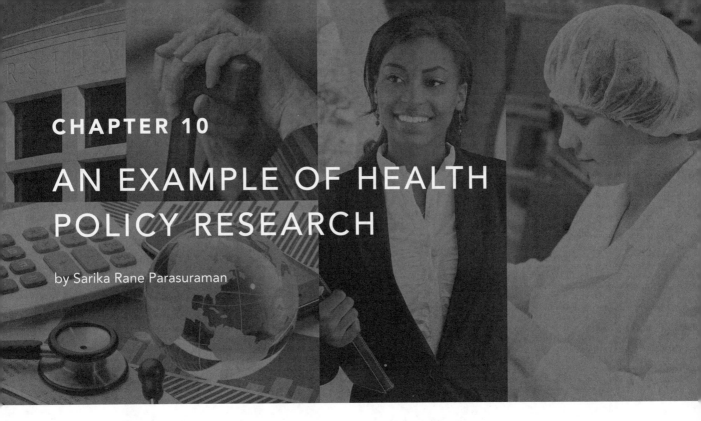

CHAPTER 10

AN EXAMPLE OF HEALTH POLICY RESEARCH

by Sarika Rane Parasuraman

Research serves to make building stones out of stumbling blocks.

— Arthur D. Little

This chapter presents an example of how policy analysis may be applied. It reproduces an actual qualifying examination completed by a student of The Johns Hopkins University Department of Health Policy & Management in 2006.

The exam requires students to choose a current public health problem and conduct a policy analysis of it. In the course of the analysis, students must present the determinants of a health problem, identify a policy intervention to address it, assess that intervention, and propose next steps in solving the health problem.

The example is presented as follows: First, the exam questions posed to the student are provided, followed by the sample exam submission. This sample policy analysis was provided by Sarika Rane Parasuraman, a graduate student at the time of the exam's completion and is used with permission (adapted for editorial style). Her selected health problem is obesity.

QUESTIONS FOR POLICY ANALYSIS

1. Briefly define the nature and scope of the public health problem chosen. Then discuss the most important individual, sociocultural, political, and economic determinants of the problem. Select what you consider to be the most important determinant or combination of determinants of the problem, and defend your choice.

2. Identify one policy intervention (e.g., changes to service delivery, prevention initiative, legislation, regulation, litigation strategy) that has been used or proposed to address the public health problem you chose. Draw from the literature, when possible, to assess the appropriateness, comprehensiveness, and effectiveness of the intervention.

3. For the sample intervention, also discuss the political and economic feasibility of implementing the policy. If considerable resources are needed to implement the program, identify the source (e.g., new taxes, fees, fines, redirected current resources).

4. For the intervention you selected, provide a summary review of previous evaluations, if available. Then you may either describe and critique an existing evaluation or suggest your own evaluation. In either case, articulate the study design, key measures, type of statistical model for your key outcome measure(s), generalizability, and notable strengths and weaknesses. Your answer should include a discussion of the strengths and weaknesses of the evaluation, including its appropriateness, the reliability and validity of key measures used, and an assessment of any threats to the validity of the findings. Be realistic in developing your evaluation plan. Do not assume unlim-

ited resources, and be mindful of standards for ethical research with human subjects.

5. On the basis of your discussion above, propose and discuss the next steps needed in the realms of research, interventions, and policy to address the problem. Of the next steps you identify, select which, in your view, is the most important next step, and justify your choice.

POLICY ANALYSIS: RESPONSES TO EXAM QUESTIONS

QUESTION 1

Introduction

Obesity in the United States is one of the most significant public health problems facing the population. The Centers for Disease Control and Prevention (CDC) estimate that more than 65 percent of adults (ages 20 and older) living in the United States are currently overweight or obese, with a body mass index [BMI] of 25 or higher (Ogden et al. 2006)—a figure that has substantially risen during the past three decades (Manson et al. 2004). The statistics describing children and adolescents are even more shocking. Over the past two decades, the proportions of youth ages 6–11 and ages 12–19 who exceed a "normal" weight has nearly doubled and tripled, respectively (Hedley et al. 2004). An estimated 18 percent of children and adolescents are at risk for becoming overweight (BMI for age at 85th percentile or higher) or are "overweight" (BMI for age at 95th percentile or higher)—a figure many experts consider an underestimate (Hedley et al. 2004; Cook et al. 2005). For the purposes of this paper, *obese* or *obesity* is used to denote all overweight conditions in adults and youth.

Researchers estimate that obesity is responsible for nearly 300,000 deaths per year; this figure will likely grow as obesity prevalence continues to rise in the population (Allison et al. 1999). Obesity could soon exceed tobacco to become the leading cause of preventable morbidity and mortality in the United States (Sturm and Wells 2001; IOM 2002) and may be responsible for reversing the trend of improvements in disability among elderly Americans over the last several decades (Sturm, Ringel, and Andreyeva 2004). Combined, overweight and obesity is one of ten leading health indicators identified by *Healthy People* (*HP*) *2010* (HHS 2000), which reinforces its significance as a public health problem (Exhibit 10.1). Obesity is also a major risk factor for, and has been linked to, the leading causes of death and disability among Americans, including heart disease, certain cancers (particularly colon and breast cancer), stroke, diabetes, hypertension, sleep apnea, pulmonary dysfunction, osteoporosis, hypercholesterolemia, and asthma (NIH 1998; National

Task Force on the Prevention and Treatment of Obesity 2000; CDC 2004a, 2004b; Ford, Williamson, and Liu 1997; Green and Kreuter 1999). Obesity experienced prior to adulthood is a significant predictor for these conditions into adulthood (Manson et al. 2004; Freedman et al. 1999; Yanovski and Yanovski 2003; Baba et al. 2007; Lawlor et al. 2006). Childhood obesity also has social and economic consequences later in life, particularly for women. One study found that women who were overweight during youth experienced low educational attainment, were less likely to be married, and had higher poverty rates (Gortmaker et al. 1993). To make matters worse, obese individuals are more likely to suffer the burden of disability throughout life in terms of fewer years free from activities of daily living limitations (Peeters et al. 2004). In fact, obesity is a major factor in the rising economic burden on the nation's healthcare system—obesity costs the United States approximately $117 billion in annual direct and indirect obesity-related medical expenditures (Daviglus 2005).

Perhaps the most alarming trends are of those conditions newly incident among youth that are traditionally associated with adulthood; for example, pediatricians now report higher incidences of asthma, hypertension, and type II diabetes in patients (Veugelers and Fitzgerald 2005; Luma and Spiotta 2006). Obese children and adolescents also experience lower health-related quality of life than their nonoverweight counterparts in the form of poor school performance, lower social functioning, poor emotional health,

Exhibit 10.1
Healthy People
2010

Leading health indicators at a glance	
Health indicator	***HP 2010* objective number**
Physical activity	22-2 and 22-7
Overweight and obesity	19-2 and 19-3c
Tobacco use	27-1a and 17-2b
Substance abuse	26-10a, 26-10c, and 26-11c
Responsible sexual behavior	13-6 and 25-11
Mental health	18-9b
Injury and violence	15-15a and 15-32
Environmental quality	8-1a and 27-10
Immunization	14-24, 14-29a, and 14-29b
Access to healthcare	1-1, 1-4a, and 16-6a

(continued)

Healthy People 2010 objectives related to nutrition and overweight in youth

Goal: Promote health and reduce chronic disease associated with diet and weight.

Objectives:

- Reduce the proportion of children and adolescents who are overweight or obese.
- Increase the proportion of persons ≥ 2 years who consume at least 2 daily servings of fruit.
- Increase the proportion of persons ≥ 2 years who consume at least 3 daily servings of vegetables, with at least one-third being dark green or orange vegetables.
- Increase the proportion of persons ≥ 2 years who consume at least 6 daily servings of grain products, with at least 3 being whole grains.
- Increase the proportion of persons ≥ 2 years who consume less than 10% of calories from saturated fat.
- Increase the proportion of persons ≥ 2 years who consume no more than 30% of calories from total fat.
- Increase the proportion of persons ≥ 2 years who consume 2,400 mg or less of sodium daily.
- Increase the proportion of persons ≥ 2 years who meet dietary recommendations for calcium.

Healthy People 2010 objectives related to physical activity and fitness in youth

Goal: Improve health, fitness, and quality of life through daily physical activity.

Objectives:

- Increase the proportion of adolescents who engage in moderate physical activity for at least 30 minutes on 5 or more of the previous 7 days.
- Increase the proportion of adolescents who engage in vigorous physical activity that promotes cardiorespiratory fitness 3 or more days per week for 20 or more minutes per occasion.
- Increase the proportion of the nation's public and private schools that require daily physical education for all students.
- Increase the proportion of adolescents who participate in daily school physical education.
- Increase the proportion of adolescents who spend at least 50 percent of school physical education class time being physically active.
- Increase the proportion of adolescents who view television 2 or fewer hours on a school day.

SOURCE: HHS (2000).

EXHIBIT 10.1
Healthy People
2010
(continued)

and depression (Williams et al. 2005; Swallen et al. 2005; Sjoberg, Nilsson, and Leppert 2005), although there is some conflicting evidence regarding these associations (Williams et al. 2005). Obesity is a severe psychosocial, medical, and economic threat to youth, which establishes it (specifically childhood obesity) as a significant public health problem that must be addressed.

Determinants of Obesity

The determinants attributed to childhood obesity are multifactorial and complex. A conceptual framework has been developed that helps to categorize determinants as proximate (biological, demographic, behavioral), mid-level distal (home, neighborhood, school), and macro-level distal (social, political, economic) (Exhibit 10.2). Sparse evidence suggests nonmodifiable causes of obesity that include genetic susceptibility, endocrine disorders, maternal diabetes, and high birth weight (American Obesity Association 2007; AACAP 2001; Mello, Rimm, and Studdert 2003; Plourde 2006). Having one or both parents who are obese is a strong and proven risk factor for childhood obesity and can be considered a proximate and distal determinant (Whitaker et al. 1997). The roles of age, gender, and race/ethnicity on obesity are more consistently proven at the population level, although the exact causal mechanisms are not completely understood (Hedley et al. 2004). The prevalence figures between males and females slightly differ. Although in recent years only males have exhibited a significant increase in obesity prevalence, females are more likely to suffer extreme obesity (Ogden et al. 2006; Manson et al. 2004). Significant differences in obesity prevalence by race/ethnicity have persisted over the years. In general, obesity is more prevalent among males and females in minority groups, but gender remains an important modifier of the relationship between race/ethnicity and obesity (Ogden et al. 2006; Freedman et al. 2006).

Proximate determinants also include behaviors, habits, and other lifestyle choices of the individual. Experts generally agree that childhood obesity mostly results from caloric intake in excess of physical activity; as previously shown, this relationship is confounded by nonmodifiable determinants. Thus, the two major behavioral determinants of childhood obesity are physical activity and dietary choices. The former is among the top ten health indicators identified in *HP 2010* (HHS 2000) and is the focus of a landmark report by the US surgeon general (HHS 1996), while the latter is a featured *HP 2010* objective related to the reduction of chronic diseases (HHS 2000). Nearly 35 percent of youth do not participate in sufficient (as defined by the CDC) physical activity (CDC 2008). Although about 50 percent are enrolled in physical education classes in schools, less than 30 percent regularly attended these classes (Grunbaum et al. 2004). Inadequate physical activity is an undisputed determinant linked to requisite energy expenditure, childhood obesity, and the development of obesity-related health conditions (Plourde 2006; Grunbaum et al. 2004; Office of the Surgeon General 2001; Duke, Huhman, and

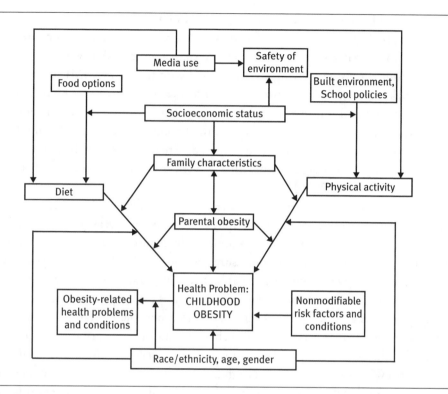

Exhibit 10.2
Conceptual Model
of Proximate
and Distal
Determinants of
Childhood Obesity

NOTE: **Proximate determinants:** race/ethnicity, age, gender, unmodifiable risk factors and conditions, diet, physical activity, family characteristics, parental obesity, and media use. **Mid-level distal determinants:** safety of environment, built environment, and food options. **Macro-level distal determinants:** socioeconomic status and school policies.

Heitzler 2003; Schneider 2000). Similarly, an unhealthy diet is a proven determinant of childhood obesity (AACAP 2001; Mello, Rimm, and Studdert 2003; Office of the Surgeon General 2001; Schneider 2000), although evidence is mixed regarding whether childhood obesity is due to excessive fat intake or excessive carbohydrate intake (Plourde 2006; Whitaker et al. 1997). One study found a dose–response relationship between the consumption of sugar-sweetened drinks and BMI in children and adolescents (Ludwig, Peterson, and Gortmaker 2001). Just one-fifth of youth nationwide consume the CDC's recommended amount of fruits and vegetables (Grunbaum et al. 2004). Both age and gender are modifying determinants between the aforementioned behavioral choices. Males are more likely to regularly engage in vigorous/moderate physical activity; in contrast, females are more likely to engage in risky behaviors aimed at trying to lose or keep from gaining weight (Grunbaum et al. 2004; University of South Australia 2004). The role of media use, particularly television viewing, is a determinant of contention. While some studies have found a link between television use and high youth BMI (Dietz and Gortmaker 1985), others have failed to prove such associations (Robinson 1993; Burdette and Whitaker 2005). Some researchers have proven an association between television use and sedentary lifestyles, reduced intake of fruits and vegetables, and reduced participation in organized sports (Dietz and Gortmaker 1985; Robinson 1993; Boynton-Jarrett et al. 2003). One early study found a dose–response relationship whereby incrementally decreasing television viewing was associated with decreasing BMI in youth (Dietz and Gortmaker 1985). A link between food choices and marketing of high-calorie food and beverages to youth on television has been posited, but little empirical evidence has emerged to support it. Finally, one study showed parental obesity to be a modifier between television use and obesity (Vandewater and Huang 2006), while another showed neighborhood safety to be significantly linked to television use but not directly to obesity (Burdette and Whitaker 2005).

Mid-level distal determinants include home, neighborhood, and school environments. The home environment includes family characteristics such as emotional well-being, marital status, and cognitive stimulation. One study quantified these home environment characteristics into one standardized measure and showed that low-scoring youth were at greater risk of developing obesity than their high-scoring counterparts (Strauss and Knight 1999). Parental obesity is a relevant determinant in this category as well (recall that it was also categorized as a personal characteristic due to a possible heritable trait of obesity). Parental obesity can interact with family characteristics (e.g., marital status, emotional well-being in the home) and can also modify the behaviors of children by influencing lifestyle choices (Whitaker et al. 1997). Neighborhood characteristics are broad and include presence of recreational facilities, number of mobility options, food choices (markets or fast-food restaurants), and other traits of the built environment. Neighborhood safety has been previously discussed, with an unproven direct link to inactivity (Burdette and Whitaker 2005). All have been linked to either sedentary lifestyles (Gordon-Larsen et al. 2006; Merchant et al. 2007; Nelson 2006) or unhealthy diets (Strauss and Knight 1999; Merchant et al. 2007; Nelson 2006; Nielsen 2002) in children, although the causal link to obesity is precarious (Merchant et al. 2007; Nelson 2006). Finally, school policies have been linked to an increasing prevalence of childhood obesity, most notably loosening standards for foods served in school cafeterias, the presence of vending machines that offer snacks and drinks with little nutritional value, and physical education requirements that are either not required or unenforced (IOM 2002; Trust for America's Health 2005). As of 2006, 49 states had some physical education requirements, although these widely varied: Just 11 states passed laws regarding school nutrition enhancement (NCSL 2007). To date, no federal laws mandate either standard.

Finally, macro-level distal determinants affect childhood obesity and include socioeconomic status (SES) as measured by income, education, and occupation. The relationship between SES and obesity is complex, and an inverse relationship between SES and BMI has been empirically determined in a number of studies (Marmot and Wilkinson

2006; Stunkard and Sorenson 1993; Janssen et al. 2006). SES and the behavioral risk factors of sedentary lifestyle, unhealthy diet, and inadequate physical activity have also been linked. However, the status of SES as a direct predictor of obesity in any of these cases is intuitively questionable (IOM 2002; Marmot and Wilkinson 2006; Janssen et al. 2006; Adler and Ostrove 1999). Experts have attempted to consolidate these factors to state that SES is likely an important modifying determinant affecting the link between home/neighborhood environment and behavioral/lifestyle determinants (Marmot and Wilkinson 2006; Stunkard and Sorenson 1993; Janssen et al. 2006). For example, SES could affect access to recreational facilities or various food options. Finally, SES is significantly associated with both family characteristics and neighborhood safety (Boynton-Jarrett et al. 2003; Gordon-Larsen et al. 2006).

Most Significant Determinant of Obesity

It is clear that behavioral and lifestyle choices of youth are the most important determinants of childhood obesity. Direct causal links between physical activity, diet, and childhood obesity have been consistently proven in the literature. Moreover, a dose–response relationship exists between physical activity and BMI; moderate physical activity results in lower BMI and a decrease in risk factor status for several obesity-related conditions (this effect is stronger after consistent vigorous physical activity) (CDC 2008). Studies also show that lifestyle habits begun during youth are likely to be continued into adulthood (CDC 2008; Rhodes, MacDonald, and McKay 2006). The link showing any effects of television viewing on these behaviors, while of interest to current experts, is still too precarious to label this factor a major determinant of obesity. Although the interaction of several more distal determinants are linked to the above primary relationships (acting to facilitate, inhibit, or confound the relationships), their association is complex and likely affected by a host of additional confounding and/or mediating determinants that are beyond the scope of this paper. In this regard, the literature can be considered limited.

A final reason that inadequate physical activity and unhealthy diets are major determinants is that they are highly actionable. As previously mentioned, many lifestyle habits begun in childhood are continued into adulthood. Primary prevention interventions that address these two determinants and affect the decision-making process of youth could have the most profound impact on reducing the prevalence of childhood obesity, regardless of intervening factors or barriers that may exist in the environment (Nelson 2006; Daviglus 2005). Recognizing that activity and diet directly affect childhood obesity, the federal government has deemed them important, actionable health areas (HHS 2000) and centerpieces of major policy objectives to reduce obesity among children and adolescents (Office of the Surgeon General 2001).

QUESTION 2

Selection of the Intervention

A hallmark of public health practice is the planning and implementation of interventions aimed at preventing a health problem. The Question 1 analysis shows that childhood obesity is a complex problem, and the major (and most actionable) determinants are those categorized as behaviors or lifestyle choices. Evidence reveals direct relationships between inadequate physical activity and unhealthy diets and childhood obesity. Because habits established during youth are likely to continue into adulthood (Rhodes, MacDonald, and McKay 2006), interventions for the primary prevention of obesity that seek to alter these risky behaviors and encourage youth to make positive and healthy lifestyle choices are most appropriate for addressing the major determinants of childhood obesity (Schneider 2000). In fact, evidence suggests that interventions aimed at behavioral modification may be more effective with youth than with adults (Yanovski and Yanovski 2003).

Schools are an ideal setting in which to administer primary obesity prevention interventions. An estimated 50 million children and adolescents attend more than 110,000 schools throughout the year (CDC 2000), so school-based interventions can reach a wide array of students. Randomized controlled trials that evaluate interventions have found that health education administered in schools can reduce risky behaviors among students, such as smoking, alcohol use, and substance abuse—behaviors that are clear determinants of adult chronic diseases (CDC 2000; Fisher et al. 2007; HHS and DOE 2000). Dietary and activity habits can be potentially risky behaviors established during school-age years (Edmunds, Waters, and Elliot 2001). Studies have underscored the potential strength of coordinated health education approaches to address childhood obesity in schools (HHS 2000; Veugelers and Fitzgerald 2005; American Obesity Association 2007; Office of the Surgeon General 2001; Nelson 2006; CDC 2000).

Clearly, childhood obesity is a salient issue, and schools are ideal settings for health education interventions; however, current results from school-based interventions are mixed. Most only show modest behavioral modifications and uneven results with regard to obesity and BMI levels. This paper considered only programs shown to be partially effective (Exhibit 10.3); Planet Health is currently one of the most effective examples of such a program.

Planet Health is a unique and ideal intervention to examine, mainly because it incorporates comprehensive health education into the standard academic curriculum. The program was applied to a broad sample of schools and among students of all demographic backgrounds. It also includes a component targeted to reducing television viewing among youth—a study outcome that had not been examined by other researchers/evaluators at the time of the pilot program. Thus, Planet Health addresses the two major determinants of childhood obesity, physical activity and diet, plus the third determinant of television

EXHIBIT 10.3
School-Based
Interventions
Considered in
Addition to Planet
Health

Child and Adolescent Trial for Cardiovascular Health (CATCH)

CATCH was a comprehensive, three-year, school-based health behavior intervention targeted to elementary school students and aimed at the primary prevention of cardiovascular disease. Program components encompassed the elementary school environment, classroom curricula, and home programs. The pilot incorporated the program through 56 intervention schools (with 40 control schools), involving more than 5,000 ethnically diverse third, fourth, and fifth graders in California, Louisiana, Minnesota, and Texas. Although the program appeared to somewhat improve the behaviors of students and lower cardiovascular risk, it did not significantly affect obesity.

SOURCE: Luepker et al. (1996).

Wellness, Academics & You (WAY)

WAY is a multidisciplinary, elementary school–based intervention focused on fourth and fifth graders. The pilot was conducted over four states (Delaware, Florida, Kansas, and North Carolina) and comprised more than 1,000 students in 16 different schools. WAY aims to reduce obesity and its concomitant diseases as well as improve academic performance. The program incorporates health content in the existing academic curriculum through rigorous and extensive modules led by teachers. It also includes activities that involve parents and families. The main areas of intended impact are obesity, fruit/vegetable consumption, and physical activity. The program showed significant changes in students' BMI and healthy food consumption, although its rigorous nature and costs are challenges to widespread implementation.

SOURCE: Spiegel (2006).

Pathways

Pathways is a two-year school-based intervention aimed at American Indian elementary school students in grades 3 through 5. The program's aim is to develop and implement an intervention to prevent obesity, promote healthy eating behaviors, and increase physical activity. It incorporates a classroom curriculum, encourages physical activity, instituted food preparation and service modifications, and includes an extensive family support component. To date the intervention has produced significant changes in students' attitudes and behaviors but no significant changes related to obesity. Furthermore, because the program's components are specific to the needs and background of American Indians, its widespread implementation and generalizability are limited.

SOURCE: Sharma (2006).

viewing, which, while more distal, is likely an important secondary, modifiable behavior and risk factor for obesity in youth that is worth incorporating into health education programs (Katz et al. 2005).

Description of the Intervention

Planet Health is an interdisciplinary program that is school based, incorporating health education into the regular, existing academic curriculum. Planet Health was developed through the Harvard Prevention Research Center on Nutrition and Physical Activity and was originally supported by the National Institute of Child Health and Human Development in 1995 as a pilot program in ten Boston public middle schools among sixth and seventh graders. Due to the initial success of the program, Boston Public Schools partnered with Planet Health researchers in 2002 to expand the pilot to 12 additional Boston middle schools. Further success of the program caught the interest of state decision makers, and in 2004, BlueCross BlueShield of Massachusetts partnered with Planet Health to implement the program statewide, expanding it to include after-school programs. Currently, 48 states and 20 countries have demonstrated interest in learning more about the program (Franks et al. 2007). The main goal of the program is to lower the prevalence of obesity among middle school students and is largely based on social cognitive theory (Gortmaker et al. 1999). The objectives of Planet Health are as follows: (1) reduce television viewing time (i.e., decrease sedentary behavior), (2) decrease consumption of unhealthy food choices, (3) increase consumption of healthy food choices, and (4) increase physical activity.

The program includes teacher training, as teachers in schools administer the program; classroom lessons in math, science, language arts, and social studies; a "media-reduction campaign"; physical education units; and wellness sessions for teachers. Classroom sessions are delivered over two years (the time duration a typical child spends attending a Boston public middle school). Sixteen sessions per year are conducted during 30- or 45-minute class periods. The time duration for teacher training is typically two to three hours. Planet Health program materials can be ordered through the program's website (Harvard Prevention Research Center 2007).

Analysis of the Intervention

It is important to first consider the appropriateness of Planet Health. The program focuses on four behavioral objectives in physical activity and diet. Health education is incorporated into 32 regular classroom lessons. Additionally, teachers lead 30 physical education "micro-units" with activity and inactivity themes. Thus, Planet Health is consistent with the primary determinants identified in question 1. The intervention also addresses television viewing with a two-week lesson entitled "Power Down," which focuses on reducing use to increase activity time. Planet Health is based on social cognitive theory, a framework that models behavior change as resulting from dynamics between psychosocial factors and individual characteristics (Glanz, Rimer, and Lewis 2002). The program encourages students to work together in modeling and practice of decision making and gives them confidence to perform behaviors with reinforcement by peers and teachers, the power of self-determination by imparting cognitive skills to alter risky behaviors, and time for self-reflection of new behaviors (Gortmaker et al. 1999; Glanz, Rimer, and Lewis 2002).

Planet Health is also appropriate when considering the participants' demographics. First, research has shown that poor eating habits, sedentary lifestyles, and even binge eating and dieting are solidified during middle childhood (Edmunds, Waters, and Elliott 2001; Tanofsky-Kraff et al. 2006). These findings indicate that the initiation of Planet Health in middle schools serves an appropriate target population of students. Furthermore, Planet Health meets standards upheld by the Massachusetts Curriculum Framework; because the program is interwoven with the standard academic curriculums, it is grade appropriate and accounts for the varying competency levels of children during middle childhood (Gortmaker et al. 1999). Studies suggest that sustained results from school-based obesity programs often originate from those focused on preadolescents, which is one potential weakness of Planet Health (although the program is being expanded to fourth and fifth graders in Massachusetts). A further weakness of the program is its lack of gender specificity. Statistics suggest that young females have different personal attitudes and sociocultural pressures than young males regarding body image and self-esteem (Grunbaum et al. 2004); the broad-based approach of Planet Health may not address such gender differences. Similarly, Planet Health does not contain educational components that are specific to minority groups who have differing levels of obesity risk (Ogden et al. 2006). Finally, a strength of Planet Health is its even application throughout most school populations, which contain both overweight students and students with normal BMI. The premise for this application lies in social cognitive theory, which espouses a population-based approach (combined with an individual approach) to effect change. Obesity, particularly among youth, often results in stigmatization and low self-esteem (Latner, Stunkard, and Wilson 2005), but Planet Health's approach avoids such stigmatization.

An assessment of Planet Health's comprehensiveness overlaps with the appropriateness analysis in terms of the target population's characteristics (i.e., age, gender, and race/ethnicity) and the breadth of obesity-related determinants it addresses. To that end, two weaknesses exist. First, the program does not attempt to address socioeconomic determinants of obesity. As previously stated, SES is a complex and distal determinant; the efficacy of actionable strategies that alter its relationship with obesity is tenuous. However, the literature does suggest the utility of school-based interventions prioritized for low-SES youth (Veugelers and Fitzgerald 2005). Furthermore, parental involvement in obesity interventions can greatly enhance the effectiveness and sustainability of behaviors, including activity levels and television viewing (Yanovski and Yanovski 2003; Vandewater and Huang 2006). The framework outlined in Question 1 identifies the moderating role of family (under family characteristics) in the relationships between physical activity, diet, and obesity. Several voluntary Planet Health lessons provide opportunities for parents and family members to participate. A strength of Planet Health with regard to comprehensiveness is its strategy incorporating health education into existing academic frameworks. Additionally, the entire school and teachers are actively involved in designing and implementing Planet Health into the curriculum. Thus, Planet Health is comprehensive in that it imparts a holistic, pedagogical approach to obesity-related health education within the target setting of schools that is widely recommended (HHS 2000; American Obesity Association 2007; Office of the Surgeon General 2001; CDC 2000; Brener et al. 2006).

To date, credible evaluations of Planet Health that report the program as effective in achieving its objectives and goals are limited. The most widely cited evaluation was conducted by program researchers during the pilot program from 1995 to 1997 (Gortmaker et al. 1999). It was a randomized controlled trial evaluating the curriculum and outcomes of the Planet Health program in ten Boston public middle schools. Students participated in the full Planet Health curriculum and were evaluated using BMI measurements, body assessments, and a food/activity survey. The evaluation found that only the amount of television viewing was reduced in both boys and girls of the intervention schools (versus control schools). The following significant outcomes were shown *only* among girls in the intervention schools: decrease in obesity prevalence, increase in consumption of fruits/vegetables, and reduction in dietary energy intake. There were no significant outcome differences among males. This evaluation is unique because it was randomized, involved a broad base of study participants, and assessed behaviors (a somewhat subjective measure) and BMI (an objective measure). Thus, this evaluation is the most useful to analyze.

A three-year diffusion analysis of this benchmark evaluation to investigate its feasibility, acceptability, and sustainability was conducted among six Boston public middle schools (Wiecha et al. 2004). During the evaluation, teachers attended training workshops on Planet Health and received instruction from trained program professionals. A majority of teachers found the curriculum to be acceptable and indicated that they would continue to use it in classrooms. Additionally, more than 90 percent found the curriculum effective and an asset to school curricula. A major weakness of this evaluation was its descriptive nature and small sample size, which prevented statistically significant assertions or power assurances. The study also depended on teacher self-report, which may have resulted in overestimates. Finally, the generalizability of the methods is questionable.

Finally, a small, two-year outcome evaluation of Planet Health was conducted in an Indiana middle school among seventh and eighth graders (Bai et al. 2006). The Planet Health curriculum was implemented in the intervention school and no intervention was administered to the control school. The School Physical Activity and Nutrition questionnaire was administered by the researchers conducting the program evaluation to students during pre- and post-intervention periods in both schools. The evaluation reported a significant decrease among all students in fat/soda intake and reduced television viewing; however, no significant change was seen in fruit/vegetable consumption or physical activity promotion. This evaluation is weakened by its small size and scope (only involving two middle schools). Furthermore, the full reliance on a self-report questionnaire by students only allows analysis of behavioral change, rather than the associated health outcome of obesity.

QUESTION 3

Organization and Financing of the Intervention

Planet Health was originally funded with grants through the National Institutes of Health (NIH) and CDC Prevention Research Centers and a monetary gift from the Harvard School of Public Health (Glanz, Rimer, and Lewis 2002). This funding helped develop the Planet Health curriculum, implement the program as a pilot, and support the subsequent benchmark randomized controlled trial study. In 2002, the US Department of Education's Physical Education for Progress grant program funded a diffusion study to assess feasibility and sustainability of the program. Results showed the Planet Health curriculum to be effective and positively viewed by teachers. Independent funding supported further efforts to expand and sustain the program in Boston schools (Glanz, Rimer, and Lewis 2002). In 2004, BlueCross BlueShield of Massachusetts announced that it would provide $3 million over four years to Massachusetts middle schools to implement and expand Planet Health programs.

The US federal government is committed to supporting initiatives aimed at childhood obesity (IOM 2002; HHS 2000; National Task Force on the Prevention and Treatment of Obesity 2000; HHS 1996; Office of the Surgeon General 2001; CDC 2008; HHS and DOE 2000). Several agencies provide avenues for obtaining funding, including the departments of Agriculture, Health and Human Services, and Education; CDC; and NIH. Recent budget constraints of health-related initiatives is indeed troubling; for example, the CDC's fiscal year (FY) 2007 budget allotment to support health promotion activities around nutrition, physical activity, and obesity decreased from FY 2006 figures by approximately 0.1 percent (CDC 2006) (Exhibit 10.4) and the president's FY 2008 budget contained a $37 million cut for CDC from FY 2007 levels. The budget request did provide $17 million for an adolescent health promotion initiative, indicating support from the administration for fighting childhood obesity (Basu 2007). The NIH also received a funding boost to reverse a continued projected budget decline for FY 2007 and was instructed by Congress to allocate part of the money to support research project grants (Endocrine Society 2007). However, it was unclear what portion of the NIH budget would be allocated to childhood obesity–related initiatives. Advocacy organizations often compile materials to assist entities in obtaining federal funding to implement obesity initiatives (Finance Project 2004).

EXHIBIT 10.4
CDC Fiscal Year
2007 Budget,
Organized by
Activity

Budget Activity/Description	FY 2005 Actual	FY 2006 Enacted	FY 2007 Estimate	FY 2007 +/- FY 2006 Dollars	Percentage
Health Promotion[1]					
Chronic Disease Prevention, Health Promotion, and Genomics	**$899,628**	**$838,664**	**$818,727**	**($19,937)**	**-2.4%**
Heart Disease and Stroke	$44,618	$44,469	$43,888	($581)	-1.3%
Diabetes	$63,457	$63,119	$62,420	($699)	-1.1%
Cancer Prevention and Control	$309,704	$307,913	$304,690	($3,223)	-1.1%
Arthritis and Other Chronic Diseases	$22,487	$22,467	$13,757	($8,710)	-38.8%
Tobacco	$104,345	$104,799	$102,685	($2,114)	-2.0%
Nutrition, Physical Activity and Obesity	$41,930	$41,520	$41,477	($43)	-0.1%
Health Promotion	$26,146	$27,443	$24,160	($3,283)	-12.0%
School Health	$56,746	$56,192	$55,820	($372)	-0.7%
Safe Motherhood/Infant Health	$44,738	$44,292	$44,009	($283)	-0.6%
Oral Health	$11,204	$11,682	$11,022	($660)	-5.7%
Prevention Centers	$29,690	$29,700	$29,206	($494)	-1.7%
Youth Media Campaign (VERB)	$58,795	$0	$0	$0	N/A
Steps to a Healthier U.S.	$44,276	$43,857	$45,255	$1,398	3.2%
Racial and Ethnic Approach to Community Health (REACH)	$34,505	$34,259	$33,942	($317)	-0.9%
Genomics	$6,987	$6,952	$6,396	($556)	-8.0%
Birth Defects, Developmental Disabilities, Disability and Health	**$124,576**	**$124,762**	**$110,481**	**($14,281)**	**-11.4%**
Birth Defects and Developmental Disabilities	$39,239	$38,659	$38,298	($361)	-0.9%
Human Development and Disability	$65,111	$66,242	$54,395	($11,847)	-17.9%
Hereditary Blood Disorders	$20,226	$19,861	$17,788	($2,073)	-10.4%
Total, Health Promotion -	**$1,024,204**	**$963,426**	**$929,208**	**($34,218)**	**-3.6%**

SOURCE: Excerpted from CDC (2006).

Federal agencies often partner with public and private organizations to support obesity initiatives, as in the case of Planet Health and its recent grant from BlueCross BlueShield. In April 2007, the Robert Wood Johnson Foundation announced that it would commit at least $500 million to initiatives (particularly school-based programs) aimed at reversing childhood obesity. Such collaborations allow different stakeholders to become engaged in the program and provide promising sources of funding for schools to implement Planet Health. Initial federal funding of Planet Health's pilots were successful in assessing positive outcomes, indicating that schools may not face onerous barriers in obtaining such funding. The fact that more than 5,000 copies of the program's textbook have been purchased by 48 states and 20 countries speaks to the large-scale implementation possibilities (Harvard Prevention Research Center 2007).

Economic Feasibility

It is important to consider the economic feasibility of implementing Planet Health in a school or school system. Avenues to obtain federal support exist, particularly considering the program's efficacy and effectiveness have been proven through evidence-based techniques. States face rising healthcare costs partly due to a rising prevalence of obesity and its concomitant conditions; more than 25 percent of growth in total US healthcare spending over the past 15 years was estimated to be attributable to obesity (Finkelstein, Fiebelkorn, and Wang 2003). An increased prevalence of childhood obesity could have profound implications on future state healthcare spending because obese individuals incur higher medical costs and have decreased quality of life compared with their nonobese counterparts (Thorpe et al. 2004). Hospital costs associated with obesity have risen nearly threefold over the past decade for youth ages 6–17 years and are largely borne by states or private insurers (Wang and Dietz 2002). These figures, while staggering, do not include intangible costs such as school absenteeism or missed days of work. Clearly, states could benefit on many levels from widespread implementation of Planet Health in schools to reduce the burden of obesity among youth and the state's future population.

Programs and policies instituted by states are not always implemented to an equal or appropriate degree by schools. Physical education requirements and school nutrition mandates are two such programs for several reasons. Schools throughout a state often serve diverse populations with different backgrounds and needs. Schools in the inner city or a rural locale may serve children of lower SES, minority students, and others who are prone to risky behaviors. Furthermore, such schools may be unable to allocate limited budgets to implementing Planet Health, purchasing didactic materials for the program, or paying for teacher training and time away from the classroom. Finally, schools may worry that funding to support activities beyond initial program implementation would be unstable and difficult to obtain.

In 2003, independent researchers conducted a cost–benefit analysis of the first randomized pilot of Planet Health (Wang et al. 2003). To date, this analysis is the only one to formally evaluate a health promotion program aimed at reducing obesity. Its strength is that it considers the benefits of Planet Health from a population perspective rather than on an individual level. The outcomes assessed were cases of adulthood obesity prevented and quality-adjusted life years saved. Tangible program costs were assessed. Due to the seamless coordination of Planet Health with existing academic curricula, additional classroom costs (monetary costs and time) are minimal. The requisite curriculum book is currently priced at about US$45.00 and includes lesson plans, micro units, the Power Down campaign, and the FitCheck self-assessment tool (Human Kinetics 2007). Wang and colleagues estimate that the program cost per student per year was $14; the program could save approximately $1.20 in medical costs and lost wages for every $1 spent. Given that states and schools have finite monetary resources, the preceding economic analysis shows that implementing Planet Health would be an "effective use of available resources and should be included in [school] portfolios" (Wang et al. 2003). However, during times of tight budgets, weak academic performance standards, or economic downturns, schools may not choose to prioritize health education or accept the relatively low program costs. Planet Health must be in part financially supported at the district, county, or state level.

Administrative Feasibility

An assessment of administrative feasibility naturally follows economic feasibility. Schools have varying levels of curriculum competencies and may face challenges in implementing Planet Health—particularly if they have little prior experience with interdisciplinary curricula or substandard existing academic curricula (Gortmaker et al. 1999). Teachers can incorporate Planet Health components in a piecemeal fashion or teach lessons in varying degrees of detail, but these approaches may compromise program efficacy. Teachers also vary in teaching competencies, and the average training time may be insufficient for those needing additional support. A strength of the program is that teachers are responsible for program implementation and administration, and they tailor Planet Health materials to their schools and classrooms. However, if the school itself is experiencing overall staffing shortages, administration of Planet Health could be threatened. The cost of teacher training is mostly a one-time cost, as teachers could pass on material and knowledge once properly trained and knowledgeable (and could volunteer if they believe it has a positive effect on students) (Wiecha et al. 2004). Planet Health requires every participating teacher to utilize the program book (Human Kinetics 2007), but as noted above, schools may not be willing or able to purchase many books. However, one book can be purchased and shared between teachers or school districts, with the only cost being the copying of materials. The technological requirements are minimal (a computer or an overhead projector for presentations during teacher training) for Planet Health and could be borrowed. Finally, because the program is diffused over the course of two years, it is not overly burdensome to deliver or administer.

Some administrative burden is placed on the human resources component associated with Planet Health. Teachers may not have the time to undergo training, although the time is designed to be minimal (an average of two to three hours). They must also spend time incorporating Planet Health components into their regular academic lessons (on the other hand, this could allow for creative adaptations). Teachers also have the option of self-training, although key components of teacher training are group activities, discussion, and expert training. They may be reluctant to participate in the voluntary program. A stipend was provided to teachers throughout the pilot program; however, schools may not be able to provide such monetary incentives even with additional funding from outside sources. School administrators could explore nonmonetary incentives to offer (e.g., the optional wellness program). Overall, Planet Health has a moderately high level of administrative feasibility and allows schools to try creative or collaborative solutions to the aforementioned challenges they may face.

Political Feasibility

A final analysis of political feasibility is critical before overall feasibility and implementation can be judged. The political environment is generally supportive of programs aimed to reduce childhood obesity. First, the American public believes obesity to be a serious health concern facing children and adolescents. A recent nationally representative survey suggests that a majority of Americans ascribe responsibility to schools with regard to addressing obesity; most also believe that it is the government's responsibility to help support health promotion programs aimed at obesity (Endocrine Society 2006; Evans 2005). Further, the program is socially acceptable due to minimal costs to the public with proven benefits (Lakdawalla, Goldman, and Shang 2005). Additional supportive stakeholders include teachers and other school administrators, community groups, family members, advocacy agencies, community healthcare providers, and private and public insurers. The cost-effectiveness of Planet Health's broad and local implementation was previously outlined, but it becomes even more striking when considered against the backdrop of costs to the federal healthcare system, which will escalate because the deleterious effects of obesity will soon eclipse those from smoking and problem drinking (Lakdawalla, Goldman, and Shang 2005; Sturm 2002). Planet Health implementation could reduce costs to the federal government and taxpayers.

As previously stated, several federal agencies already support initiatives targeting childhood obesity. Some federal lawmakers have championed the issue and pushed it onto Congress's agenda with the introduction of legislation, such as the Improved Nutrition and Physical Activity Act and the Childhood Obesity Reduction Act. Such bills offer comprehensive approaches to prevention but are slow to garner attention. State-level policies are similarly slow to develop. A critical point is thus revealed: Planet Health, which is evidence based, generally feasible in its implementation and delivery, cost-effective, and socially acceptable presents a unique alternative that is palatable to a wide range of stakeholders. This demonstrates the unique role of what John Kingdon (2003) terms *specialists*—hidden participants in the generation of policy/program alternatives who are often responsible for unique yet grounded ideas. Lawmakers may view policies structured in a similar manner as Planet Health to be characterized as "client politics"—politically attractive to lawmakers on both sides of the aisle, large in scope, having a clear and measured objective(s), and targeting a group deemed deserving (Oliver 2006). The ultimate political success of Planet Health lies in the formation of coalition groups comprising a wide array of stakeholders; such collaborations would increase buy-in to the program, enable the generation of creative strategies and solutions that are personalized to the community's needs, and encourage program sustainability.

QUESTION 4

Selection of the Evaluation

Few outcome evaluations of Planet Health exist for one main reason. As outlined in Question 3, conducting outcome evaluations is a challenge for many schools with limited human and financial resources or expertise. One evaluation was a diffusion analysis aimed at evaluating feasibility, acceptability, and sustainability of Planet Health. The descriptive study used a relatively small sample size (Wiecha et al. 2004). Another evaluation was performed between two Indiana middle schools using a quasi-experimental design but was small in sample size and collected data completely through self-report questionnaires from students (Bai et al. 2006).

The evaluation chosen avoids many of these weaknesses (Gortmaker et al. 1999). When it was conducted, little evidence showed a causal link between program objectives, target behaviors, and obesity. In addition, few studies had been conducted on school-based interventions for broad populations of adolescents (such studies were mostly on obese/ high-risk individuals). The evaluation used a population deemed demographically and ethnically diverse. Its objective was to evaluate the impact of Planet Health on obesity among boys and girls in grades 6–8. Completion of this evaluation produced a benchmark that is widely used in the implementation of Planet Health and related programs.

Study Design

This evaluation employed a randomized pretest–posttest control group experimental design (Gliner and Morgan 2000) (Exhibit 10.5). At the start in 1995, schools were matched by town, or school size and ethnic composition, after which ten schools from four communities were randomly assigned as either intervention or control schools. The Planet Health curriculum was administered to students whose school enrollments in grades 6 or 7 began in fall 1995. Intervention school students received two years of Planet Health teaching within schools. In contrast, control schools did not receive the Planet Health curriculum—they only received the standard health education and/or existing physical education classes. Baseline data were collected in fall 1995 and follow-up data were collected in spring 1997. Planet Health didactic materials were provided to each teacher in the intervention schools, and the curriculum was applied during teacher trainings, classroom lessons, and other activities.

Study Population

The target or theoretical population from which researchers hoped to generalize results included all male and female students in grades 6–8. Researchers recruited schools to participate, choosing them on the basis of their willingness to implement the classroom/physical education curriculum, understanding of possible random assignment to a control or intervention group, and having an ethnically diverse student body. A cluster sampling technique was employed—schools were first matched in a nonrandom way and later randomly assigned to a study group. The selected sample had divided ten schools into an intervention group ($N_I = 5$) and control group ($N_C = 5$). Students within each school (cluster) were not randomized. The study sample was an appropriate target for the intervention.

This study met ethical considerations to ensure protection of study participants and was approved by the Committee on Human Subjects at the Harvard School of Public Health. Five schools used active informed consent, which required parents to return a consent form whether or not they wanted the child to participate. The other five schools used passive consent; parents had to sign and return a form only if they did *not* want their child to participate. Forms were translated into seven different languages to accommodate the schools' multiethnic compositions.

Researchers collected baseline data from 1,560 students after considering exclusion criteria; sample size calculations for precision were not performed. Students were excluded

---

EXHIBIT 10.5

Study Design of Planet Health

Randomized experimental design: pretest–posttest control design

Assignment	Group	Fall 1995 (pretest)	I.V.	Spring 1997 (posttest)
R	E:	O_1	X	O_3
R	C:	O_2	~X	O_4

Key
I.V. = Active independent variable
R = Random
E: = Experimental/intervention group
C: = Control or comparison group
O = Observation/measurement (anthropometric and behavioral assessments)
X = Intervention (Planet Health)
~X = Control or other treatment

if they had transferred schools during 1995, attended special education classes, or were in the "wrong" grade (either skipped a grade or were held back). Baseline analysis showed that the intervention and control students were similar in terms of gender, age, and ethnic composition.

Key Measures

Several types of variables and measures were used in this analysis (see Exhibit 10.6 for variable analysis and measure assessment). The active independent variable was the Planet Health intervention. Attribute independent variables were assessed by program staff and included age, sex, and race/ethnicity. Dependent variables included BMI (as a function of height and weight), triceps skinfold (TSF), television and video viewing, moderate/vigorous physical activity levels, intake of fruits/vegetables, proportion of energy from fat/saturated fat, and total energy intake. Several measures were used to assess these variables, including assessment by program staff and student self-report on a food and activity survey.

The main outcome measure was obesity, defined as a "BMI and TSF measure greater than or equal to the 85th percentile of age- and sex-specific reference data" (Gortmaker et al. 1999). Researchers cited limitations in previous obesity assessment using solely

Exhibit 10.6

Key Variables and Measures

Category of variable	Variables	Levels of measures	Data collection (instruments, etc.)	Instrument and measure assessment
(1) Attribute independent variables	Age (years)	Continuous	Calculated by program staff on the basis of birthdate and date of baseline examination.	Generally reliable. In cases of missing birthdate, data from the Food and Activity Survey were used (questionable reliability).
	Sex (M/F)	Dichotomous, categorical	Classified by program staff during baseline examination.	Reliable; in cases of missing data, data from school records were obtained.
	Race/ethnicity (White, African American, Hispanic, Asian/Pacific Islander, Other)	Nominal, categorical	Reported by students; based on responses to baseline surveys.	Generally reliable although weakened due to reliance on self-report and student discretion.
(2) Active independent variable	Planet Health intervention	N/A	N/A	Not available at time of evaluation.

(continued)

(3) Dependent variables	BMI (kg/m2)*	Continuous	Height and weight were obtained by program staff. Height was measured using a Shorr stadiometer; weight was measured using a calibrated electronic scale.	The electronic scale for measuring weight was calibrated using a standard test. It is unclear whether the instrument used to measure height was calibrated.	**EXHIBIT 10.6** Key Variables and Measures *(continued)*
	TSF (mm)	Continuous	Program staff measured TSF using Holtain calipers.	Measurements of TSF were performed twice to ensure precision. When measurements differed substantially, an average measure was calculated.	
	Television and video viewing (hours/day)	Continuous	Students answered 11 questions pertaining to a television and video measure.	The study cited high test-retest reliability of youth self-reports for television viewing.	
	Moderate and vigorous physical activity levels (hours/day)	Continuous	Students answered 16 questions on a youth activity questionnaire.	The questionnaire was excerpted from a larger survey that had been proven reliable and valid in adults **only**.	
	Intake of fruits and vegetables (servings/day)	Continuous	Students answered questions on a youth food frequency questionnaire.	The questionnaire was excerpted from a larger survey that had been validated for use in ethnically and socio-economically diverse populations. It is unclear whether validation occurred only among children.	
	Proportion of energy from fat and saturated fat (%)	Continuous			
	Total energy intake (kJ/day)	Continuous			
	Dieting to lose weight (%)	Continuous	Students answered questions on the Food and Activity Survey related to these measures.	These questions were adapted from the Youth Risk Behavior Surveillance Survey (YRBSS), which is widely recognized and used among youth. The measures used in the YRBSS have been shown to be associated with obesity in youth (Grunbaum et al. 2004).	
	Exercising to lose weight (%)	Continuous			
	Vomiting/taking laxatives to lose weight (%)	Continuous			
	Taking diet pills to lose weight (%)	Continuous			

*BMI has high specificity but low sensitivity for identifying adolescents who are overweight or obese. BMI has a high degree of correlation with laboratory measures of body fat composition but may differ by age, sex, and race/ethnicity. The use of BMI alone is also weak because it does not account for an individual's body frame size (Freedman et al. 2006).

BMI or TSF (see Exhibit 10.6) and chose to use this definition to ensure methodological soundness. Baseline data to assess demographics, anthropometry, and diet/activity were collected in fall 1995 from students in both intervention and control schools. Follow-up data on anthropometry and diet/activity were collected in spring 1997 from students in both intervention and control schools.

Analytic Strategy

Researchers employed the generalized estimating equation (GEE) regression method (Zeger and Liang 1986) to adjust for individual-level confounders within clusters (schools) and account for correlations between responses within schools. GEE is an appropriate regression model to use because it works well in analyses of multivariate, longitudinal data; assumes independence of between-cluster responses; assumes that a correlation pattern exists within cluster responses; and can control for the matched-pair design of this study. Researchers also accounted for school matching by including indicator variables in the regression analysis to represent randomization pairs. A further strength of the strategy used by Zeger and Liang was that it accounted for differences between boys and girls—running separate regressions by gender. The following variables were controlled for in the regression models: race/ethnicity, age, BMI, TSF, intervention status, and randomization pair indicators.

Regression analyses were run not only to predict changes in behavioral measures but also to assess to what level the intervention could be attributed to significant changes in behavior. Neither power calculations to ensure sufficient ability to detect statistical change nor α and β levels were reported in the analysis.

Threats to Internal Validity

The randomized design granted a high degree of internal validity to this study, which helped ensure that any observed outcomes were actually due to the active independent variables. Researchers controlled for most threats to internal validity by ensuring equivalence of intervention and control schools through their particular sampling methods and assessment of baseline characteristics. Regarding instrumentation, steps were taken for all measures to ensure measurement validity and reliability, through proper calibration of instruments or objective survey results assessment (i.e., Scantron) (see Exhibit 10.6). Randomization averted threats from regression—groups were similar throughout the study and did not appear to have extreme characteristics at the outset—and selection bias in this study. (An additional note: Neither schools nor students self-selected into either group.) Attrition initially appeared to be a threat. At baseline, the participation rate of students was 65 percent; rates were lower at follow-up due to school transfers, school absences during data collection times, or refusal to participate. However, participation rates at test points were similar between intervention and control schools, suggesting that any effects from attrition are likely to be controlled in the study.

Because this was a field-based design, particularly one being conducted in schools, researchers had a low level of control over extraneous variables in the students' environment (Gliner and Morgan 2000). While Planet Health's ultimate goal is to enable adolescents to make healthy choices in any scenario, the lack of control for such factors in the analysis threatened internal validity. As an example, a major advocacy group could have launched a nationwide campaign aimed at reducing child obesity during this study's time period, rendering any significant results solely attributed to Planet Health questionable. Finally, the use of self-report on dietary intake and physical activity is a major threat to validity. Students could have overestimated their actual behaviors to paint themselves in a positive light or simply reported results that they thought researchers would want to see. These self-report responses also have questionable reliability due to the young age of study participants—a measurement error that could have biased outcome measures.

Threats to External Validity

External validity refers to the generalizability of the study. Study populations were determined to be a good representation of adolescents across the country; because the actual sample was a good representation of the theoretical target population, a high level of population external validity exists (Gliner and Morgan 2000). A high degree of ecological external validity also exists, as a "natural" setting for Planet Health was used (Gliner and Morgan 2000). External validity was threatened by reactive/situational effects of testing. Students' awareness of learning from the Planet Health program may have been heightened during the study time—particularly after their baseline characteristics were gathered and the food and activity survey was administered. Their responsiveness may also have changed after taking the pretest—this could have occurred in both the intervention and control groups. Finally, threats from multiple treatments were small but may have existed. Although additional interventions were not administered in the schools, health promotion campaigns could have existed in the community or at parents' workplaces. Such situations could have biased the results of the study to make them less generalizable to the general population. A final source of bias could have been inherent in the researchers' initial active recruitment of the ten schools. Researchers sought schools that had experience with multidisciplinary curriculums and whose academic standards were at least minimally being met with adequate resources. These schools also received financial assistance. Such assistance may not exist in many other schools; thus, results may be tempered if Planet Health is applied in other settings.

Appropriateness of the Evaluation

Overall, the use of a randomized design for this evaluation strengthened the design and validity of the study. Randomization reduced bias and ensured equivalence among control and intervention schools; the initial matching of school pairs only served to enhance sampling efficiency and did not appear to affect outcomes. The main outcome measure was a reliable and valid indicator of obesity change because it incorporated both BMI and TSF measures. Furthermore, although the behavioral measures were assessed via self-report, they were compiled using valid and reliable survey instruments. The large sample populations taking the surveys overcame any inaccuracies of survey results. Possible confounding characteristics of the obesity–behavior relationship were controlled by both randomization and sampling as well as within regression analyses. When considering recommended program evaluation standards (CDC 1999), this Planet Health evaluation scored high—having great utility (properly served the needs of participants), good feasibility (practicality), high propriety (fair application of the intervention to students along appropriate ethical protocols), and high accuracy (addressed every hypothesis and research question it posited). It showed that Planet Health achieved many of its goals and objectives. Thus, although the generalizability of Planet Health was moderate, both the program and proper evaluations must continue to occur. Such evaluations will increase knowledge about the reliability and validity of program measures and continue to build an evidence base for Planet Health.

QUESTION 5

Consideration of the Intervention

As shown, Planet Health is a school-based primary prevention program that uniquely addresses childhood obesity by weaving health education through a school's academic curriculum. It addresses the major proximate and most actionable determinants of obesity (physical activity/diet) through comprehensive classroom lessons. Planet Health also incorporates the theory that television viewing among youth is an important and actionable determinant of obesity with the inclusion of a two-week campaign aimed at limiting television use and encouraging physical activity.

Planet Health targets a population on the basis of evidence that supports the efficacy of such programs in focusing on risky health behaviors. It also addresses the alarming increased prevalence, noting that it becomes more difficult for aging, overweight children to return to normal weight, who are then at risk for developing a host of obesity-related conditions. Thus, middle-aged adolescents are at a critical age for interventions such as Planet Health, strengthening the potential effectiveness of such a program. It is encouraging to learn that researchers are expanding Planet Health programs for fourth and fifth graders throughout Massachusetts. Per Question 3, schools, policymakers, and other stake-holders may perceive advantages to Planet Health implementation due to its low startup and subsequent costs, cost-effectiveness, and high administrative feasibility. That it is a school- and community-wide collaborative effort—requiring active participation from teachers and families—only ensures that the program is likely to be sustained. Finally, per Question 4, Planet Health was scientifically proven to deliver on several program goals and objectives: lowering obesity rates in schools, decreasing time of television viewing, and increasing quality of diet. Clearly, this program can deliver tangible results within just one program cycle (two years) when fully implemented.

Next Steps in Research

Perhaps the biggest strength of Planet Health—its randomized outcome evaluation—also reveals an inherent weakness. The evaluation is one of the first to assess a school-based program targeting obesity among this age bracket, and while its results are strong, it may have limited impact (particularly to policymakers). Sound evaluative research is a challenge to conduct, although Planet Health is relatively simple to implement. Schools may lack the human and financial resources necessary to conduct an evaluation. School staff may be busy with school-related responsibilities, with little time for or interest in evaluation. The absence of long-term cohort data is another area of major concern. This data would show that Planet Health is effective well beyond the middle school years, but its collection would require a large commitment of resources. There is also little data showing the effectiveness of Planet Health on other age groups or populations (e.g., elementary school students, minority populations). However, this information may be forthcoming with the recent expansion of Planet Health throughout the state of Massachusetts and among different grades. As alluded to in Question 3, political feasibility is often swayed by evidence-based arguments proving the efficacy and financial soundness of policy and program alternatives. Furthermore, policymakers and school administrators alike look to best practices when considering the implementation of new and innovative programs. In this regard, "best practices" databases that compile data on various school-based health promotion programs would be useful. The widespread implementation of Planet Health and similar programs may be stymied due to such current limitations.

In broader terms, there is a clear need for research on the relationships between other mid-level distal obesity determinants outlined in Question 1, including demographics, family characteristics, and home environment. Planet Health is successful in reducing obesity and certain behavioral measures *only* among females. These results suggest that mediating forces exist in the direct relationship between gender and obesity—a hypothesis that is mostly unsupported in the scientific literature and merits further research. Further research would be prudent to elucidate the association between obesity and risk in ethnically/culturally diverse populations (Freedman et al. 2006). The federal government has identified this as a crucial area of obesity research, but evidence for adults or children still lacks substance (National Task Force on the Prevention and Treatment of Obesity 2000). Finally, SES remains a complex yet distal determinant tied to obesity. Little evidence exists that adds to better understanding of this relationship; thus, there exists a need for research in this area.

Next Steps in Interventions

To date, the Planet Health program has been implemented in a number of demographically and socioeconomically diverse schools. As stated, the relatively simple implementation strategy is a major draw for school administrators interested in adding health education to school curriculums. However, a potential limitation of the current program is that it is only available in one form, which could hamper widespread implementation. Race/ethnicity/culture plays a potentially large role in obesity development, and expansion of Planet Health's curriculum could account for a variety of community needs. Multiple versions of the didactic materials specific to various cultures, ethnicities, languages, and even religions could be produced. The development of culturally competent materials need not be overly burdensome. Planet Health seems to thrive on school and community involvement; thus, different stakeholders throughout a community could collaborate to tailor the program to the specific needs of students served by community schools in keeping with the broad programmatic goals.

Planet Health is effective in helping students overcome risks associated with obesity by giving them the competencies to make healthy decisions in schools and beyond. However, the framework in Question 1 showed that distal factors, such as neighborhood safety, availability of food choices, and built environments, can have an effect on obesity. The program is somewhat limited by forces that exist beyond the school walls. The CDC supports and funds interventions designed to fall within one or more parts of the Coordinated School Health Program—a systematic model aimed at promoting student health through a multifaceted approach (Fisher et al. 2007). Thus, many possible interventions can be implemented throughout the school and community to address these distal determinants, such as initiatives to add or enhance the presence of community recreational facilities or to deliver comprehensive after-school programs for students and families. To this end, Planet Health is ahead of the curve through the addition of coordinated after-school programs throughout Massachusetts.

Next Steps in Policy

Per Question 3, the Planet Health program has a high degree of political feasibility, mostly due to its low cost and simple administration and the high salience of the problem among lawmakers and the American public. The program has important implications for targeted policy initiatives. The first is regarding research support. Question 3 outlined mechanisms from federal sources that exist to fund programs such as Planet Health. Clearly, federal financial support is critical to most schools that are interested in implementing Planet Health; the precarious nature of federal grants for health promotion programs reinforces the need for policies that ensure sustained support to states and communities. Similarly, the challenges to conducting valid, reliable, and long-term evaluations of Planet Health are questionable. Many grant mechanisms for health promotion programs fail to support long-term goals, indicating the need for policies that ensure sustained funding. Finally, one weakness of Planet Health concerned its implementation and sustainability within schools that may have limited budgets or serve poor socioeconomic populations. Priority funding could be allocated to such schools to implement Planet Health and similar programs (Veugelers and Fitzgerald 2005).

A unique strength of Planet Health is its effect on television viewing. Question 1 hypothesized the effect of commercial messaging on obesity. Policy options to this end include a ban on food product advertising targeted to children, mandatory marketing about nutrition and fitness that is equal in time to junk food ads, or a prohibition of the use of children's characters to promote unhealthy food (Mello, Rimm, and Studdert 2003; KFF 2004). Advocacy groups are persistent in pushing this issue, but Congress has been slow to act in regulating either the food manufacturing industry or media corporations. In 1990, Congress passed the Children's Television Act, mandating advertising limits during children's programming. This action is a step in the right direction but likely not enough to strengthen the effects of a program such as Planet Health. Finally, schools across the United States are decreasing or eliminating physical or health education from curriculums, partly due to financial constraints. Public schools also face pressures in meeting academic standards to obtain funding. Few states require the recommended level of physical education for students, and of these states, many either lack the resources for implementation or freely grant participation waivers to excuse students. School nutrition standards suffer from similar circumstances—nutritious foods are often expensive for schools and difficult to prepare. Moreover, many schools depend on subsidies from food or vending machine manufacturers that provide unhealthy food options to students. The Planet Health program could fall victim to this circumstance, thereby confusing students in schools that provide lessons on healthy eating yet offer unhealthy food options. Federal or state policies that mandate physical education or set standards for school food options would address these problems. Advocates continue to push this issue at both levels, although states have been more receptive to such policies than Congress has.

Most Important Next Step

The most crucial step in addressing childhood obesity relates to research—to develop and evaluate initiatives focused on gender and certain sociodemographic groups. The link between gender, SES, race/ethnicity, and obesity is poorly understood, yet these are powerful confounders affecting the pathways between many other determinants and obesity. Females, youth of low SES, and racial/ethnic minorities still disparately suffer from obesity and its concomitant conditions. Strong research findings could feed the political "problem stream" (Kingdon 2003) and drive broad-based policy changes, such as increased funding toward initiatives for certain marginalized populations. This point is particularly important when considering that issues related to the above groups typically have moderate social or political acceptability (although issues related to children are much more salient). A further important step is federal, state, or local financial support of health promotion programs and accompanying evaluations among these groups. As stated, evidence proving the efficacy of such programs—particularly among youth—is sparse. Policymakers need to know which types of interventions are successful and a prudent use of public funds. Childhood obesity is a major health problem that is complex in its origin and the potential avenues for solutions, which warrants continued research to understand its determinants. Such research drives development of evidence-based health promotion interventions aimed at primary prevention in youth. Research and the development of interventions aimed at certain marginalized groups, set in either schools or communities, appear to be the most important steps when considering how best to address the problem. While entities face many challenges in how they choose to address childhood obesity, the growing magnitude and salience of the problem will continue to drive science and practice solutions.

REFERENCES

Adler, N. E., and J. M. Ostrove. 1999. "Socioeconomic Status and Health: What We Know and What We Don't." *Annals of the New York Academy of Sciences* 896: 116–19.

Allison, D. B., K. R. Fontaine, J. E. Manson, J. Stevens, and T. B. VanItallie. 1999. "Annual Deaths Attributable to Obesity in the United States." *Journal of the American Medical Association* 282 (16): 1530–38.

American Academy of Child & Adolescent Psychiatry (AACAP). 2001. "Facts for Families: Obesity in Children and Teens." Updated in January. http://aacap.org/page.ww?name=Obesity+in+Children+and+Teens&section=Facts+for+Families.

American Obesity Association [renamed Obesity Society]. 2007. "Childhood Obesity." Accessed June 11. www.obesity.org/subs/childhood/.

Baba, R., M. Koketsu, M. Nagashima, H. Inasaka, M. Yoshinaga, and M. Yokota. 2007. "Adolescent Obesity Adversely Affects Blood Pressure and Resting Heart Rate." *Circulation Journal* 71: 722–26.

Bai, Y., D. A. Tanner, V. A. Caine, N. Omoiele, and A. D. Fly. 2006. "Evaluation of the Planet Health Intervention in an Indiana Middle School." *The FASEB Journal* 20: A1011.

Basu, S. 2007. "CDC FY '08 Budget Request $37 Million Less than Current Funding Level." *U.S. Medicine*. Published in March. www.usmedicine.com/article.cfm?article ID=1528&issueID=97.

Boynton-Jarrett, R., T. N. Thomas, K. E. Peterson, J. Wiecha, A. M. Sobol, and S. L. Gortmaker. 2003. "Impact of Television Viewing Patterns on Fruit and Vegetable Consumption Among Adolescents." *Pediatrics* 112: 1321–26.

Brener, N. D., L. Kann, S. Lee, M. L. McKenna, H. Wechsler, J. E. Fulton, and D. A. Galuska. 2006. "Secondary School Health Education Related to Nutrition and Physical Activity— Selected Sites, United States, 2004." *Morbidity and Mortality Weekly Report* 55 (30): 821–24.

Burdette, H. L., and R. C. Whitaker. 2005. "A National Study of Neighborhood Safety, Outdoor Play, Television Viewing, and Obesity in Preschool Children." *Pediatrics* 116: 657–62.

Centers for Disease Control and Prevention (CDC). 2008. "Physical Activity and Good Nutrition: Essential Elements to Prevent Chronic Diseases and Obesity, 2008." Published in February. www.cdc.gov/nccdphp/publications/aag/pdf/dnpa.pdf.

———. 2006. "FY 2007 CDC/ATSDR Funding Table, 2006." Accessed June 13, 2007. www .cdc.gov/fmo/PDFs/FY07/FundFunctAreaTable.pdf.

———. 2004a. "Indicators for Chronic Disease Surveillance." *Morbidity and Mortality Weekly Report* 53 (RR-11): 1–6.

———. 2004b. "Prevalence of Overweight and Obesity Among Adults with Diagnosed Diabetes—United States, 1988–1994 and 1999–2002." *Morbidity and Mortality Weekly Report* 53 (45): 1066–68.

———. 2000. "School Health Programs: An Investment in Our Nation's Future." Accessed June 11, 2007. www.cdc.gov/nccdphp/dash.

———. 1999. "Framework for Program Evaluation in Public Health." *MMWR Recommendations and Reports* 48 (No. RR-11).

Cook, S., M. Weitzman, P. Auinger, and S. E. Barlow. 2005. "Screening and Counseling Associated with Obesity Diagnosis in a National Survey of Ambulatory Pediatric Visits." *Pediatrics* 116: 112–16.

Daviglus, M. L. 2005. "Health Care Costs in Old Age Are Related to Overweight and Obesity Earlier in Life." *Health Affairs* 5: 97–100.

Dietz, W. H., and S. L. Gortmaker. 1985. "Do We Fatten Our Children at the Television Set? Obesity and Television Viewing in Children and Adolescents." *Pediatrics* 75: 807–12.

Duke, J., M. Huhman, and C. Heitzler. 2003. "Physical Activity Levels Among Children Aged 9–13 Years—United States, 2002." *Morbidity and Mortality Weekly Report* 52 (33): 785–88.

Edmunds, L., E. Waters, and E. J. Elliott. 2001. "Evidence-Based Management of Childhood Obesity." *BMJ* 323: 916–19.

Endocrine Society. 2007. "NIH FY 2007 Budget Finally Set; President Signs Joint Funding Resolution." *Endocrine Insider.* Published February 21. www.endo-society.org/publicpolicy/insider/.

Endocrine Society, Research America. 2006. "Obesity Cited Number One Kids' Health Issue." Published December 13. www.endo-society.org/news/press/2006/upload/Rls_Endocrine_Poll_FINAL.pdf.

Evans, W. D. 2005. "Public Perceptions of Childhood Obesity." *American Journal of Preventive Medicine* 28 (1): 26–32.

Finance Project. 2004. "Financing Childhood Obesity Prevention Programs: Federal Funding Sources and Other Strategies." Published in September. www.financeproject.org/Publications/obesityprevention.pdf.

Finkelstein, E. A., I. C. Fiebelkorn, and G. Wang. 2003. "National Medical Spending Attributable to Overweight and Obesity: How Much, and Who's Paying?" *Health Affairs* W3: 219–26.

Fisher, C., P. Hunt, L. Kann, L. Kolbe, B. Patterson, and H. Wechsler. 2007. "Building a Healthier Future Through School Health Programs." CDC Health Youth Publications. Accessed June 11. www.cdc.gov/HealthyYouth/publications/pdf/PP-Ch9.pdf.

Ford, E. S., D. F. Williamson, and S. Liu. 1997. "Weight Change and Diabetes Incidence: Findings from a National Cohort of U.S. Adults." *American Journal of Epidemiology* 146 (3): 214–22.

Franks, A. L., S. H. Kelder, G. A. Dino, K. A. Horn, S. L. Gortmaker, J. L. Wiecha, and E. J. Simoes. 2007. "School-Based Programs: Lessons Learned from CATCH, Planet Health, and Not-on-Tobacco." *Preventing Chronic Disease*. Published April 6. www.cdc.gov/pcd/issues/2007/apr/06_0105.htm.

Freedman, D. S., W. H. Dietz, S. R. Srinivasan, and G. S. Berenson. 1999. "The Relation of Overweight to Cardiovascular Risk Factors Among Children and Adolescents: The Bogalusa Heart Study." *Pediatrics* 103: 1175–82.

Freedman, D. S., L. K. Khan, M. K. Serdula, C. L. Ogden, and W. H. Dietz. 2006. "Racial and Ethnic Differences in Secular Trends for Childhood BMI, Weight, and Height." *Obesity* 14 (2): 301–8.

Glanz, K., B. K. Rimer, and F. M. Lewis. 2002. *Health Behavior and Health Education: Theory, Research, and Practice*. San Francisco: Jossey-Bass.

Gliner, J. A., and G. A. Morgan. 2000. *Research Methods in Applied Settings: An Integrated Approach to Design and Analysis.* Mahwah, NJ: Lawrence Erlbaum.

Gordon-Larsen, P., M. C. Nelson, P. Page, and B. M. Popkin. 2006. "Inequality in the Built Environment Underlies Key Health Disparities in Physical Activity and Obesity." *Pediatrics* 117: 417–24.

Gortmaker, S. L., A. Must, J. M. Perrin, A. M. Sobol, and W. H. Dietz. 1993. "Social and Economic Consequences of Overweight in Adolescence and Young Adulthood." *New England Journal of Medicine* 329 (14): 1008–12.

Gortmaker, S. L., K. Peterson, J. Wiecha, A. M. Sobol, S. Dixit, M. K. Fox, and N. Laird. 1999. "Reducing Obesity via a School-Based Interdisciplinary Intervention Among Youth." *Archives of Pediatrics & Adolescent Medicine* 53: 409–18.

Green, L. W., and M. W. Kreuter. 1999. *Health Promotion Planning: An Educational and Ecological Approach*, 3rd ed. Boston: McGraw Hill.

Grunbaum, J. A., L. Kann, S. Kinchen, J. Ross, J. Hawkins, R. Lowry, W. A. Harris, T. McManus, D. Chyen, and J. Collins. 2004. "Youth Risk Behavior Surveillance—United States, 2003." *MMWR CDC Surveillance Summary* 53 (2): 1–96.

Harvard Prevention Research Center on Nutrition and Physical Activity. 2007. Planet Health home page. Accessed June 11. www.hsph.harvard.edu/prc/proj_planet.html.

Hedley, A. A., C. L. Ogden, C. L. Johnson, M. D. Carroll, L. R. Curtin, and K. M. Flegal. 2004. "Prevalence of Overweight and Obesity Among US Children, Adolescents, and Adults, 1999–2002." *Journal of the American Medical Association* 291 (23): 2847–50.

Human Kinetics. 2007. "Planet Health—an Interdisciplinary Curriculum for Teaching Middle School Nutrition and Physical Activity." Accessed June 12. www.humankinetics.com/products/showproduct.cfm?isbn=0736031057.

Institute of Medicine (IOM). 2002. *The Future of the Public's Health in the 21st Century.* Washington, DC: National Academies Press.

Janssen, I., W. F. Boyce, K. Simpson, and W. Pickett. 2006. "Influence of Individual- and Area-Level Measures of Socioeconomic Status on Obesity, Unhealthy Eating, and Physical Inactivity in Canadian Adolescents." *American Journal of Clinical Nutrition* 83: 139–45.

Kaiser Family Foundation (KFF). 2004. "The Role of Media In Childhood Obesity." [Issue brief.] Published in February. www.kff.org/entmedia/entmedia022404pkg.cfm.

Katz, D. L., M. O'Connell, M.-C. Yeh, H. Nawaz, V. Njike, L. M. Anderson, S. Cory, and W. Dietz. 2005. "Public Health Strategies for Preventing and Controlling Overweight and Obesity in School and Worksite Settings: A Report on Recommendations of the Task Force on Community Preventive Services." *Morbidity and Mortality Weekly Report* 54 (No. RR10): 1–12.

Kingdon, J. W. 2003. *Agendas, Alternatives, and Public Policies*, 2nd ed. New York: Longman.

Lakdawalla, D. N., D. P. Goldman, and B. Shang. 2005. "The Health and Cost Consequences of Obesity Among the Future Elderly." *Health Affairs* W5: R30–R40.

Latner, J. D., A. J. Stunkard, and G. T. Wilson. 2005. "Stigmatized Students: Age, Sex, and Ethnicity Effects in the Stigmatization of Obesity." *Obesity Research* 13 (7): 1226–31.

Lawlor, D. A., R. M. Martin, D. Gunnell, B. Galobardes, S. Ebrahim, J. Sandhu, Y. Ben-Shlomo, P. McCarron, and G. Davey Smith. 2006. "Association of Body Mass Index Measured in Childhood, Adolescence, and Young Adulthood with Risk of Ischemic Heart Disease and Stroke: Findings from 3 Historical Cohort Studies." *American Journal of Clinical Nutrition* 83: 767–73.

Ludwig, D. S., K. E. Peterson, and S. L. Gortmaker. 2001. "Relation Between Consumption of Sugar-Sweetened Drinks and Childhood Obesity: A Prospective, Observational Analysis." *Lancet* 357: 505–8.

Luepker, R. V., C. L. Perry, S. M. McKinlay, P. R. Nader, G. S. Parcel, E. J. Stone, L. S. Webber, J. P. Elder, H. A. Feldman, C. C. Johnson, et al. 1996. "Outcomes of a Field Trial to Improve Children's Dietary Patterns and Physical Activity. The Child and Adolescent Trial for Cardiovascular Health. CATCH Collaborative Group." *Journal of the American Medical Association* 275 (10): 768–76.

Luma, G. B., and R. T. Spiotta. 2006. "Hypertension in Children and Adolescents." *American Family Physician* 73 (9): 1558–68.

Manson, J. E., P. J. Skerrett, P. Greenland, and T. B. VanItallie. 2004. "The Escalating Pandemics of Obesity and Sedentary Lifestyle: A Call to Action for Clinicians." *Archives of Internal Medicine* 164: 249–57.

Marmot, M., and R. G. Wilkinson (eds.). 2006. *Social Determinants of Health*, 2nd ed. New York: Oxford University Press.

Mello, M. M., E. B. Rimm, and D. M. Studdert. 2003. "The McLawsuit: The Fast-Food Industry and Legal Accountability for Obesity." *Health Affairs* 22 (6): 207–16.

Merchant, A. T., M. Dehghan, D. Behnke-Cook, and S. S. Anand. 2007. "Diet, Physical Activity, and Adiposity in Children in Poor and Rich Neighborhoods: A Cross-Sectional Comparison." *Nutrition Journal* 6 (1): 1–7.

National Conference of State Legislatures (NCSL). 2007. "Childhood Obesity—2006 Update and Overview of Policy Options." Updated April 30. www.ncsl.org/programs/health/ ChildhoodObesity-2006.htm.

National Institutes of Health (NIH). 1998. *Clinical Guidelines on the Identification, Evaluation, and Treatment of Overweight and Obesity in Adults: The Evidence Report*. Published in September. www.nhlbi.nih.gov/guidelines/obesity/ob_gdlns.pdf.

National Task Force on the Prevention and Treatment of Obesity. 2000. "Overweight, Obesity, and Health Risk." *Archives of Internal Medicine* 160: 898–904.

Nelson, M. C. 2006. "Body Mass Index Gain, Fast Food, and Physical Activity: Effects of Shared Environments over Time." *Obesity* 14 (4): 701–9.

Nielsen, S. J. 2002. "Trends in Food Locations and Sources Among Adolescents and Young Adults." *Preventive Medicine* 35: 107–13.

Office of the Surgeon General. 2001. "The Surgeon General's Call to Action to Prevent and Decrease Overweight and Obesity." Published December 13. www.surgeongeneral.gov/topics/obesity/calltoaction/toc.htm.

Ogden, C. L., M. D. Carroll, L. R. Curtin, M. A. McDowell, C. J. Tabak, and K. M. Flegal. 2006. "Prevalence of Overweight and Obesity in the United States, 1999–2004." *Journal of the American Medical Association* 295 (13): 1549–55.

Oliver, T. R. 2006. "The Politics of Public Health Policy." *Annual Review of Public Health* 27: 195–233.

Peeters, A., L. Bonneux, W. J. Nusselder, C. De Laet, and J. J. Barendregt. 2004. "Adult Obesity and the Burden of Disability Throughout Life." *Obesity Research* 212 (7): 1145–51.

Plourde, G. 2006. "Preventing and Managing Pediatric Obesity." *Canadian Family Physician* 52: 322–28.

Rhodes, R. E., H. M. MacDonald, and H. A. McKay. 2006. "Predicting Physical Activity Intention and Behaviour Among Children in a Longitudinal Sample." *Social Science & Medicine* 62: 3146–56.

Robert Wood Johnson Foundation (RWJF). 2007. "Robert Wood Johnson Foundation Announces $500-Million Commitment to Reverse Childhood Obesity in U.S." Published April 4. www.rwjf.org/newsroom/newsreleasesdetail.jsp?id=10483.

Robinson, T. N. 1993. "Does Television Viewing Increase Obesity and Reduce Physical Activity? Cross-Sectional and Longitudinal Analyses Among Adolescent Girls." *Pediatrics* 91: 273–80.

Schneider, M. 2000. *Introduction to Public Health*. Gaithersburg, MD: Aspen.

Sharma, M. 2006. "School-Based Interventions for Childhood and Adolescent Obesity." *Obesity Reviews* 7 (3): 261–69.

Sjoberg, R. L., K. W. Nilsson, and J. Leppert. 2005. "Obesity, Shame, and Depression in School-Aged Children: A Population-Based Study." *Pediatrics* 116: e389–e392.

Spiegel, S. A. 2006. "Reducing Overweight Through a Multidisciplinary School-Based Intervention." *Obesity* 14 (1): 88–96.

Strauss, R. S., and J. Knight. 1999. "Influence of the Home Environment on the Development of Obesity in Children." *Pediatrics* 103: 85–92.

Stunkard, A. J., and T. I. Sorenson. 1993. "Obesity and Socioeconomic Status—A Complex Relation." *New England Journal of Medicine* 328: 1036–37.

Sturm, R. 2002. "The Effects of Obesity, Smoking, and Drinking on Medical Problems and Costs." *Health Affairs* 21 (2): 245–53.

Sturm, R., J. S. Ringel, and T. Andreyeva. 2004. "Increasing Obesity Rates and Disability Trends." *Health Affairs* 23 (2): 199–205.

Sturm, R., and K. B. Wells. 2001. "Does Obesity Contribute as Much to Morbidity as Poverty or Smoking?" *Public Health* 115 (3): 229–35.

Swallen, K. C., E. N. Reither, S. A. Haas, and A. M. Meier. 2005. "Overweight, Obesity, and Health-Related Quality of Life Among Adolescents: The National Longitudinal Study of Adolescent Health." *Pediatrics* 115: 340–47.

Tanofsy-Kraff, M., M. L. Cohen, S. Z. Yanovski, C. Cox, K. R. Theim, M. Keil, J. C. Reynolds, and J. A. Yanovski. 2006. "A Prospective Study of Psychological Predictors of Body Fat Gain Among Children at High Risk for Adult Obesity." *Pediatrics* 117: 1203–9.

Thorpe, K. E., C. S. Florence, D. H. Howard, and P. Joski. 2004. "The Impact of Obesity on Rising Medical Spending." *Health Affairs* W4: 480–86.

Trust for America's Health. 2005. "F as in Fat: How Obesity Policies Are Failing in America." [Issue report.] Published in August. http://healthyamericans.org/reports/obesity2005/Obesity2005Report.pdf.

University of South Australia. 2004. "Children and Sports: An Overview." Australian Sports Commission. Accessed June 11, 2007. www.ausport.gov.au/research/documents/ChildrenSportOverview.pdf.

US Department of Health and Human Services (HHS). 2000. *Healthy People 2010.* Washington, DC: HHS.

———. 1996. *Physical Activity and Health: A Report of the Surgeon General.* Accessed June 11, 2007. www.cdc.gov/nccdphp/sgr/pdf/sgrfull.pdf.

US Department of Health and Human Services (HHS) and US Department of Education (DOE). 2000. "Promoting Better Health for Young People Through Physical Activity and Sports: A Report to the President." Accessed June 11, 2007. www.cdc.gov/nccdphp/dash/presphysactrpt.

Vandewater, E. A., and X. Huang. 2006. "Parental Weight Status as a Moderator of the Relationship Between Television Viewing and Childhood Overweight." *Archives of Pediatrics & Adolescent Medicine* 60: 425–31.

Veugelers, P. J., and A. L. Fitzgerald. 2005. "Prevalence of and Risk Factors for Childhood Overweight and Obesity." *Canadian Medical Association Journal* 173 (6): 607–13.

Wang, G., and W. H. Dietz. 2002. "Economic Burden of Obesity in Youth Aged 6 to 17 Years: 1979–1999." *Pediatrics* 109: 81–87.

Wang, L. Y., Q. Yang, R. Lowry, and H. Wechsler. 2003. "Economic Analysis of a School-Based Obesity Prevention Program." *Obesity Research* 11 (11): 1313–24.

Whitaker, R. C., J. A. Wright, M. S. Pepe, K. D. Seidel, and W. H. Dietz. 1997. "Predicting Obesity in Young Adulthood from Childhood and Parental Obesity." *New England Journal of Medicine* 337 (13): 869–73.

Wiecha, J. L., A. M. El Ayadi, B. F. Fuemmeler, J. E. Carter, S. Handler, S. Johnson, N. Strunk, D. Korzec-Ramirez, and S. L. Gortmaker. 2004. "Diffusion of an Integrated Health Education Program in an Urban School System: Planet Health." *Journal of Pediatric Psychology* 29 (6): 467–74.

Williams, J., M. Wake, K. Hesketh, E. Maher, and E. Waters. 2005. "Health-Related Quality of Life of Overweight and Obese Children." *Journal of the American Medical Association* 293 (1): 70–76.

Yanovski, J. A., and S. Z. Yanovski. 2003. "Treatment of Pediatric and Adolescent Obesity." *Journal of the American Medical Association* 289 (14): 1851–53.

Zeger, S., and K. Liang. 1986. "Longitudinal Data Analysis for Discrete and Continuous Outcomes." *Biometrics* 42: 121–30.

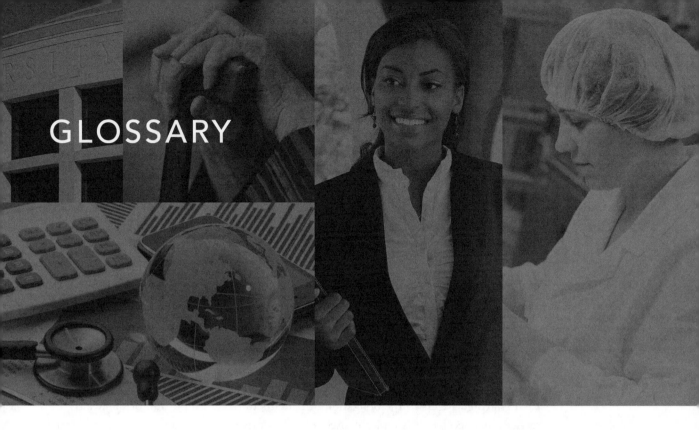

GLOSSARY

Activities of daily living (ADLs): Measure of functioning that includes six basic activities: eating; bathing; dressing; using a toilet; maintaining bowel and bladder control; and transferring, such as getting out of bed or moving into a chair.

Administrative simplification: Provision in the Health Insurance Portability and Accountability Act and the Affordable Care Act that aims to reduce administrative costs through the adoption of electronic transactions and standardization of operating rules.

Agency relationship: The consumer, or the patient in healthcare, delegates some authority to make decisions and perform actions on his behalf to an expert agent (in the case of healthcare, the physician or other healthcare provider).

Agenda/agenda setting: In this context, agenda refers to issues targeted for policy consideration. Agenda setting refers to the ability to influence the priorities of issues for policy consideration.

Amendment: Change or addition to a current law or piece of legislation.

Attrition: Loss of participants during a study that measures outcomes over time.

Avian influenza: A type-A influenza viral infection in wild or domestic birds. The avian flu virus can become a public health danger if a change (mutation) allows it to more easily infect humans, and it can potentially start a worldwide epidemic.

Capitation: A fixed fee for each patient.

Clinical practice guidelines: Evidence-based and systematically developed protocols (statements) used to assist healthcare providers in making appropriate healthcare and clinical decisions regarding specific conditions or circumstances.

Communicable diseases: Also called infectious diseases; refer to illnesses caused by organisms such as bacteria, viruses, fungi, and parasites. Communicable diseases may be transmitted by one infected person to another, from an animal to a human, or from some inanimate object to an individual, depending on the disease.

Conditions of Participation: Health and safety standards defined by CMS as the minimum requirements that hospitals and medical centers must meet to be eligible to serve publicly insured patients.

Corporate America: An informal term referring to the corporations based and operating in the United States; they are not under direct governmental control.

Cost sharing: Refers to the obligation of patients to pay for a portion of the healthcare services they receive. It is typically used as an incentive to avoid excessive or unnecessary utilization. However, it may also deter appropriate utilization.

Cross-sectional survey: A descriptive research method used to examine characteristics of a population within a short time frame.

Culturally appropriate services: Efforts by healthcare organizations and providers to increase understanding and produce effective interventions for patients by taking into account patients' cultural and linguistic characteristics.

Deductible: The amount an insured patient must pay out-of-pocket for his medical care per year before the insurance plan covers the costs.

Defensive medicine: The practice of medicine in which the main goal is to avoid malpractice claims, not to ensure good health for the patient or maximum medical efficiency.

Democratic: The term *democratic* ("small-d") refers to processes carried out in the democratic, representative tradition. It is not the same as *Democratic* ("big-D"), which often refers to the Democratic political party in the United States.

Dependent variable: The variable that is examined to determine whether its observed value changes when the independent variable is present or when exposed to the independent variable.

Determinants of health: Factors that influence one's health status. Typically, they include one's socioeconomic status, environment, behaviors, heredity, and access to medical care.

Disability: A physical or mental condition that limits an individual's ability to perform functions generally characterized as normal.

Disability-adjusted life year (DALY): A measure of the loss of healthy life. This measurement is intended to capture the economic, social, and functional realities that a person with a disability will face and the corresponding loss in health status and quality of life.

Discounted fee-for-service: A fee agreed on between an insurance plan and physicians to provide medical services at a lower cost than is common for the area in exchange for access to the insurance plan's pool of patients.

Distributive policy: Regulations that provide benefits or services to targeted populations or subpopulations, typically as entitlements.

Efficiency analysis: Analysis of the overall direct and indirect costs and benefits of an intervention; can be used to compare interventions or programs with similar goals.

Enabling services: Services (e.g., transportation, interpretation, education, community outreach) that enhance access to medical care.

Evidence-based medicine: Using the best available evidence acquired through the scientific method to guide clinical decision making.

Fast food: Refers to the ready-to-eat, often portable and inexpensive foods available through many outlets in the United States. This type of food tends to be less healthy than homemade food and has been criticized for contributing to the obesity epidemic in the United States.

Federal poverty level (FPL): A calculation reflecting a set of federal government guidelines related to income that is based on the cost of living (the amount of income needed by families of different sizes to be self-supportive). Many federal assistance programs use a percentage of FPL as part of their eligibility criteria.

Federal Register: A public-access source that publishes presidential and federal agency documents. A daily publication of the US federal government.

Gatekeeper: A qualified health professional, usually a primary care physician, who must approve specialist visits before they are covered by an insurance program.

General interview guide approach: An approach to conducting interviews that provides an outline of subjects the interviewer is required to cover but allows the interviewer flexibility with regard to the type and order of questions asked.

Global health: An area of study, research, and practice that focuses on improving health and achieving health equity for all people worldwide (Koplan et al. 2009).

Globalization: Worldwide changes in many aspects of people's lives driven by the exchange of information across borders and characterized by (1) increased production of goods and services by developing countries and (2) the expanded interdependence of developed and emerging economies (Shi and Singh 2011).

Gross domestic product: Refers to the value of all goods and services produced within a country for a given period; a key indicator of the country's economic activity and financial well-being.

H1N1 (swine) flu: A respiratory disease caused by influenza type-A viruses first detected in 2009. The new strain of influenza A (H1N1) virus is a mix of swine, human, and/or avian influenza viruses that is contagious and can cause seasonal flu.

Health maintenance organization (HMO): A managed care organization that focuses on wellness care and requires use of a specified panel of providers.

Health policy: Legislation over individuals, organizations, or the society whose goal is to improve health for the population or subpopulations.

Healthcare policy: Part of health policy but with a focus on healthcare. Specifically, it is related to the financing, delivery, and governance of health services for the populations or subpopulations within a jurisdiction.

Heterogeneous: Consisting of different types; a term used to describe a sample or a population composed of subjects that have dissimilar characteristics.

Independent variable: The variable representing the treatment, characteristic, exposure, or other intervention that is being examined to determine its effect on the dependent variable.

Informal conversational interview: An interview conducted in observational studies that does not follow a prescribed set of questions.

Institutional review board (IRB): A committee that examines the ethical implications of research to protect study subjects from physical or psychological harm.

Instrumental activities of daily living (IADLs): Measure of an individual's ability to perform activities that are necessary to live independently in noninstitutional settings, such as driving a car, shopping, preparing meals, and performing light housework.

Interest group: A collective of individuals or entities that hold a common set of preferences on a particular health issue and often seek to influence policymaking or public opinion.

Jurisdiction: The authority to interpret and apply the law.

Legislation: Law made by government to achieve a particular objective.

Legislator: Individual responsible for making or enacting laws.

Life expectancy: Anticipated number of years of life remaining.

Lobbying: Activities seeking to influence an individual or organization with decision-making authority.

Longitudinal survey: A survey administered to the same sample or similar samples at repeated intervals over a predetermined length of time.

Managed care: A care model characterized by a designated provider network, standardized review and quality improvement measures, an emphasis on preventive rather than acute care, and financial incentives for doctors and patients to reduce unnecessary medical care use.

Managed care organizations (MCOs): Organizations that seek to apply the components of managed care to a population in the hope of providing high-quality care at a lower cost than that incurred by the provision of fee-for-service care.

Marginalization: A process in which a person or an idea is pushed aside in favor of another. A marginalized subject typically receives few resources and little attention.

Matching: The process of ensuring equal representation among experimental and control groups by matching participants or proportions of participants on the basis of selected characteristics.

Measurement reliability: The extent to which results are similar if the measurement tool is reapplied in a consistent way.

Measurement validity: The extent to which the measurement tool accurately measures the intended concepts.

Medicaid: Joint federal and state insurance plan for the indigent.

Medical outcomes research: Research that examines the comparative effectiveness of available treatments for a patient with specified characteristics.

Medicare: Federal government insurance plan for persons aged 65 years or older, disabled individuals who are entitled to Social Security benefits, and people who have end-stage renal (kidney) disease.

Morbidity: Incidence or prevalence of diseases in a given population within a specified period.

Mortality: Number of deaths in a given population within a specified period.

Noncommunicable diseases: Refer to noninfectious medical conditions or illnesses; typically of long duration and slow progression.

Nongovernmental organizations: Organizations that are operated independent of the government.

Office of Management and Budget: The largest component of the Executive Office; implements and enforces the commitments and priorities of the president and assists executive departments and agencies across the federal government.

Oversight: Activities to review, monitor, or supervise the process of formulating, implementing, and modifying public policy.

Panel study: A study in which data are collected repeatedly over time from the same sample selected from the overall population to examine how individuals change over time.

Pay for performance: Payment-related incentives often used by insurance companies or government payers to reward healthcare providers, such as physicians and hospitals, for meeting preestablished performance measures for quality and efficiency.

Policy analysis: A systematic approach by which to assess problems and guide decision making.

Policy entrepreneur: Public innovator who, from outside the formal positions of government, introduces, translates, and implements new ideas into public practice.

Policy position: The stand taken regarding a particular issue. Policy position often influences the focus and orientation of legislation.

Preferred provider organization (PPO): A managed care organization that offers unrestricted provider options to enrollees and discounted fee arrangements to providers.

Premium: The amount an enrollee must pay to join the managed care plan. It serves as a membership fee and is typically adjusted annually.

Privatization: The movement of an industry in a country from the public to the private sphere.

Purposive (quota) sampling: A nonprobability sampling technique whereby the investigator selects among accessible sites or participants to establish proportions of characteristics in the sample that are similar to the proportions found in the population.

Quality-adjusted life years (QALYs): A combined mortality–morbidity index that reflects years of life free of disability and symptoms of illness.

Random selection: Methods by which subjects from a sampling frame are randomly selected to create a representative sample.

Redistributive policy: Deliberate efforts to alter the distribution of benefits by taking money or property from one group and giving it to another.

Regular source of care (RSC): A usual place where, or a usual provider from whom, an individual receives healthcare services.

Regulatory policies: Regulations or rules that impose restrictions and are intended to control the behavior of a target group by monitoring the group and imposing sanctions if it fails to comply.

Republican: A type of democratic government in which the head of state is not a monarch; governmental activities and affairs are open to all interested citizens.

Safety net providers: As defined by the Institute of Medicine, "providers that by mandate or mission organize and deliver a significant level of health care and other health-related services to the uninsured, Medicaid, and other vulnerable patients" (IOM 2006).

Sampling frame: The population from which a sample is selected.

Senate majority leader: Senate leader elected by the party that holds majority in the Senate. He or she serves as the chief Senate spokesperson for his or her party and is responsible for scheduling the legislative and executive business of the Senate.

Social contacts: The frequency of social activities a person undertakes within a specified period.

Social resources: Interpersonal relationships with social contacts and the extent to which the individual can rely on them for support.

Speaker of the House: The presiding officer of the US House of Representatives, typically chosen from the majority party of the House.

Standardized open-ended interview: A structured interview that is conducted by reciting predetermined open-ended questions verbatim in a specified order.

State executives: Officials in the executive branch of state government. Examples include the governor, who is chief executive of a state or territory, and the attorney general, who serves as the main legal adviser to the state government and has executive responsibility for law enforcement.

State legislature: A generic term referring to the legislative body of a US state. It may also be called the Legislature, General Assembly, or Legislative Assembly.

Statutory authority: The capacity to enforce legislation on behalf of the government as granted by the US Constitution.

Strata: Levels into which a population or a sample is divided on the basis of selected characteristics.

Stratified random sampling: A random selection of individual subjects from sampling frame subgroups, where each subgroup is made up of individuals who share a characteristic of interest.

Tabling legislation: An action undertaken by Congress to postpone consideration of the legislation.

Trend study: A series of cross-sectional studies examining how a characteristic or set of characteristics changes over time through repeated sampling from the overall population.

Veto: Unilaterally stopping an official action; as a noun, the authority to do so.

World Health Assembly: The decision-making and policymaking body of WHO, composed of delegations from all WHO member states.

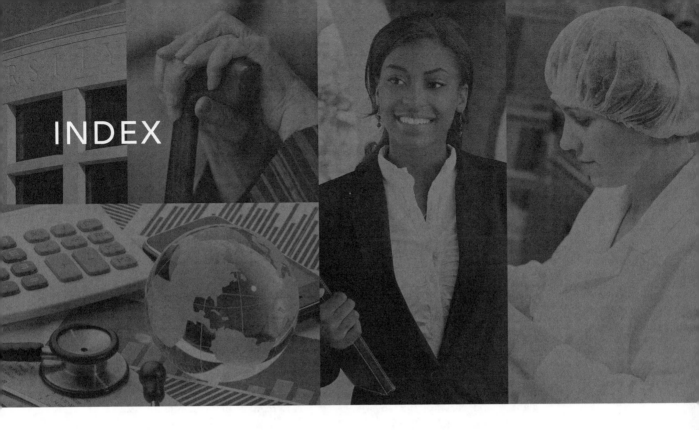

INDEX

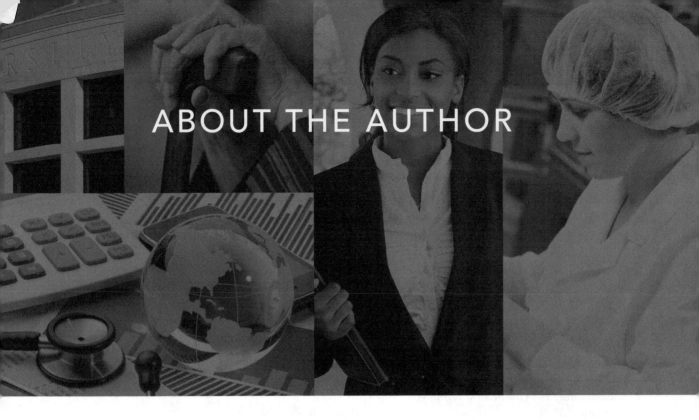

ABOUT THE AUTHOR

Leiyu Shi, DrPH, is professor of health policy and health services research at the Johns Hopkins University Bloomberg School of Public Health in the Department of Health Policy and Management. He also serves as director of the Johns Hopkins Primary Care Policy Center. He received his doctoral education from the University of California, Berkeley, majoring in health policy and services research. He also has a master's degree in business administration focusing on finance. Dr. Shi's research focuses on primary care, health disparities, and vulnerable populations. He has conducted extensive studies related to the association between primary care and health outcomes, particularly on the role of primary care in mediating the adverse impact of income inequality on health outcomes. Dr. Shi is also well known for his extensive research on vulnerable populations in the United States, in particular community health centers that serve vulnerable populations in the areas of sustainability, provider recruitment and retention experiences, financial performance, experience under managed care, and quality of care. Dr. Shi is the author of nine textbooks and more than 150 scientific journal articles.